Obstetrics & Gynaecology

Lawrence Impey

BA, FRCOG
Consultant in Obstetrics and Fetal Medicine
The John Radcliffe Hospital
Headington, Oxford

Tim Child

MA, MD, MRCOG
Associate Professor in Reproductive Medicine
University of Oxford
Honorary Consultant Gynaecologist
The John Radcliffe Hospital
Headington, Oxford

5th edition

WILEY Blackwell

Library of Congress Cataloging-in-Publication Data

Names: Impey, Lawrence, author. | Child, Tim, author.
Title: Obstetrics & gynaecology / Lawrence Impey and Tim Child.
Other titles: Obstetrics and gynaecology
Description: 5th edition. | Chichester, West Sussex : John
    Wiley & Sons Ltd., 2017. | Includes bibliographical references and index.
Identifiers: LCCN 2016030548| ISBN 9781119010791 (pbk.) | ISBN 9781119010807
    (Adobe PDF) | ISBN 9781119010838 (ePub)
Subjects: | MESH: Pregnancy | Genital Diseases, Female | Pregnancy
    Complications | Outlines
Classification: LCC RG101 | NLM WQ 18.2 | DDC 618.02/02—dc23 LC record available at
https://lccn.loc.gov/2016030548

A catalogue record for this book is available from the British Library.

Obstetrics &
Gynaecology

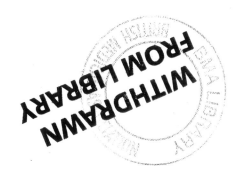

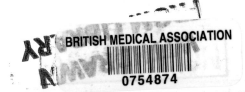

This title is also available as an e-book. For more details, please see

www.wiley.com/buy/9781119010791

or scan this QR code:

Contents

Preface to the fifth edition

In this 5th edition, we hold to the same principles as the first: to be concise with words not facts, with the emphasis on clarity, principles of management and easy access to the information. However, the text has been completely updated to reflect new information and practice. This book is primarily meant to help medical students pass and even do really well in their exams, but its clarity and emphasis on management should also prove useful to practising doctors to structure their knowledge and improve their practice.

Lawrence Impey
Tim Child 2016

Preface to the first edition

This book is written for the UK medical student, in line with changes in medical education and the advent of the core curriculum. The level of information is enough to allow a high mark in the final obstetrics and gynaecology examinations. But its strong emphasis on management should also be useful for practising doctors and those about to take postgraduate examinations.

As a student and then a lecturer, I was always surprised at the deficiencies of many textbooks: how they failed to emphasize what was common or important, how little emphasis they placed on 'what to do' in a real situation, and how little they allowed understanding of the subject. Problem-based learning is in part a backlash against this. Yet there remains a need for a comprehensive yet straightforward textbook. In this, the space given to each topic reflects its importance. The information is up to date, evidence based where possible, and referenced, at least for important, new or contentious issues. At the end of each chapter, summaries of all the major topics should aid revision and prevent the need for a separate revision text. At the end of the book, separate management sections describe what to do in all the common clinical situations, from the management of slow progress in labour to the management of the subfertile couple.

Lawrence Impey
1999

Acknowledgements

I am grateful to the many friends and colleagues in the UK and Ireland who have made criticisms in their areas of expertise and have helped with the preparation of this book. These are Mr Mike Bowen, Dr Bill Boyd, Dr Patricia Boyd, Dr Bridgette Byrne, Dr Paul Dewart, Dr Valerie Donnelly, Dr Anne Edwards, Dr Michael Foley, Miss Michelle Fynes, Mr Mike Gillmer, Miss Catharine Greenwood, Dr Jonathan Hobson, Mr James Hopkisson, Miss Pauline Hurley, Mr Simon Jackson, Dr Catherine James, Dr Declan Keane, Mr Sean Kehoe, Mr Stephen Kennedy, Dr Peter Lenehan, Dr Graham Lloyd-Jones, Dr Graz Luzzi, Dr Dermott MacDonald, Dr Pamela MacKinnon, Dr Peter McParland, Mr Enda McVeigh, Miss Kathryn MacQuillan, Dr Jane Mellanby, Miss Jo Morrison, Miss Jane Moore, Miss Alice Nelson, Miss Brenda O'Kelly, Miss Meghana Pandit, Dr John Picard, Miss Charlotte Porter, Professor Chris Redman, Miss Margaret Rees, Dr Robin Russell, Miss Susan Sellers, Dr Sarah Sheikh, Dr Orla Sheil, Mr Alex Slack, Mr Alexander Smarason, Mr Kevin Smith, Professor Philip Steer, Mr Alex Swanton, and Dr Mary Wingfield. I am indebted to Blackwell Science, particularly Ms Rebecca Huxley, Dr Andrew Robinson and Dr Michael Stein for their faith, help and encouragement, and to the medical students of the Royal College of Surgeons in Ireland and of Oxford University for their criticisms. And I am particularly grateful to Ms Jane Fallows for her illustrations. Most of all, however, I thank Susan and Cicely Impey for their support and patience during the writing of this book.

Acknowledgements for the fifth edition

In addition to the many people who helped with the first edition, we would like to thank Miss Natalia Price, Dr Jackie Sherrard, Miss Catharine Greenwood, Dr Michael Yousif, Mr Simon Jackson, Prof Margaret Rees, Dr Lucy Mackillop, Miss Ruth Houlden, Prof Ahmed Ahmed, Mr Richard Clayton and Mr Charles Muteshi.

Lawrence Impey
Tim Child

List of abbreviations

ACA	anticardiolipin antibody		CRL	crown–rump length
ACE	angiotensin-converting enzyme		CRP	C-reactive protein
ACT	artemisin combination therapy		CSF	cerebrospinal fluid
ACTH	adrenocorticotrophic hormone		CT	computed tomography
AD	Alzheimer's disease		CTG	cardiotocography
AEDF	absent end-diastolic flow		CVA	cerebrovascular accident
AFC	antral follicle count		CVD	cardiovascular disease
AFP	alpha fetoprotein		CVP	central venous pressure
AIDS	acquired immune deficiency syndrome		CVS	chorionic villus sampling
AIS	androgen insensitivity syndrome		D&C	dilatation and curettage
ALP	alkaline phosphatase		DCDA	dichorionic diamniotic
ALT	alanine aminotransferase		DES	diethylstilboestrol
AMH	antimullerian hormone		DEXA	dual-energy X-ray absorptiometry
AP	antero-posterior		DI	donor insemination
APH	antepartum haemorrhage		DIC	disseminated intravascular coagulation
APS	antiphospholipid syndrome		DLE	diathermy loop excision
ARDS	adult respiratory distress syndrome		DNA	deoxyribonucleic acid
ARM	artificial rupture of membranes		DVT	deep vein thrombosis
ASD	atrial septal defect		DZ	dizygotic
AST	aspartate aminotransferase		ECG	electrocardiogram
AUB	abnormal uterine bleeding		ECMO	extracorporeal membrane oxygenation
AV	aerobic vaginitis		ECV	external cephalic version
BCG	Bacille bilié de Calmette–Guérin		EDD	expected day of delivery
β-hCG	human chorionic gonadotrophin beta-subunit		EFM	electronic fetal monitoring
			EIA	enzyme immunoassay
BMD	bone mineral density		EPAU	early pregnancy assessment unit
BMI	body mass index		EPDS	Edinburgh Postnatal Depression Scale
BP	blood pressure			
BSO	bilateral salpingo-oophorectomy		ERPC	evacuation of retained products of conception
BV	bacterial vaginosis			
CA	carcinoma		eSET	elective single embryo transfer
CA 125	serum cancer antigen 125		ESR	erythrocyte sedimentation rate
CCAM	congenital cystic adenomatous malformation		EUA	examination under anaesthetic
			FBC	full blood count
CGH	comparative genomic hybridization		FBS	fetal blood sampling
CGIN	cervical glandular intraepithelial neoplasia		FDA	Food and Drug Administration
			FER	frozen embryo replacement
CHC	combined hormonal contraception		FFP	fresh frozen plasma
CIN	cervical intraepithelial neoplasia		FGM	female genital mutilation
CMV	cytomegalovirus		FGR	fetal growth restriction
CNS	central nervous system		FHR	fetal heart rate
CNST	Clinical Negligence Scheme for Trusts		FIGO	International Federation of Gynaecology and Obstetrics
COC	combined oral contraceptive			
CPP	chronic pelvic pain		FISH	fluorescence in situ hybridization
CPR	cerebroplacental ratio; cardiopulmonary resuscitation		FPR	false-positive rate
			FSD	female sexual dysfunction

FSH	follicle-stimulating hormone	LBC	liquid-based cytology
G&S	group and save	LDA	low-dose aspirin
GBS	group B streptococcus	LDH	lactic dehydrogenase
GFR	glomerular filtration rate	LFT	liver function test
GMC	General Medical Council	LH	luteinizing hormone
GnRH	gonadotrophin-releasing hormone	LLETZ	large loop excision of transformation zone
GSI	genuine stress incontinence	LMP	last menstrual period
GTD	gestational trophoblastic disease	LMWH	low molecular weight heparin
GTT	glucose tolerance test	LN	lymph node
HAART	highly active antiretroviral therapy	LSCS	lower segment caesarean section
Hb	haemoglobin	LUNA	laparoscopic uterine nerve ablation
HbF	fetal haemoglobin	MC	monochorionic
hCG	human chorionic gonadotrophin	MCA	middle cerebral artery
HCV	hepatitis C virus	MCDA	monochorionic diamniotic
HELLP	(syndrome of) haemolysis, elevated liver enzymes and low platelets	MCHC	mean cell haemoglobin concentration
HFEA	Human Fertilization and Embryology Authority	MCMA	monochorionic monoamniotic
		MCV	mean cell volume
HIV	human immunodeficiency virus	MDT	multidisciplinary team
HMB	heavy menstrual bleeding	MHT	menopausal hormone therapy
HNPCC	hereditary non-polyposis colorectal cancer	MOH	massive obstetric haemorrhage
		MRI	magnetic resonance imaging
HPV	human papilloma virus	MSAFP	maternal serum alpha fetoprotein
HRT	hormone replacement therapy	MSU	mid-stream urine
HSG	hysterosalpingogram	MZ	monozygotic
HSV	herpes simplex virus	NAAT	nucleic acid amplification test
HVS	high vaginal swab	NEC	necrotizing enterocolitis
IA	intermittent auscultation	NGS	next generation sequencing
IBS	irritable bowel syndrome	NHS	National Health Service
ICAS	Independent Complaints Advocacy Service	NICE	National Institute for Health and Care Excellence
ICSI	intracytoplasmic sperm injection	NIPT	non-invasive prenatal testing
Ig	immunoglobulin	NPV	negative predictive value
IM	intramuscular	NRT	nicotine replacement therapy
IMB	intermenstrual bleeding	NSAID	non-steroidal anti-inflammatory drug
IPT	intermittent preventive treatment	NTD	neural tube defect
IUD	intrauterine device	NVP	nausea and vomiting of pregnancy
IUGR	intrauterine growth restriction	OA	occipito-anterior
IUI	intrauterine insemination	OAB	overactive bladder
IUS	intrauterine system	OCD	obsessive compulsive disorder
IV	intravenous	OCP	oral contraceptive pill
IVF	*in vitro* fertilization	OHSS	ovarian hyperstimulation syndrome
IVP	intravenous pyelogram	OP	occipito-posterior
JVP	jugular venous pressure	OT	occipito-transverse
LARC	long-acting reversible contraceptive	PAPPA	pregnancy-associated plasma protein A
LAVH	laparoscopic-assisted vaginal hysterectomy	PBS	painful bladder syndrome
		PCA	patient-controlled analgesia

PCB	postcoital bleeding		SROM	spontaneous rupture of membranes
PCO	polycystic ovary		SSR	surgical sperm retrieval
PCOS	polycystic ovary syndrome		SSRI	selective serotonin reuptake inhibitor
PCP	*Pneumocystis carinii* pneumonia		STI	sexually transmitted infection
PCR	protein:creatinine ratio		STV	short-term variability
PDA	patent ductus arteriosus		T3	triiodothyronine
PET	pre-eclamptic toxaemia		T4	thyroxine
PFMT	pelvic floor muscle training		TAH	total abdominal hysterectomy
PGD	preimplantation genetic diagnosis		TAPS	twin anaemia polycythaemia sequence
PGE_2	prostaglandin E_2		TB	tuberculosis
PGF_{2a}	prostaglandin F_{2a}		TCRE	transcervical resection of endometrium
PGS	preimplantation genetic screening		TCRF	transcervical resection of fibroid
PI	Pearl Index; pulsatility index		TEDS	thromboembolic disease stockings
PID	pelvic inflammatory disease		TENS	transcutaneous electrical nerve stimulation
PlGF	placental growth factor			
PM	postmortem		TFT	thyroid function test
PMB	postmenopausal bleeding		TLH	total laparoscopic hysterectomy
PMS	premenstrual syndrome		TOP	termination of pregnancy
POP	progestogen-only pill		TOT	transobdurator tape
PPH	postpartum haemorrhage		TRAP	twin reversed arterial perfusion
PPV	positive predictive value		TSH	thyroid-stimulating hormone
PSTT	placental site trophoblastic tumour		TTN	transient tachypnoea of the newborn
PSV	peak velocity in systole		TTTS	twin–twin transfusion syndrome
PTSD	post-traumatic stress disorder		TURP	transurethral resection of prostate
PTU	propylthiouracil		TVS	transvaginal sonography
PUL	pregnancy of unknown location		TVT	tension-free vaginal tape
PV	per vaginam		U&E	urea and electrolytes
RCT	randomized controlled trial		UAE	uterine artery embolization
REDF	reversed end-diastolic flow		UDCA	ursodeoxycholic acid
RMI	risk of malignancy index		UmbA	umbilical artery
SARA	sexually acquired reactive arthritis		USI	urodynamic stress incontinence
SBR	serum bilirubin		USS	ultrasound scan
SD	standard deviation		UTI	urinary tract infection
SERM	selective estrogen receptor modulator		VBAC	vaginal delivery after a previous caesarean section
SFD	small for dates			
SFH	symphysis–fundal height		VDRL	Venereal Disease Research Laboratories
SGA	small for gestational age		VE	vaginal examination
SHBG	steroid hormone-binding globulin		VEGF	vascular endothelial growth factor
SIDS	sudden infant death syndrome		VH	vaginal hysterectomy
SLE	systemic lupus erythematosus		VIN	vulvar intraepithelial neoplasia
SLNB	sentinel lymph node biopsy		VMA	vanillylmandelic acid
SMM	surgical management of miscarriage		VQ	ventilation/perfusion
SNRI	serotonin and noradrenaline reuptake inhibitor		VSD	ventricular septal defect
			VTE	venous thromboembolism
SPRM	selective progesterone receptor modulator		WBC	white blood cell count
			WHO	World Health Organization

About the companion website

Don't forget to visit the companion website for this book:

http://www.impeyobgyn.com

There you will find valuable material designed to enhance your learning, including:

- Interactive MCQs and EMQs (prepared by Miss Ruth Houlden BSc, MBBS, MRCOG)
- Revision notes
- Figures from the book

Scan this QR code to visit the companion website:

Gynaecology

CHAPTER 1

The history and examination in gynaecology

The remit of the doctor is to improve quality of life, not just to treat life-threatening disease: if a symptom is causing distress, treatment should be considered. The type and extent of treament are determined largely by the patient; the doctor gives information and advice, so the patient can give her *informed* consent. The patient's history should be used not only to help make a diagnosis but also to discover how much her symptom(s) is/are affecting her. Or she may simply be cocerned as to the cause of her symptoms (e.g. malignancy) and reassurance is enough.

The gynaecological history

Personal details

Ask her name, age and occupation.

Presenting complaint(s)

How long has the problem been present and how much does it affect her? If it is pain, what alleviates and what exacerbates it, where is it and what is its nature? Allow the patient to elaborate as there may be more than one problem, initially without asking direct questions, perhaps asking her to rate her problems in order of severity. Has she ever consulted a doctor about this problem before and, if so, what has been done? If there are multiple presenting complaints, these should be put in order of severity/effect on her life.

Specific gynaecological questions

These are asked next, starting with ones that are relevant to this presenting complaint. For example, if it is a menstrual problem, the most appropriate next questions concern menstruation; if it is a urinary problem, one should ask all the appropriate urinary tract questions next.

Menstrual questions: How often does she menstruate (how many days from the first day of bleeding to the next first day?) and how long does menstruation last? (4/28 means bleeding lasts for 4 days and occurs every 28 days.) Is it regular or irregular? Is it heavy? (Number of pads/tampons used or the presence of clots can be useful.) Is it or the days leading up to it painful? Is there ever intermenstrual bleeding (IMB)? Is there ever postcoital bleeding (PCB)? Is there ever vaginal discharge and, if so, what is it like? Does she experience premenstrual tension? When was her last menstrual period (LMP)? If postmenopausal, has there been postmenopausal bleeding (PMB)?

Sexual/contraceptive questions: Is she sexually active? If so, is it painful? If so, is it on penetration (superficial dyspareunia) or deep inside (deep dyspareunia) and is it during and/or after (delayed)? What contraceptive (if appropriate) does she use and what has she used in the past?

Obstetrics & Gynaecology, Fifth Edition. Lawrence Impey, Tim Child.
© 2017 John Wiley & Sons, Ltd. Published 2017 by John Wiley & Sons, Ltd.

Cervical smear questions: When was her last cervical smear? (This should be done every 3 years between the ages of 25 and 49 years, every 5 years between 50 and 64 years, and not performed thereafter unless never screened or history of recent abnormal tests.) Has she ever had an abnormal smear? If so, what was done?

Urinary/prolapse questions: Does she experience frequency (normal is 4–7 times per day), nocturia (micturition at night) or urgency (a severe desire to void)? Does she ever leak urine, including when asleep (nocturnal enuresis)? If so, how severe is it and with what is it associated (e.g. coughing, lifting/straining or urgency)? Is there ever dysuria (pain on micturition) or haematuria (blood in the urine)? Does she ever get a dragging sensation or feel a mass in or at the vagina?

Menstrual questions

How often and for how long?
Heavy or painful?
Regularity?
Intermenstrual bleeding (IMB) or postcoital bleeding (PCB)?
When was her last menstrual period (LMP)?

Other history

Past obstetric history: This should be brief. Start with 'Have you ever been pregnant?' If the answer is 'No', go on to past medical history. If 'Yes', ask for details about previous pregnancies in chronological order. See Chapter 16 for explanation of parity and gravidity. Of deliveries, ask when, what weight, how was the infant born and how the infant is now. Ask about any major complications in the pregnancy or labour.

Past medical history: First ask about any previous, particularly gynaecological, operations, however distant. Then directly ask about venous thrombosis, diabetes, lung and heart disease, hypertension, jaundice, etc. as in any medical history. If you elicit no significant history, ask 'Have you ever been in hospital?'

Systems review: Ask the usual cardiovascular, respiratory and neurological questions. In particular, ask about urinary and gastrointestinal symptoms in view of the close pelvic relationship.

Drugs: Does she take any regular medication including prescribed, over-the-counter or complementary? Consider asking about illegal drug use if relevant.

Family history: Is there a family history of breast or ovarian carcinoma, of diabetes, venous thromboembolism, heart disease or hypertension?

Personal/social history: Does she smoke? Does she drink alcohol? If either, how much? Is she married or in a stable relationship and, if not, is there support at home? Where does she live and what sort of accommodation is it?

Allergies: Ask specifically about penicillin and latex.

Presenting the history

Start by summing up the important points, including relevant gynaecological questions:

This is . . . , who is a . . . year-old . . . (parity), with a . . . (time) history of . . . , who . . . (most significant findings in history).

Example: This is Mrs X, who is a 38-year-old nulliparous woman, with a 3-month history of postcoital bleeding (PCB), who has a normal menstrual cycle and last had a cervical smear 7 years ago.

N.B. By mentioning the last smear, you have shown understanding that PCB may be a symptom of cervical carcinoma.

Now go through the history in some detail.
Then sum up again, in one sentence.

Gynaecological history: specific essential questions

Presenting complaint, its history
Menstrual questions: last menstrual period (LMP), cycle, flow, intermenstrual bleeding (IMB), postcoital bleeding (PCB)
Urinary/prolapse questions
Sexual/contraceptive questions
Cervical smear history
Past obstetric history

Other questions

Now ask 'Is there anything else you think I ought to know?'. This gives her the opportunity to help you if you have not discovered all the important facts.

Summarizing the history

1 Could the symptoms be a manifestation of underlying disease that needs to be treated? (For example, erratic menstrual bleeding may be a sign of malignancy.)
2 Are the symptoms themselves causing physical damage? (For example, erratic menstrual bleeding may lead to severe anaemia.)
3 Are the symptoms themselves causing distress? (For example, erratic menstrual bleeding may disrupt a woman's life such that she may feel unable to leave the home.) Or is she unconcerned?

The gynaecological examination

General examination

This is to:
1 seek the effects (e.g. secondary spread of malignancy) or, more rarely, the causes (e.g. thyroid abnormalities cause menstrual disturbances) of gynaecological problems
2 assess general health and incidental disease, particularly if an anaesthetic may be needed.
General appearance and weight, temperature, blood pressure and pulse, and possible anaemia, jaundice or lymphadenopathy should be noted. More detailed examination of the rest of the body is often perfunctory in the young, fit patient, but is important in the older or more sick patient, or in those about to have an anaesthetic.

Breast and axillary examination

This can be performed as a screening test for breast cancer, although breast examination is not routinely undertaken in UK gynaecological practice unless investigating a potentially malignant pelvic mass (Fig. 1.1). The patient sits back, the breasts are inspected for irregularities and all four breast quadrants are palpated as the patient lies supine with her hands behind her head. The axilla, a principal area for lymph drainage, is then palpated with the patient's arm resting on the examiner's shoulder.

Abdominal examination

The patient lies comfortably on her back with her head on a pillow, discreetly exposed from the xiphisternum to the symphysis pubis. The bladder should be empty.

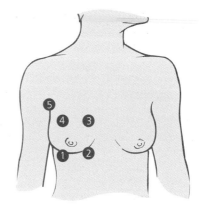
Fig. 1.1 Examination of the breast.

Inspect

Look for scars, particularly just above the symphysis pubis and in the umbilicus. Look at the distribution of body hair, for irregularities, striae and hernias.

Palpate

Ask about tenderness first, then palpate gently around the abdomen looking for masses or tenderness. Then palpate specifically for masses from above the umbilicus down to the symphysis pubis (Fig. 1.2). If any masses are present, do they arise from the pelvis (i.e. can you get below them)?

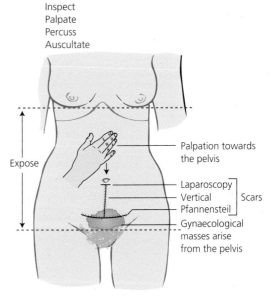
Fig. 1.2 Abdominal examination.

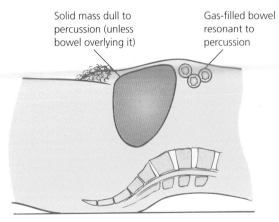

Solid mass dull to percussion (unless bowel overlying it)

Gas-filled bowel resonant to percussion

Fig. 1.3 Percussion of the abdomen.

Percuss

Go around the abdomen. The bowel is resonant; fluid-filled and solid cavities (e.g. masses, full bladder) are dull (Fig. 1.3). Look for shifting dullness (free fluid).

Auscultate

Listen to the bowel sounds.

Gynaecological examination
General
(Breast)
Abdomen
Pelvic palpation: digital
Cervical/vaginal inspection: speculum

Vaginal examination

Ensure privacy, explain simply what you intend and ask for the patient's permission. Offer her the opportunity to use the bathroom first. A chaperone must be offered, whether you are male or female, and the presence and name of the chaperone documented in the notes. Use lubricating jelly. A metal speculum should be warmed. Internal examination is often uncomfortable, but severe tenderness is abnormal.

Inspect

The vulva and the vaginal orifice are inspected first. Are there any coloured areas, ulcers or lumps on the vulva? Is a prolapse evident at the introitus? Three types of examination have different purposes.

Digital bimanual examination

This assesses the pelvic organs. The patient lies flat, with her ankles together drawn up towards her buttocks and knees apart. Warn the patient before you touch her and ask her to let you know if she finds the examination too uncomfortable. The left hand is placed on the abdomen above the symphysis pubis and is pushed down into the pelvis, so that the organs are palpated between it and two fingers are gently inserted into the vagina (Fig. 1.4).

The uterus is normally the size and shape of a small pear. Size, consistency, regularity, mobility, anteversion or retroversion and tenderness are assessed.

The cervix is normally the first part of the uterus to be felt vaginally and the os is felt as an opening like a toy car tyre. Is the cervix hard or irregular?

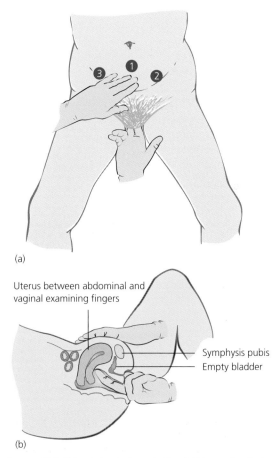

(a)

Uterus between abdominal and vaginal examining fingers

Symphysis pubis

Empty bladder

(b)

Fig. 1.4 Digital bimanual vaginal examination: (a) bimanually palpate areas 1, 2, 3 in order; (b) digital bimanual palpation of the pelvis.

The adnexa (lateral to the uterus on either side, containing tube and ovary): tenderness and size and consistency of any mass are assessed. Is it separate from the uterus?

The pouch of Douglas (behind the cervix): the uterosacral ligaments should be palpable. Are these even, irregular or tender, or is there a mass?

Cusco's speculum examination

This allows inspection of the cervix and vaginal walls. The patient lies as for the digital examination. With the blades closed and parallel to the labia and the opening mechanism pointing to the patient's right, gently insert the speculum (Fig. 1.5a). Then rotate it 90° anteriorly and insert it as far as it will go without causing discomfort (Fig. 1.5b). Open it slowly under direct vision and the cervix will come into view (Fig. 1.5c). Common

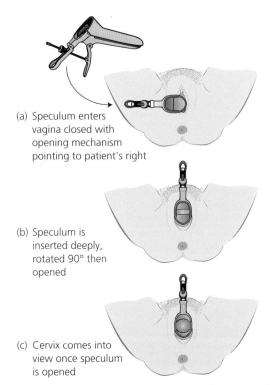

(a) Speculum enters vagina closed with opening mechanism pointing to patient's right

(b) Speculum is inserted deeply, rotated 90° then opened

(c) Cervix comes into view once speculum is opened

Fig. 1.5 Cusco's speculum examination of the cervix and vaginal walls. (a) Speculum enters vagina closed with opening mechanism pointing to patient's right. (b) Speculum is inserted deep, rotated 90°, then opened. (c) The cervix comes into view once the speculum is opened.

mistakes include not inserting the speculum sufficiently deep and/or posterior with an anteverted uterus. The cervix may be very anterior with a retroverted uterus. Look for ulceration, spontaneous bleeding or irregularities. A cervical smear can be taken. Now slightly withdraw the speculum under direct vision and partly close it without catching the cervix. Slowly withdraw it just open, allowing inspection of the vaginal walls to the introitus, and then close the speculum and remove it, rotating the speculum through 90° on the way out.

Sims' speculum

This allows better inspection of the vaginal walls and, specifically, the prolapse. The patient should be positioned in the left lateral position with the legs partly curled up. Insert the curved speculum into the vagina from behind, with one end pressing against the posterior wall to allow inspection of the anterior wall. Then reverse the speculum, pressing back the anterior wall so that the posterior wall can be seen (Fig. 1.6). If the patient is asked to bear down, the prolapse of either wall and the cervix or vaginal vault can be assessed.

Rectal examination

This is occasionally appropriate if there is posterior wall prolapse, to distinguish between an enterocoele and a rectocoele, and in assessing malignant cervical disease. It may also be necessary if the woman complains of cyclical rectal bleeding, possibly due to rectovaginal endometriosis.

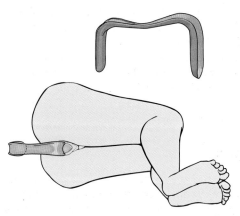

Fig. 1.6 Sims' speculum examination of the vaginal walls.

Presenting the examination

Present the examination findings, including relevant positive or negative findings:

Mrs X is . . . (describe general appearance sensitively), her blood pressure, temperature and pulse are . . . and abdominal and pelvic examination reveals. . . . There is . . . (mention important positive and negative findings).

Example: Mrs X looks thin and clinically anaemic, her blood pressure is 120/60 mmHg, temperature is normal and pulse is 90 beats/min; abdominal examination reveals a mass arising from the pelvis up to the level of the umbilicus, with no obvious ascites. There is no lymphadenopathy or breast abnormality.

N.B. By mentioning ascites, lymphadenopathy and the breasts, you demonstrate your understanding of the possible aetiology and effects of a pelvic mass.

Management plan. Now decide on a course of action. Plan what investigations (if any) are needed and what course of action (if any) is most appropriate.

Gynaecological history at a glance

Personal details	Name, age, occupation	
Presenting complaint	Details, time-scale, any previous treatment. Prioritize	
Gynaecological questions	(Start with most relevant to complaint)	
	Menstrual:	Last menstrual period (LMP), cycle, heaviness, intermenstrual bleeding (IMB), postcoital bleeding (PCB)
	Sex/contraceptive:	Sexually active, dyspareunia, contraception?
	Cervical smear:	Last smear, ever abnormal?
	Urinary/prolapse	Frequency, incontinence, lump at introitus
Other history	Past obstetric history:	Ever pregnant? If so, details
	Past medical history:	Operations, major illnesses. Ever in hospital?
	Systems review, drugs, personal (smoking, alcohol), social, family history (particularly breast/ovarian/heart disease), allergies	
Summarize	Presenting complaint and relevant history findings	

Gynaecological examination at a glance

General	Appearance, anaemia, lymph nodes, blood pressure, pulse
(Breasts/axillae)	Inspect, palpate
Abdomen	Inspect, palpate (particularly suprapubically), percuss, auscultate
Vaginal	Inspect vulva; digital examination; Cusco's speculum, Sims' speculum if prolapse
Summarize	Positive and important negative findings; consider management

CHAPTER 2
The menstrual cycle and its disorders

Physiology

Puberty

This is the onset of sexual maturity, marked by the development of secondary sex characteristics. The *menarche*, or onset of menstruation, is normally the last manifestation of puberty in the female, and in the West occurs on average at 13 years of age. Normal puberty is controlled centrally. The hypothalamic–pituitary axis can be considered as 'waking' and then 'waking up' the ovaries. After the age of 8 years, hypothalamic gonadotrophin-releasing hormone (GnRH) pulses increase in amplitude and frequency, such that pituitary follicle-stimulating hormone (FSH) and then luteinizing hormone (LH) release increases. These stimulate oestrogen release from the ovary (Figs 2.1, 2.2).

Oestrogen is responsible for the development of secondary sexual characteristics: the *thelarche*, or beginning of breast development, occurs first at 9–11 years; the *adrenarche*, or growth of pubic hair (also dependent on adrenal activity), starts at 11–12 years; the final stage is the *menarche* (see Fig. 2.2). Menstruation may be irregular at first; as oestrogen secretion rises, it will become regular. Pregnancy is now possible. These changes are accompanied by the growth spurt, due to increased growth hormone release. By the age of 16 years, most growth has finished and the epiphyses fuse. The average age of the menarche is reducing.

The menstrual cycle

The hormonal changes of the menstrual cycle cause ovulation and induce changes in the endometrium that prepare it for implantation should fertilization occur.

Days 1–4: menstruation

At the start of the menstrual cycle (designated as the first day of menstruation), the endometrium is shed as its hormonal support is withdrawn. Myometrial contraction, which can be painful, also occurs.

Days 5–13: proliferative phase

Pulses of GnRH from the hypothalamus stimulate LH and FSH release which induce follicular growth. The follicles produce oestradiol and inhibin which suppress FSH secretion in a 'negative feedback', such that (normally) only one follicle and oocyte mature. As oestradiol levels continue to rise and reach their maximum, however, a 'positive-feedback' effect on the hypothalamus and pituitary causes LH levels to rise sharply: ovulation follows 36 hours after the LH surge. The oestradiol also causes the endometrium to re-form and become 'proliferative': it thickens as the stromal cells proliferate and the glands elongate.

Days 14–28: luteal/secretory phase

The follicle from which the egg was released becomes the corpus luteum. This again produces oestradiol, but relatively more progesterone, levels of which peak around a week later (day 21 of a 28-day cycle). This induces 'secretory' changes in the endometrium, whereby the stromal cells enlarge, the glands swell and the blood supply increases. Towards the end of the luteal phase, the corpus luteum starts to fail if the egg is not fertilized, causing progesterone and oestrogen levels to fall. As its hormonal support is withdrawn, the

Obstetrics & Gynaecology, Fifth Edition. Lawrence Impey, Tim Child.
© 2017 John Wiley & Sons, Ltd. Published 2017 by John Wiley & Sons, Ltd.

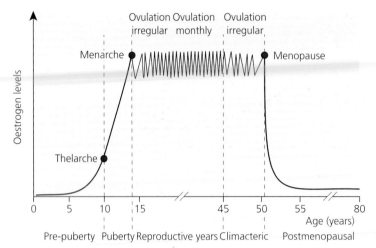

Fig. 2.1 Oestrogen levels in a lifetime.

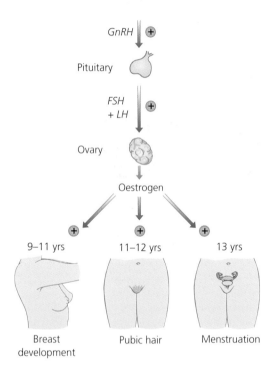

Fig. 2.2 Endocrine changes during puberty. FSH, follicle-stimulating hormone; GnRH, gonadotrophin-releasing hormone; LH, luteinizing hormone.

Normal menstruation
Menarche <16 years
Menopause >45 years
Menstruation 3–8 days in length
Blood loss <80 mL
Cycle length 24–38 days
No intermenstrual bleeding (IMB)

Abnormal uterine bleeding (AUB)

Definition

Abnormal uterine bleeding is a common condition affecting women of reproductive age that has significant social and economic impact. It is defined as any variation from the normal menstrual cycle, and includes changes in regularity and frequency of menses, in duration of flow, or in amount of blood loss. Heavy menstrual bleeding (HMB) is the most common complaint of AUB. FIGO has established a new classification system for the terminology, definitions and causes of AUB (*J Obstet Gynaecol Can* 2013; **35(5 eSuppl)**: S1–S28).

Causes of AUB

The acronym PALM-COEIN ('palm-coin'), developed by FIGO (*Int J Gynaecol Obstet* 2011; **113**: 3–13), describes the nine main categories of causes of AUB.

endometrium breaks down, menstruation follows and the cycle restarts (Fig. 2.3). Continuous administration of exogenous progestogens maintains a secretory endometrium. This can be used to delay menstruation.

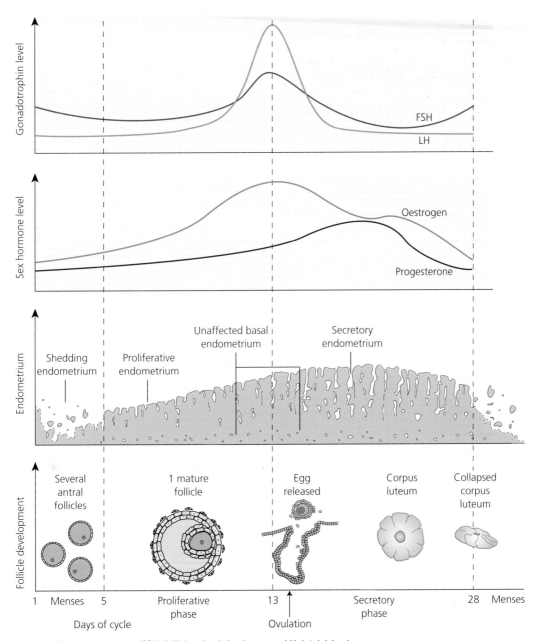

Fig. 2.3 The menstrual cycle. FSH, follicle-stimulating hormone; LH, luteinizing hormone.

Abnormal uterine bleeding and definitions of terms (FIGO)

Characteristic	Terminology	Description
Volume	Heavy menstrual bleeding	Excessive menstrual blood loss which interferes with the woman's physical, emotional, social and material quality of life, and which can occur alone or in combination with other symptoms
Regularity (cycle-to-cycle variation)	Irregular menstrual bleeding Absent menstrual bleeding (amenorrhoea)	Cycle-to-cycle variation >20 days No bleeding in a 6-month interval
Frequency (normal every 24–38 days)	Infrequent menstrual bleeding (previously oligomenorrhoea) Frequent menstrual bleeding	Bleeding at intervals >38 days apart Bleeding at intervals <24 days apart
Duration (normal 3–8 days)	Prolonged menstrual bleeding Shortened menstrual bleeding	Bleeding >8 days duration Bleeding <3 days duration
Irregular, non-menstrual bleeding	Intermenstrual Postcoital Premenstrual and postmenstrual spotting	Irregular episodes of bleeding, often light and short, occurring between otherwise normal menstrual periods Bleeding post intercourse Bleeding for one or more days before or after the recognized menstrual period
Bleeding outside reproductive age	Postmenopausal bleeding Precocious menstruation	Bleeding occurring more than 1 year after the acknowledged menopause Bleeding before the age of 9 years

The PALM side of the classification refers to structural causes that could be evaluated and diagnosed on imaging and/or biopsy. The COEIN side allows consideration of underlying medical disturbances that could result in AUB. More than one cause may be present.

Structural causes	Non-structural causes
Polyps	**C**oagulopathy
Adenomyosis	**O**vulatory dysfunction
Leiomyomas (fibroids) –Submucosal –Other	**E**ndometrial (primary disorder of mechanisms regulating *local* endometrial haemostasis)
Malignancy and hyperplasia	**I**atrogenic
	Not yet specified

Heavy menstrual bleeding (HMB)

Definition

Heavy menstrual bleeding (HMB; previously called menorrhagia).

Clinical definition: Excessive menstrual blood loss that interferes with the woman's physical, emotional, social and material quality of life, and which can occur alone or in combination with other symptoms.

Objective definition: This is blood loss of >80 mL in an otherwise normal menstrual cycle. This value corresponds to the maximum amount that a woman on a normal diet can lose per cycle without becoming iron deficient. In practice, actual blood loss is rarely measured.

Epidemiology

One-third of women complain of heavy periods although most do not seek medical help.

Aetiology

The majority of women with HMB have no histological abnormality that can be implicated in its causation. Most women with regular cycles are ovulatory, and HMB may result from subtle abnormalities of endometrial haemostasis or uterine prostaglandin levels. Uterine fibroids (approximately 30% of women with HMB) and polyps (approximately 10% of women with HMB) are the most common form of pathology found. Chronic pelvic infection, ovarian tumours and endometrial and cervical malignancy (Fig. 2.4) usually cause irregular bleeding. Thyroid disease, haemostatic disorders, such as von Willebrand's disease, and anticoagulant therapy are rare causes of HMB. A coagulopathy may be suggested by a family or personal history of excessive bleeding after surgery/trauma or easy bruising.

Clinical features

History: This should assess both the amount and timing of the bleeding. A menstrual calendar is helpful. 'Flooding' and the passage of large clots indicate excessive loss. Any method of contraception should be ascertained.

Examination: Anaemia is common. Pelvic signs are often absent. Irregular enlargement of the uterus suggests fibroids; tenderness with or without enlargement suggests adenomyosis. An ovarian mass or fibroids may be felt.

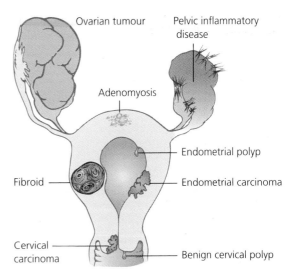

Fig. 2.4 Anatomical causes of menorrhagia.

Investigations

To assess the effect of blood loss and fitness, the patient's haemoglobin is checked.

To exclude systemic causes, coagulation and thyroid function are checked only if the history is suggestive of a problem.

To exclude local structural causes, a transvaginal ultrasound of the pelvis is performed (Fig. 2.5). This

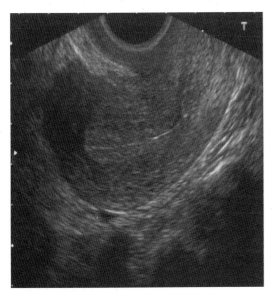

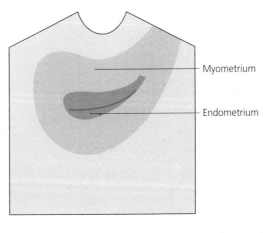

Fig. 2.5 Transvaginal ultrasound of a normal uterus and mid-cycle endometrium.

will assess endometrial thickness, exclude a uterine fibroid or ovarian mass and detect intrauterine polyps. The normal endometrium in a premenopausal woman varies in thickness according to the menstrual cycle from 4 mm in the follicular phase up to 16 mm in the luteal phase. A *saline ultrasound scan* involves the introduction of 5–15 mL of saline through the cervix into the uterine cavity during the transvaginal scan and improves the diagnosis of intrauterine pathology, in particular polyps and submucosal fibroids.

Endometrial biopsy should be considered in women with HMB over age 40 or in those with bleeding not responsive to medical therapy, or with significant intermenstrual bleeding, as well as in younger women with risk factors for endometrial cancer, to exclude both endometrial hyperplasia and cancer. Risk factors for endometrial cancer in younger women include obesity, diabetes, nulliparity, history of polycystic ovary syndrome (PCOS) and family history of hereditary nonpolyposis colorectal cancer (HNPCC). The biopsy can be undertaken with a Pipelle (Fig. 2.6) in the outpatient clinic or in combination with an outpatient or inpatient hysteroscopy. Focal lesions of the endometrium (such as endometrial focal thickening or a polyp) that require biopsy are managed through hysteroscopy-guided evaluation. A dilatation and curettage (D&C) is not a treatment for HMB.

Management

Treatment can be instigated once pathology has been excluded and depends on the woman's contraceptive needs (Fig. 2.7). Thus, while intrauterine progestogens are very effective and recommended as a first line by the National Institute for Health and Care Excellence (NICE), this is not an option for a woman who wishes to conceive (NICE Clinical Knowledge Summaries 2012: http://cks.nice.org.uk/menorrhagia#!scenario).

Medical treatment

First line

Intrauterine system (IUS): This progestogen-impregnated intrauterine device (IUD; Fig. 2.8) is a 'coil' that reduces

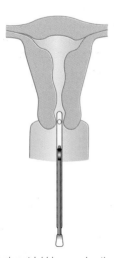

Fig. 2.6 Pipelle endometrial biopsy going through the cervix.

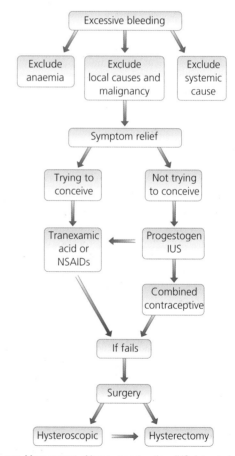

Fig. 2.7 Management of heavy menstruation. IUS, intrauterine system; NSAIDs, non-steroidal anti-inflammatory drugs.

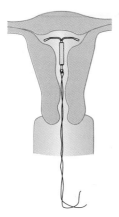

Fig. 2.8 Progestogen-impregnated intrauterine system (IUS) *in situ* in the uterus.

menstrual flow by >90% with considerably fewer side effects than systemic progestogens (*Cochrane* 2015; CD002126). It is a highly effective alternative to both medical and surgical treatment of menorrhagia with outcomes similar to endometrial ablation. It is a contraceptive and also provides the progestogen component of hormone replacement. It should be distinguished from copper IUDs which may increase menstrual loss.

Second line

Antifibrinolytics (tranexamic acid) are taken during menstruation only. By reducing fibrinolytic activity, this can reduce blood loss by about 50%. There are few side effects and in the UK it is available without prescription.

Non-steroidal anti-inflammatory drugs (NSAIDs, e.g. mefenamic acid) inhibit prostaglandin synthesis, reducing blood loss in most women by about 30%. They are also useful for dysmenorrhoea. Side effects are similar to those of aspirin. Ibuprofen and aspirin are available without prescription.

The combined oral contraceptive usually induces lighter menstruation, but is less effective if pelvic pathology is present. Its role is more limited because its complications are more common in older patients and it is these patients who have the most menstrual problems.

Third line

Progestogens taken in high doses orally or by intramuscular injection will cause amenorrhoea, but bleeding will follow withdrawal.

Gonadotrophin-releasing hormone agonists produce amenorrhoea. Unless add-back hormone replacement therapy (HRT) is used, duration is limited to 6 months. Bleeding will follow withdrawal.

Pharmacological treatments for menorrhagia
First line Intrauterine system (IUS)
Second line Antifibrinolytics (tranexamic acid) Non-steroidal anti-inflammatory drugs (NSAIDs) Combined oral contraceptive
Third line Progestogens (high-dose oral or intramuscular) Gonadotrophin-releasing hormone (GnRH) analogues

Surgical treatment

Hysteroscopic

Polyp removal: If localized abnormalities such as polyps are seen, they can be resected. This can be performed under general or local anaesthesia though the latter is associated with lower rates of successful polyp removal and patient acceptability (*BMJ* 2015; **350**: h1398).

Endometrial ablation techniques involve removal or destruction of endometrium. Amenorrhoea or lighter periods usually follow. Long-term patient satisfaction with endometrial destructive techniques is less than with hysterectomy, although surgical complications and hospital stay are less (BMJ Clin Evid 2015; **2015**. pii: 0805). Endometrial ablation is most appropriate in older women with pure menorrhagia and when the uterus is <10 weeks' size. The procedures reduce fertility but are non-sterilizing and so effective contraception should be advised.

Earlier ('first-generation') techniques include transcervical resection of endometrium (TCRE) and transcervical rollerball ablation. These use monopolar diathermy with electric current passing down the hysteroscope into either a cutting loop (TCRE) or a rollerball to excise or ablate the endometrium. Newer ('second-generation') techniques involve the use of thermal balloons, microwave, cryotherapy or radiotherapy energy delivered via the cervix to heat (or cool) and destroy the endometrium. They have similar success rates to first-generation techniques and a lower risk of uterine perforation.

Transcervical resection of fibroid (TCRF) uses the same hysteroscopic equipment as for a TCRE. Submucosal fibroids up to 3 cm diameter are resected to reduce menstrual flow and improve fertility. If fertility is not desired then a TCRE can be performed at the same time as the TCRF.

More radical

Myomectomy is the removal of fibroids from the myometrium. It can be open or laparoscopic (if <4 fibroids of <8 cm diameter, depending on surgeon's experience) and is used if fibroids are causing symptoms but fertility is still required. GnRH agonists or ulipristal acetate are often used preoperatively to reduce the size of fibroids.

Hysterectomy should be the last resort in the treatment of abnormal uterine bleeding and the numbers of women undergoing this procedure are falling in the UK. The operation can be vaginal, abdominal or laparoscopic. The uterus is found to be normal in about half of women having hysterectomy for menorrhagia.

Uterine artery embolization (UAE) treats menorrhagia due to fibroids and is suitable for women who want to retain their uterus and avoid surgery. The effects of UAE on fertility are not clear (*Maturitas* 2014; **79**: 106–116).

When to do an endometrial biopsy (Pipelle or hysteroscopy)

Age >40 years
HMB with intermenstrual bleeding (IMB)
Risk factors for endometrial cancer
HMB unresponsive to medical therapy
If ultrasound suggests a polyp or focal endometrial thickening (perform hysteroscopy)
Prior to endometrial ablation/diathermy as tissue will not be available for pathology (unlike TCRE)
If abnormal uterine bleeding has resulted in acute admission

Irregular menstruation and intermenstrual bleeding

Epidemiology

This may coexist with heavy menstrual bleeding and is more common at extremes of reproductive age.

Causes

Anovulatory cycles are common in the early and late reproductive years (i.e. just after the menarche and before the menopause).

Pelvic pathology: Non-malignant causes include fibroids, uterine and cervical polyps, adenomyosis, ovarian cysts and chronic pelvic infection. However, with older women, particularly if there has been a recent change, the chances of malignancy, ovarian and cervical, and most particularly endometrial, are slightly increased.

Clinical features

Women should be assessed as for HMB. Speculum examination may reveal a cervical polyp.

Investigations

To assess the effect of blood loss and fitness, the patient's haemoglobin is checked.

Investigations should exclude malignancy, except in young women where malignancy is rare, and exclude local treatable pathology. A cervical smear is taken if required. An *ultrasound* examination of the cavity is performed for women over the age of 35 years with irregular or intermenstrual bleeding, and in younger women if medical treatment has failed, and will also detect a uterine fibroid or ovarian mass. *Endometrial biopsy* is then performed if the endometrium is either focally or very thickened, a polyp is suspected (combine with hysteroscopy), the woman is over 40 years of age, IMB is significant, there are risk factors for endometrial cancer, or if endometrial ablation surgery or the IUS are to be used.

Management

Drugs

This is appropriate where no anatomical cause is detected; cycles are considered anovulatory. *The IUS or the combined oral contraceptive* are first-line treatment options. The contraceptive pill usually induces regular and lighter menstruation. Its role is limited because its complications are more common in older patients (although it can be used until the menopause in suitable women). *Progestogens* in high doses will cause amenorrhoea, but bleeding will follow withdrawal. They induce secretory changes in the endometrium and so, when given on a cyclical basis, can mimic normal menstruation. HRT may regulate erratic uterine bleeding during the perimenopause. *Other treatments* that are second-line treatments for HMB may also be used.

Surgery

A cervical polyp can be avulsed and sent for histological examination. Surgery is as for women with HMB, except that ablative techniques tend to be less helpful as some endometrium often remains and so irregular but light bleeding may continue.

Absent and infrequent menstrual bleeding (amenorrhoea and oligomenorrhoea)

Definitions

Amenorrhoea is the absence of menstruation. *Primary amenorrhoea* is when menstruation has not started by the age of 16 years. It may be a manifestation of *delayed puberty*, which is when secondary sex characteristics are not present by the age of 14 years. Amenorrhoea may also occur in girls with otherwise normal secondary sexual characteristics, when a problem of menstrual outflow is likely. *Secondary amenorrhoea* is when previously normal menstruation ceases for 3 months or more (Fig. 2.9). *Oligomenorrhoea* is when menstruation occurs every 35 days to 6 months.

Classification of causes

Physiological amenorrhoea occurs during pregnancy, after the menopause and, usually, during lactation. Constitutional delay is common and often familial.
Pathological causes may lie in the hypothalamus, pituitary, thyroid, adrenals, ovary or uterus and 'outflow tract'. Drugs such as progestogens, GnRH analogues and, sometimes, antipsychotics (through increasing prolactin levels) cause amenorrhoea.

Where pathological, primary amenorrhoea is due either to rare congenital abnormalities or acquired disorders that arise before the normal time of puberty.

Secondary amenorrhoea or oligomenorrhoea is due to acquired disorders that arise later. The most common causes of secondary amenorrhoea or oligomenorrhoea are the premature menopause, PCOS and hyperprolactinaemia.

Hypothalamus

Hypothalamic hypogonadism is common and is usually due to psychological factors, low weight/anorexia nervosa or excessive exercise. Tumours are an uncommon cause and are excluded by brain magnetic resonance imaging (MRI). GnRH and therefore FSH, LH and oestradiol are reduced. Treatment is supportive; bone density is reduced if there has been prolonged hypo-oestrogenism and requires monitoring. Oestrogen replacement is required (plus progesterone for endometrial protection) using either the combined oral contraceptive or HRT. Anorexia nervosa is life-threatening and requires psychiatric treatment.

Pituitary

Hyperprolactinaemia is usually caused by pituitary hyperplasia or benign adenomas. Treatment is with bromocriptine, cabergoline or, occasionally, surgery. Rare pituitary causes include other pituitary tumours and Sheehan's syndrome, in which severe postpartum haemorrhage causes pituitary necrosis and varying degrees of hypopituitarism.

Adrenal or thyroid gland

Overactivity or underactivity of the thyroid can cause amenorrhoea. Hypothyroidism leads to raised prolactin levels and amenorrhoea. Congenital adrenal hyperplasia or virilizing tumours are rare.

Ovary

Acquired disorders: The most common is *polycystic ovary syndrome*. This can cause primary or secondary amenorrhoea, although oligomenorrhoea is more common. It is extremely important as it is common, is also associated with subfertility and has long-term health consequences. *Premature menopause* occurs in 1 in 100 women. Rare *virilizing tumours* can arise in the ovary.

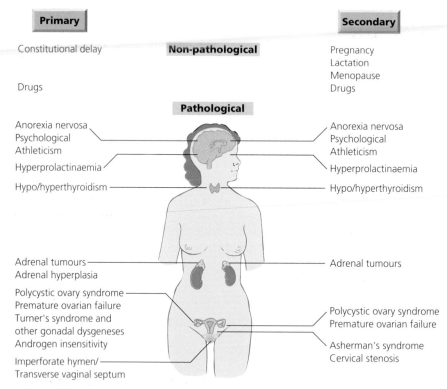

Primary | Secondary

Non-pathological

Constitutional delay

Pregnancy
Lactation
Menopause
Drugs

Drugs

Pathological

Anorexia nervosa
Psychological
Athleticism

Anorexia nervosa
Psychological
Athleticism

Hyperprolactinaemia

Hyperprolactinaemia

Hypo/hyperthyroidism

Hypo/hyperthyroidism

Adrenal tumours
Adrenal hyperplasia

Adrenal tumours

Polycystic ovary syndrome
Premature ovarian failure
Turner's syndrome and
other gonadal dysgeneses
Androgen insensitivity

Polycystic ovary syndrome
Premature ovarian failure

Asherman's syndrome
Cervical stenosis

Imperforate hymen/
Transverse vaginal septum

Fig. 2.9 Causes of amenorrhoea.

Congenital causes: The most common is *Turner's syndrome*, in which one X chromosome is absent, producing the 45 XO genotype. These women have short stature and poor secondary sexual characteristics, but normal intelligence. In other forms of *gonadal dysgenesis*, the ovary is imperfectly formed due to mosaic abnormalities of the X chromosomes. Gonadal agenesis and androgen insensitivity are extremely rare.

Outflow tract problems: menstrual flow is obstructed or absent

Congenital problems cause primary amenorrhoea with normal secondary sexual characteristics. The *imperforate hymen* and the *transverse vaginal septum* obstruct menstrual flow, which therefore accumulates over the months in the vagina (haematocolpos) or uterus (haematometra), which may be palpable abdominally. Treatment is surgical. Rarer causes include absence of the vagina with or without (Rokitansky's syndrome) a functioning uterus.

Acquired problems usually cause secondary amenorrhoea. *Cervical stenosis* prevents release of blood from the uterus, causing a haematometra. *Asherman's syndrome* is an uncommon consequence of excessive curettage at evacuation of retained products of conception (ERPC) performed following miscarriage or delivery; *endometrial resection* or *ablation* produces this effect intentionally.

Management

The important conditions of premature menopause, PCOS and hyperprolactinaemia are discussed elsewhere.

Postcoital bleeding

Definition

Vaginal bleeding following intercourse that is not menstrual loss. Except for first intercourse, this is always abnormal and cervical carcinoma must be excluded.

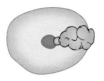

Fig. 2.10 Cervical carcinoma.

Aetiology

When the cervix is not covered in healthy squamous epithelium, it is more likely to bleed after mild trauma. Cervical ectropions, benign polyps and invasive cervical cancer account for most cases. The bleeding occasionally comes from the vaginal wall, usually if it is atrophic.

Causes of postcoital bleeding
Cervical carcinoma (Fig. 2.10)
Cervical ectropion
Cervical polyps
Cervicitis, vaginitis

Management

The cervix is carefully inspected and a smear is taken. If a polyp is evident, it is avulsed and sent for histology; this is normally possible without anaesthesia. If the smear is normal, an ectropion can be frozen with cryotherapy. If not, colposcopy is undertaken to exclude a malignant cause.

Dysmenorrhoea

This is painful menstruation. It is associated with high prostaglandin levels in the endometrium and is due to contraction and uterine ischaemia.

Causes and their management

Primary dysmenorrhoea is when no organic cause is found. It usually coincides with the start of menstruation and is very common (50% of women, 10% severe), particularly in adolescents. Pain usually responds to NSAIDs or ovulation suppression (e.g. the combined oral contraceptive). Reassurance in the young adolescent is important. Pelvic pathology is more likely if medical treatment fails.

Secondary dysmenorrhoea is when pain is due to pelvic pathology. Pain often precedes and is relieved by the onset of menstruation. Deep dyspareunia and menorrhagia or irregular menstruation are common. Pelvic ultrasound and laparoscopy are useful. The most significant causes are fibroids, adenomyosis, endometriosis, pelvic inflammatory disease and ovarian tumours, which should be treated appropriately. *Laparoscopic uterine nerve ablation* (LUNA) is not beneficial (*Cochrane* 2005; CD001896).

Precocious puberty

This is when menstruation occurs before the age of 9 years or other secondary sexual characteristics are evident before the age of 8 years. It is very rare. The growth spurt occurs early, but final height is reduced due to early fusion of the epiphyses. Investigation is essential, as it may be a manifestation of other disorders. Treatment is essential to arrest sexual development and allow normal growth.

Causes and their management

In 80% of cases, no pathological cause is found. GnRH agonists are used to inhibit sex hormone secretion, causing regression of secondary sex characteristics and cessation of menstruation.

Central causes: increased GnRH secretion: Meningitis, encephalitis, central nervous system tumours, hydrocephaly and hypothyroidism may prevent normal prepubertal inhibition of hypothalamic GnRH release.

Ovarian/adrenal causes: increased oestrogen secretion: Hormone-producing tumours of the ovary or adrenal glands will also cause premature sexual maturation. Regression occurs after removal. The McCune–Albright syndrome consists of bone and ovarian cysts, *café au lait* spots and precocious puberty. Treatment is with cyproterone acetate (an antiandrogenic progestogen).

Ambiguous development and intersex

There are many causes and degrees of ambiguous genitalia. Psychological support is important and gender assignation should be consistent.

Increased androgen function in a genetic female

Congenital adrenal hyperplasia is recessively inherited. Cortisol production is defective, usually as a result of 21-hydroxylase deficiency; adrenocorticotrophic hormone (ACTH) excess causes increased androgen production. The condition normally presents at birth with ambiguous genitalia; glucocorticoid deficiency may cause Addisonian crises. Occasionally, it presents at puberty with an enlarged clitoris and amenorrhoea. Treatment involves cortisol and mineralocorticoid replacement; lack of these can be fatal. Androgen-secreting tumours and other causes of Cushing's syndrome are rare.

Reduced androgen function in a genetic male

Androgen insensitivity syndrome (AIS) occurs when a male has cell receptor insensitivity to androgens, which are converted peripherally to oestrogens. The individual appears to be female; the diagnosis is only discovered when 'she' presents with amenorrhoea. The uterus is absent and rudimentary testes are present. These are removed because of possible malignant change and oestrogen replacement therapy is started.

Premenstrual syndrome

Premenstrual syndrome (PMS) encompasses psychological, behavioural and physical symptoms that are experienced on a regular basis during the luteal phase of the menstrual cycle and often resolve by the end of menstruation.

Epidemiology

Ninety-five per cent of women experience some premenstrual symptoms; in about 5% they are severely debilitating (Fig. 2.11).

Aetiology

This is unknown, but is dependent on normal ovarian function and the hormone progesterone. Exogenous progestogens are known to cause PMS-like symptoms.

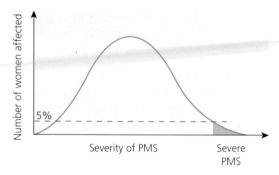

Fig. 2.11 Distribution of premenstrual syndrome (PMS) in the population.

Differing neurochemical responses to ovarian function (certain neurotransmitter levels may be altered during the luteal phase in severely affected women) may account for the differing severities of the syndrome.

Clinical features

History: These vary and it is the cyclical nature rather than the symptoms themselves that enable diagnosis. Behavioural changes include 'tension', irritability, aggression, depression and loss of control. In addition, a sensation of bloatedness, minor gastrointestinal upset and breast pain can occur.

Examination: Psychological evaluation may be helpful as depression and neurosis can present as PMS. There are no biochemical markers for PMS. Women should be asked to complete menstrual diaries, recording their moods and other symptoms for at least two cycles.

Management

Drugs

Selective serotonin reuptake inhibitors (SSRIs) are effective, given either continuously or intermittently in the second half of the cycle. Because true PMS is in some way caused by the fluctuation of hormones in the second half of the cycle, ablating the cycle may be effective. If the woman needs contraception, continuous oral contraception should help; 100 μg oestrogen HRT patches may be effective. If this is unsuccessful and symptoms are extreme, a trial of

GnRH agonists and add-back oestrogen therapy to induce a pseudomenopause may be undertaken. If this is successful, then agonists with add-back HRT can be continued or, as a final resort, bilateral oophorectomy considered (although combined HRT or the contraceptive pill would then be required for bone and endometrial protection). The role of progesterone is uncertain.

Other

Supplements: Evening primrose oil is good for breast tenderness. Pyridoxine (vitamin B6) 50 mg twice daily helps in mild PMS, but can cause a neuropathy in excessive doses. Vitex agnus-castus extract can help PMS.
Cognitive–behavioural therapy aims to change the way a woman copes with her life.

Further reading

BMJ Point of Care/Best Practice. *Premenstrual Syndrome and Dysphoric Disorder*. Available at: http://bestpractice.bmj.com/best-practice/monograph/419.html (accessed 5 July 2016).

Clinical Knowledge Summaries (CKS). *Amenorrhea*. Available at: http://cks.nice.org.uk/amenorrhoea#!topicsummary (accessed 5 July 2016).

Clinical Knowledge Summaries (CKS). Menorrhagia. Available at: http://cks.nice.org.uk/menorrhagia (accessed 5 July 2016).

National Institute for Health and Care Excellence (NICE). *Heavy Menstrual Bleeding*. NICE Clinical Guideline 44. London: NICE, 2007.

SOGC Clinical Practice Guideline. Abnormal uterine bleeding in pre-menopausal women. *Journal of Obstetrics and Gynaecology Canada* 2013; **35(5 eSuppl)**: S1–S28 (open access paper).

Menstrual cycle disorders at a glance

Types	Heavy menstrual bleeding (menorrhagia), irregular menstruation, intermenstrual bleeding (IMB)
Epidemiology	One-third of women describe heavy periods (not age related), most do not seek help
Aetiology	*HMB*: Usually ovulatory cycles. Cause not usually found. May be anatomical
	Irregular bleeding: Often anovulatory, polycystic ovary syndrome (PCOS) most common cause. Sometimes anatomical
	Structural causes: PALM, i.e. polyp, adenomyosis, leiomyoma, malignancy, and hyperplasia (endometrial or cervical)
	Non-structural causes: COEIN, i.e. coagulopathy, ovulatory dysfunction, endometrial (problems with local regulatory mechanisms), iatrogenic, not yet published
Investigations	Full blood count (FBC), pelvic ultrasound, ± endometrial biopsy (sometimes combined with hysteroscopy) if IMB, or thickened or irregular endometrium, or age >40 years, or risk factors for endometrial cancer
Treatment	Treat systemic disease appropriately. Then symptom relief
	Medical: To reduce volume: intrauterine system (IUS), tranexamic acid, mefenamic acid, combined contraceptive pill
	To regulate timing: IUS (amenorrhoea in most), combined contraceptive or cyclical/continuous progestogens
	Surgical: Hysteroscopic surgery: resection or ablation, hysterectomy occasionally, myomectomy/embolization of fibroids

CHAPTER 3
The uterus and its abnormalities

Anatomy and physiology of the uterus

Anatomy and function

The uterus nourishes, protects and, ultimately, expels the fetus. Inferiorly, it is continuous with the cervix, which acts as its neck and communication with the vagina. The superior part is the fundus; on either side of this, the uterus communicates with the fallopian tubes at the cornu. It is supported predominantly at the inferior end, at the cervix, by the uterosacral and cardinal ligaments. In 80% of women, it tilts up towards the abdominal wall, which is called anteversion. In 20% of women, it is retroverted, tilting back into the pelvis. The wall is made of smooth muscle (the tissue of origin of the benign tumours *fibroids*) that encloses the uterine cavity. This is lined by glandular epithelium – the endometrium (the tissue of origin of *endometrial carcinoma*). The outside coat of the uterus, or serosa, is the peritoneum posteriorly. This also covers the uterus anteriorly down to the bladder, which is in front of the lower uterus, the cervix and the vagina. (The proximity of the bladder to the lower uterus and vagina explains the ease with which it can be damaged at surgery or in childbirth.) Laterally, this peritoneum is continuous with the broad ligaments that run between the uterus and pelvic side wall. These have little function as supports but are continuous with the fallopian tubes and round ligaments superiorly, and contain the uterine blood supply, ureters and parametrium inferiorly (Fig. 3.1).

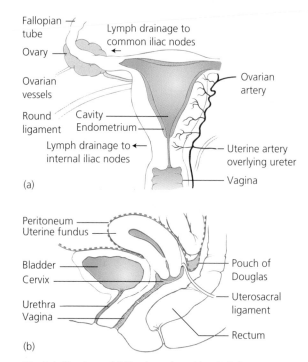

Fig. 3.1 The uterus. (a) Blood supply and lymph drainage. (b) Relations of the pelvic organs.

Blood and lymph

The uterine blood supply (see Fig. 3.1) is from the uterine arteries, which cross over the ureters lateral to the cervix and pass inferiorly and superiorly, supplying the myometrium and endometrium. At the cornu, there is an arterial anastomosis with the ovarian blood

Obstetrics & Gynaecology, Fifth Edition. Lawrence Impey, Tim Child.
© 2017 John Wiley & Sons, Ltd. Published 2017 by John Wiley & Sons, Ltd.

supply. Inferiorly, there is an anastomosis with the vessels of the upper vagina. Lymph drainage of the uterus (see Fig. 3.1) is mostly via the internal and external iliac nodes.

The endometrium

The endometrium is supplied by the spiral and basal arterioles. The former are important in menstruation and in nourishment of the growing fetus. The endometrium is responsive to oestrogen and progesterone. In the first 14 days of the menstrual cycle, it proliferates: the glands elongate and the endometrium thickens, largely under the influence of oestrogens (proliferative phase). After ovulation, under the influence of progesterone, the glands swell and the blood supply increases (luteal or secretory phase; see Fig. 2.3). Towards the end of this phase, progesterone levels drop, the secretory endometrium disintegrates as its blood supply can no longer support it and menstruation occurs. Poor hormonal control commonly causes erratic bleeding patterns.

Fibroids

Definition and epidemiology

Also known as leiomyomata, these are benign tumours of the myometrium. By age 50, nearly 70% of white women and more than 80% of black women have had at least one fibroid. They are more common with increasing age during reproductive years, in black and Asian women (who are also more likely to have multiple fibroids), in obese women, those with an early menarche (before age 11) and in women with an affected first-degree relative. They are less common in parous women and those who have taken the combined oral contraceptive or injectable progestogens.

Pathology and sites of fibroids

Fibroids can be single or multiple and range in size from a few millimetres to massive tumours filling the abdomen. The fibroid may be intramural, subserosal or submucosal (Fig. 3.2). Submucosal fibroids occasionally form intracavity polyps. Smooth muscle and fibrous elements are present, and in transverse section the fibroid has a 'whorled' appearance.

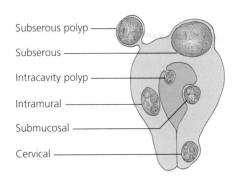

Subserous polyp
Subserous
Intracavity polyp
Intramural
Submucosal
Cervical

Fig. 3.2 Sites of fibroids showing intramural, subserosal and submucosal placement.

Aetiology

Fibroid growth is oestrogen and progesterone dependent. During pregnancy, fibroids are equally likely to grow, shrink or show no change. Fibroids regress after the menopause due to the reduction in circulating sex hormones. Each fibroid is of monoclonal origin.

Clinical features

History: Fifty per cent are asymptomatic and discovered only at physical or ultrasound examination. Symptoms are related more to the site than the size. For example, a 2 cm diameter submucosal fibroid will often lead to abnormal menstrual bleeding whereas a 2 cm diameter subserosal fibroid will usually be aymptomatic.
- Menstrual problems: heavy menstrual bleeding occurs in 30%, although the timing of menses is usually unchanged. Intermenstrual loss may occur if the fibroid is submucosal or polypoid. Fibroids are common in the perimenopausal woman and may be incidental; menstrual problems may also be the result of hormonal irregularities or malignancy.
- Pain: fibroids can cause dysmenorrhoea. They seldom cause pain, unless torsion, red degeneration or, rarely, sarcomatous change occurs.
- Other symptoms: large fibroids pressing on the bladder can cause frequency and occasionally urinary retention, those pressing on the ureters can cause hydronephrosis; other pressure effects may also be felt. Fertility can be impaired if the tubal ostia are blocked or submucous fibroids prevent implantation. Intramural fibroids not distorting the cavity also reduce fertility though the mechanism is unclear.

Examination: A solid mass may be palpable on pelvic or even abdominal examination. It will arise from the pelvis and be continuous with the uterus. Multiple small fibroids cause irregular 'knobbly' enlargement of the uterus.

Symptoms of fibroids
None (50%)
Menorrhagia (30%)
Erratic/bleeding (IMB)
Pressure effects
Subfertility

Natural history/complications of fibroids

Enlargement can be very slow. Fibroids stop growing and often calcify after the menopause, although the oestrogen in hormone replacement therapy (HRT) may stimulate further growth. In mid-pregnancy they may enlarge. Pedunculated fibroids occasionally undergo torsion, causing pain.

'Degenerations' are normally the result of an inadequate blood supply: 'red degeneration' is characterized by pain and uterine tenderness; haemorrhage and necrosis occur. In 'hyaline degeneration' and 'cystic degeneration', the fibroid is soft and partly liquefied.

Malignancy: Around 0.1% of fibroids are leiomyosarcomata. This may be the result of malignant change or *de novo* malignant transformation of normal smooth muscle. Usually diagnosed only on histology, the potential diagnosis should be considered when there is fibroid growth in postmenopausal women or rapidly enlarging fibroids or sudden onset of pain in women of any age. The risks of tumour spread by intraabdominal morcellation of an unsuspected leiomyosarcoma during laparoscopic myomectomy should be considered.

Complications of fibroids		
Torsion of pedunculated fibroid		
Degenerations	Red (particularly in pregnancy)	
	Hyaline/cystic	
	Calcification (postmenopausal and asymptomatic)	
Malignancy	Leiomyosarcoma	

Fibroids and pregnancy

Premature labour, malpresentations, transverse lie, obstructed labour and postpartum haemorrhage can occur. Red degeneration is common in pregnancy and can cause severe pain. Fibroids should not be removed at caesarean section as bleeding can be heavy. Pedunculated fibroids may tort postpartum.

Hormone replacement therapy and fibroids

Hormone replacement therapy can cause continued fibroid growth after the menopause. Treatment is as for premenopausal women or the HRT is withdrawn.

Investigations

To establish diagnosis: Ultrasound is the initial screening method and determines the number, size and position of fibroids. Magnetic resonance imaging (MRI) is sometimes used if the diagnosis is unclear or if greater accuracy is required, particularly when deciding the mode of treatment (Figs 3.3, 3.4). Adenomyosis can exist as a fibroid-like mass, differentiated by MRI. Hysteroscopy, saline transvaginal ultrasonography or hysterosalpingogram (HSG) is used to assess distortion of the uterine cavity, particularly if fertility is an issue.

To establish fitness: The haemoglobin concentration may be low as a result of vaginal bleeding, but also high as fibroids can secrete erythropoietin.

Treatment

Fibroids only require treatment when they cause symptoms. If a woman's quality of life is affected by fibroids then her desire for fertility, preservation of her uterus or both will likely guide decision making on whether to observe or proceed to medical, radiological or surgical treatment.

Medical treatment

Tranexamic acid, non-steroidal anti-inflammatory drugs or *progestogens* are often ineffective when menorrhagia is due to fibroids but may be worth trying as a simple first-line treatment. Whilst the *progesterone intrauterine system (IUS)* is an excellent treatment for

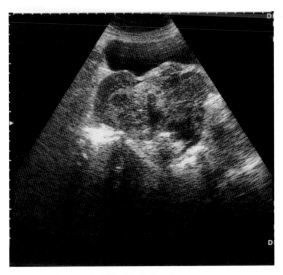
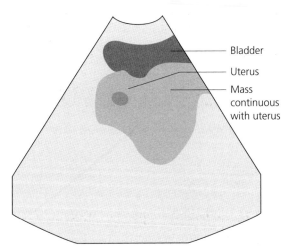

Fig. 3.3 Ultrasound of fibroids in the uterus.

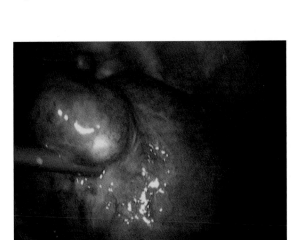

Fig. 3.4 Laparoscopic view of a uterus containing intramural and subserosal fibroids.

women with HMB in the absence of fibroids, evidence for its efficacy in women with fibroids is limited, it cannott be used if the uterine cavity is distorted, and submucosal fibroids can cause explusion.

Gonadotrophin-releasing hormone (GnRH) agonists cause temporary amenorrhoea and fibroid shrinkage by inducing a temporary menopausal state. Side effects and bone density loss restrict their use to only 6 months, usually near the menopause or to make surgery easier and safer. However, concomitant use of 'add-back'

HRT may prevent such effects without causing enlargement, allowing longer administration. Once the GnRH agonist is stopped and hormone levels return to normal then fibroids will return to their previous size. GnRH agonist treatment is not appropriate for women trying to conceive due to the induced anovulation and return of the fibroids with drug cessation. Consequently, surgery is usually used to manage fibroids under these circumstances.

Selective progesterone receptor modulators (SPRMs) (e.g. oral *ulipristal acetate*) are a new class of drug that reduce HMB, commonly cause reversible amenorrhoea and shrink fibroids (volume reduced by 50%, similar to GnRH agonists) without causing bone density loss and menopausal side effects. They can be used short term in preparation for surgery or long term intermittently to control fibroid symptoms and avoid surgery altogether (*Fertil Steril* 2015; **103**: 519–527). They cause reversible benign endometrial changes.

Is the fibroid malignant?

Uncommon, but more likely if there is:
- pain and rapid growth
- growth in postmenopausal woman not on HRT
- poor response to GnRH agonists or ulipristal acetate

Surgical treatment

Hysteroscopic surgery

The fibroid polyp or small (up to 3 cm) submucous fibroid that is causing menstrual problems or subfertility can be resected at hysteroscopy (transcervical resection of fibroid (TCRF)). Pretreatment with a GnRH agonist for 1–2 months will shrink the fibroid, reduce vascularity and thin the endometrium, so making resection easier and safer.

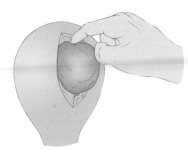

Fig. 3.5 Myomectomy.

Myomectomy

Fibroids can be removed from the uterus by open or laparoscopic myomectomy (Fig. 3.5). Blood loss may be heavy (risk of blood transfusion, or hysterectomy to save life) and small fibroids can be missed or new ones develop, causing problems to recur. Myomectomy is performed if medical treatment has failed but preservation of reproductive function is required and uterine artery embolization is not desired (see below). Myomectomy can be preceded by 2–3 months' treatment with GnRH analogues or ulipristal acetate to shrink the fibroid and reduce vascularity. Perioperative injection of vasopressin directly into the myometrium reduces blood loss (*Cochrane* 2014: CD005355). Adhesions can form at the site of myomectomy which, if affecting the endometrial cavity or fallopian tubes/ovaries, significantly reduce fertility.

Endometrial cavity adhesions can be very difficult to treat. If the endometrial cavity is opened during myomectomy or if the fibroids are multiple and/or large, then caesarean section is indicated in future pregnancies because of an increased risk of uterine rupture during labour.

During laparoscopic myomectomy, fibroids are usually removed via powered morcellation in which the morcellator instrument, introduced through one of the laparoscopic ports, 'apple cores' the fibroid. If an unrecognized leiomyosarcoma is morcellated, there is a risk of malignancy spread. The risk of an unexpected leiomyosarcoma at surgery for presumed benign fibroid is estimated to be 2–3 per 1000 in women aged <50 years (*Oncologist* 2015; **20**: 433–439). Though the risk is relatively low, this led to the US Food and Drug Administration (FDA) warning in 2014 against morcellation of fibroids, though the advice is contentious since the main alternative to laparoscopic myomectomy (laparotomy) carries other increased surgical risks and,

overall, may lead to more deaths (*Am J Obstet Gynecol* 2015; **212**: 591).

Radical: hysterectomy

Fibroids are a common indication for hysterectomy, performed laparoscopically, vaginally or abdominally. Patient satisfaction scores are high and hysterectomy is cost effective but clearly not suitable for women wanting to preserve fertility. Pretreatment with GnRH agonist or ulipristal acetate for 2–3 months will shrink the fibroids and uterine size and possibly allow a less invasive operation, for instance, a laparoscopic or vaginal approach rather than open.

Other treatments

Embolization: Uterine artery embolization (UAE) by radiologists has an 80% success rate and is an alternative to hysterectomy or myomectomy. The volume of embolized fibroids reduces by around 50%. The hospital stay is shorter with a quicker return to normal activities. However, pain may get worse, readmission and further surgical intervention rates are higher than with myomectomy, and hysterectomy may still be required. As the effects of UAE on uterine function are unclear, most fertility specialists do not offer it to women desiring future pregnancy (*J Obstet Gynaecol Can* 2015; **37**: 277–285). However, the results of randomized controlled trials (RCTs) comparing UAE against myomectomy are awaited since both uterine-sparing treatments have advantages and disadvantages.

Ablation: Novel methods of treating fibroids include ablation by MRI-guided transcutaneous focused ultrasound. The safety and efficacy remain to be fully determined.

Adenomyosis

Definition and epidemiology

Previously called 'endometriosis interna', this is the presence of endometrium and its underlying stroma within the myometrium (Fig. 3.6). Its true incidence is unknown, but it occurs in up to 40% of hysterectomy specimens. It is most common around the age of 40 years and is associated with endometriosis and fibroids. Symptoms subside after the menopause.

Pathology and aetiology

The endometrium appears to grow into the myometrium to form adenomyosis. The extent is variable but in severe cases, pockets of menstrual blood can be seen in the myometrium of hysterectomy specimens. Occasionally, endometrial stromal tissue in the myometrium displays varying degrees of atypia or even invasion.

Clinical features

History: Symptoms may be absent, but painful, regular, heavy menstruation is common.
Examination: The uterus is mildly enlarged and tender.

Investigations

Adenomyosis can be suspected on ultrasound but clearly diagnosed on MRI.

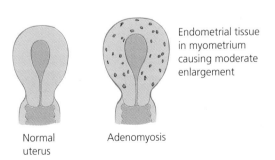

Endometrial tissue in myometrium causing moderate enlargement

Normal uterus   Adenomyosis

Fig. 3.6 Adenomyosis. Source: Sutton CJ et al. *Fertil Steril* 1994; **62**: 696–700. Reproduced with permission of Elsevier

Treatment

Medical treatment with the progesterone IUS or the combined oral contraceptive pill with or without NSAIDs may control the menorrhagia and dysmenorrhoea, but hysterectomy is often required. For some women, a trial of GnRH analogue therapy may determine if symptoms attributed to adenomyosis are likely to improve with hysterectomy. The condition is oestrogen dependent, but why it occurs is unknown. The effects on fertility are unclear.

Other benign conditions of the uterus

Endometritis

This often occurs secondary to sexually transmitted infections, as a complication of surgery, particularly caesarean section and intrauterine procedures (e.g. surgical termination), or because of foreign tissue, particularly intrauterine devices (IUDs) and retained products of conception. Infection in the postmenopausal uterus is commonly due to malignancy. The uterus is tender and pelvic and systemic infection may be evident. Pyometra is when pus accumulates and is unable to escape. Antibiotics and occasionally evacuation of retained products of conception (ERPC) are required.

Intrauterine polyps

These are small, usually benign tumours that grow into the uterine cavity. Most are endometrial in origin (Fig. 3.7), but some are derived from submucous fibroids. They are common in women aged 40–50 years and when oestrogen levels are high. In the postmenopausal woman, they are often found in patients on tamoxifen for breast carcinoma. Occasionally, they contain endometrial hyperplasia or carcinoma. Although sometimes asymptomatic, they often cause menorrhagia and intermenstrual bleeding and very occasionally prolapse through the cervix. They are normally diagnosed at ultrasound or when a hysteroscopy is performed because of abnormal bleeding. Resection of the polyp with cutting diathermy or avulsion normally cures bleeding problems.

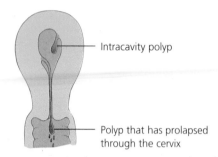

Fig. 3.7 Endometrial polyps.

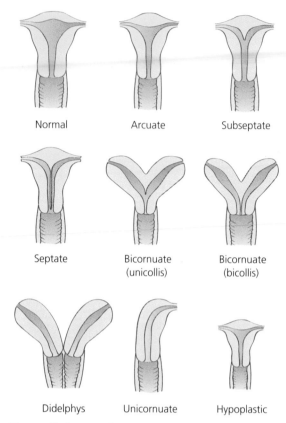

Fig. 3.8 Uterine anomalies.

Haematometra

This is menstrual blood accumulating in the uterus because of outflow obstruction. It is uncommon. The cervical canal is usually occluded by fibrosis after endometrial resection, cone biopsy or by a carcinoma. Congenital abnormalities, for example imperforate hymen or blind rudimentary uterine horn, present in adolescence as primary amenorrhoea.

Congenital uterine malformations

Abnormalities result from differing degrees of failure of fusion of the two Mullerian ducts at about 9 weeks (Fig. 3.8). These are common but are seldom clinically significant. Total failure of fusion leads to two uterine cavities and cervices (didelphys) with sometimes a longitudinal vaginal septum; or one duct may fail, causing a 'unicornuate' uterus. If one duct develops better than the other one, a smaller 'rudimentary horn' is formed. Its cavity can be blind or continuous with the dominant horn. At the other end of the spectrum, there may simply be a small septum at the fundus. Women with a congenital uterine anomaly have an increased incidence of renal anomalies and should undergo renal tract imaging.

About 25% cause pregnancy-related problems that lead to their discovery. These include malpresentations or transverse lie, preterm labour, recurrent miscarriage (<5% of these) or retained placenta. Treatment for pregnancy-related problems, however, should not be undertaken lightly as congenital abnormalities may be incidental. Simple septa can be resected hysteroscopically; rudimentary horns need removal at either open or laparoscopic surgery. Bicornuate uteri are no longer treated surgically as the complication rates were too high.

Endometrial carcinoma

Epidemiology

This is now the most common gynaecological cancer, with women having a cumulative risk of 1% of developing endometrial cancer by the age of 75 (Fig. 3.9).

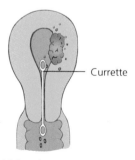

Fig. 3.9 Endometrial carcinoma.

Prevalence is highest at the age of 60 years, with only 15% of cases occurring premenopausally and <1% in women under 35 years of age. Because it usually presents early, it is often incorrectly considered to be relatively benign, but stage for stage the prognosis is similar to ovarian malignancy.

Pathology

Endometrial cancer is classified into two subtypes on the basis of histology. *Type 1* (the majority) consists of low-grade endometrioid cancers which are oestrogen sensitive, associated with obesity and usually less aggressive. They often have atypia as a precursor. *Type 2* cancers include high-grade endometrioid, clear cell, serous or carcinosarcoma cancers which tend to be more aggressive and not oestrogen sensitive. These tend not to be related to obesity.

Aetiology

Risk factors

The main risk factor is exposure to endogenous and exogenous oestrogens associated with obesity, diabetes, early age at menarche, nulliparity, late-onset menopause, older age (>55 years), unopposed oestrogen HRT and use of tamoxifen. Although an oestrogen antagonist in the breast and used in the treatment of breast cancer, tamoxifen is mainly an agonist in the postmenopausal uterus. It is possible that the link with diabetes is related to body mass index (BMI). The combined oral contraceptive and pregnancy are protective.

Premalignant disease: endometrial hyperplasia with atypia

Oestrogen acting unopposed or erratically can cause 'hyperplasia' of the endometrium. Further stimulation predisposes to abnormalities of the cellular and glandular architecture or 'atypical hyperplasia'. This may cause menstrual abnormalities or postmenopausal bleeding and is premalignant. Hyperplasia with atypia often coexists (40%) with carcinoma elsewhere in the uterine cavity but is seldom recognized prior to the diagnosis of malignancy. Endometrial hyperplasia with atypia is uncommon in women of reproductive age. If this diagnosis is

made, hysterectomy should be discussed. If fertility is a concern, progestogens (IUS or continuous oral) and 3–6-monthly hysteroscopy and endometrial biopsy are used along with referral to a fertility specialist for consideration of treatment.

Risk factors for endometrial carcinoma	
Endogenous oestrogen excess	Polycystic ovary syndrome (PCOS) (if prolonged amenorrhoea leading to unopposed oestrogen) and obesity Nulliparity, early menarche and late menopause Obesity
Exogenous oestrogens	Unopposed oestrogen therapy Tamoxifen therapy
Miscellaneous	Diabetes (due to raised BMI?) Lynch type II syndrome (familial non-polyposis, colonic, ovarian and endometrial carcinoma)

Clinical features

History: Postmenopausal bleeding (PMB; 10% risk of carcinoma) is the most common presentation. The likelihood that PMB is due to endometrial cancer rather than benign or unknown causes increases with age. Premenopausal patients have irregular or intermenstrual bleeding (IMB) or, occasionally, only recent-onset menorrhagia.

Examination: The pelvis often appears normal and atrophic vaginitis may coexist.

Spread and staging

The tumour spreads directly through the myometrium to the cervix and upper vagina (Fig. 3.10). The ovaries may be involved. Lymphatic spread is to pelvic and then para-aortic lymph nodes. Blood-borne spread occurs late. Staging (FIGO 2009) is surgical and histological and, in contrast to cervical carcinoma, includes lymph node involvement.

Histological grade: G1–3 is also included for each stage, G1 being a well-differentiated tumour.

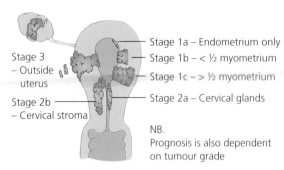

Stage 3 – Outside uterus

Stage 2b – Cervical stroma

Stage 1a – Endometrium only
Stage 1b – < ½ myometrium
Stage 1c – > ½ myometrium
Stage 2a – Cervical glands

NB.
Prognosis is also dependent on tumour grade

Fig. 3.10 Stages of endometrial carcinoma.

Spread and staging for endometrial carcinoma	
Stage 1	*Lesions confined to uterus*:
1a	<½ of myometrial invasion
1b	>½ of myometrial invasion
Stage 2	*As above but in cervix also*:
2	Cervical stromal invasion, but not beyond uterus
Stage 3	*Tumour invades through the uterus*:
3a	Invades serosa or adnexae
3b	Vaginal and/or parametrial involvement
3Ci	Pelvic node involvement
3cii	Para-aortic involvement
Stage 4	*Further spread*:
4a	In bowel or bladder
4b	Distant metastases

Investigations

Abnormal vaginal bleeding is investigated as discussed for premenopausal women (see Chapter 2) and for post-menopausal women (see Chapter 13). Depending on age, menopausal status and symptoms (i.e. likelihood of underlying cancer), an ultrasound scan and/or endometrial biopsy with a Pipelle or hysteroscopy is performed. Endometrial biopsy is required to make the diagnosis. Staging is only possible following hysterectomy. An MRI may be used to give an estimate of myometrial invasion and, therefore, guide appropriate referral to a cancer centre in cases with deep invasion. A chest X-ray is required to exclude rare pulmonary spread.

To assess the patient's fitness, full blood count (FBC), renal function, glucose testing and an electrocardiogram (ECG) are normally required as most patients are elderly.

Treatment

Surgery

Seventy-five per cent of patients present with stage 1 disease. Unless the patient is unfit or has disseminated disease, a total laparoscopic (abdominal if not possible) hysterectomy and bilateral salpingo-oophorectomy (BSO) is performed. The value of pelvic and para-aortic lymphadenectomy is debatable but it may be useful in high-risk cases (e.g. high-grade endometrioid carcinoma) to select patients for external beam radiotherapy. As staging is surgico-pathological, disease that appears to be stage 1 at surgery may subsequently turn out to be stage 3 if lymph nodes are involved. However, routine lymphadenectomy is not beneficial in early stage disease (*Cochrane* 2015; **373**: 125–136) and is associated with the development of limb lymphoedema, but an estimate of stage and risk should be made to determine further management.

Adjuvant therapy

External beam radiotherapy: This is used following hysterectomy in patients with, or considered at 'high risk' for, lymph node involvement, but not in those with early-stage disease. Risk factors from pathological examination of the uterus are deep myometrial spread, poor tumour histology or grade, or cervical stromal involvement (i.e. stage 2). It is also used for pelvic recurrence, when it is most beneficial if it has not been given previously.

Vaginal vault radiotherapy is also used where the above risk factors are present. Its usage reduces local recurrence but does not prolong survival.

Chemotherapy: Recently completed and current trials are assessing the role of chemotherapy, radiation therapy, or a combination of both in women with high risk and advanced endometrial cancer (*Lancet* 2016; Morice P).

Progestogens are now seldom used.

General indications for radiotherapy
High risk for extrauterine disease: deep myometrial or cervical stromal spread, poor grade
Proven extrauterine disease
Inoperable and recurrent disease
Palliation for symptoms, e.g. bleeding

Prognosis of endometrial carcinoma	
Stage	*Five-year survival rate (%)*
1	90
2	75
3	60
4	25
Overall	75

Prognosis

Recurrence is most common at the vaginal vault, normally in the first 3 years. Poor prognostic features are older age, advanced clinical stage, deep myometrial invasion in stage 1 and 2 patients, high tumour grade and adenosquamous histology.

Uterine sarcomas

These are rare tumours, accounting for only 150 cases per year in the UK.

Leiomyosarcomas are 'malignant fibroids' and present with rapid, painful uterine ('fibroid') enlargement.

Treatment is with hysterectomy but early recurrence is common due to haematogenous spread. Radiotherapy or chemotherapy can be used following hysterectomy, but overall survival is only 30% at 5 years.

Endometrial stromal tumours are tumours of the stroma beneath the endometrium. Histological types vary from the benign endometrial stromal nodule to the highly malignant endometrial stromal sarcoma. These are most common in the perimenopausal woman.

Further reading

Cancer Research UK. *Uterine (Womb) Cancer Statistics – UK*. Available at: http://info.cancerresearchuk.org/cancerstats/types/uterus/ (accessed 7 July 2016).

Lumsden MA, Hamoodi I, Gupta J, Hickey M. Fibroids: diagnosis and management. *BMJ* 2015; **315**: h4887.

Morice P, Leary A, Creutzberg C, Abu-Rustum N, Darai E. Endometrial cancer. *Lancet* 2016; **387**:1094–1108.

RCOG. Management of Endometrial Hyperplasia. Green-top Guideline No. 67. Available at: www.rcog.org.uk/en/guidelines-research-services/guidelines/gtg67/ (accessed 7 July 2016).

Fibroids at a glance

Epidemiology	25% of women, older, nulliparous, Afro-Caribbean or Asian
Pathology	Benign tumours of myometrium
Aetiology	Monoclonal, oestrogen and progesterone dependent
Clinical features	None (50%) Menstrual problems, dysmenorrhoea, pressure effects, subfertility and pain
Complications	Torsion of pedunculated fibroid. Degenerations: red or hyaline degeneration. Sarcomatous change Complicates pregnancy
Investigations	Full blood count, hysteroscopy, ultrasound Magnetic resonance imaging or laparoscopy if diagnosis unsure
Treatment	Observation or … *Conservative*: Symptomatic relief, ulipristal acetate *Surgical*: Hysteroscopic resection if intrauterine. Myomectomy (fertility preserving), embolization or hysterectomy

Endometrial carcinoma at a glance

Epidemiology	Most common gynaecological carcinoma, usually over 60 years of age
Pathology	>90% adenocarcinomas. Type 1 (less aggressive, oestrogen dependent) and type 2 (more aggressive, not oestrogen dependent) subtypes
Aetiology	High oestrogen:progesterone ratio. Nulliparity, late menopause, polycystic ovary syndrome if long-term amenorrhoea, obesity. Unopposed oestrogens and tamoxifen Combined pill and pregnancy protective
Clinical features	Postmenopausal bleeding (PMB) (10% risk of endometrial cancer) Premenopausal women see a 'change': irregular, intermenstrual or heavier bleeding
Screening	Not routine. Presents early. Probably worthwhile if taking tamoxifen
Investigations	If PMB then ultrasound scan plus, if endometrium >4 mm thick or multiple episodes, biopsy by Pipelle or during hysteroscopy If premenopausal, do ultrasound scan then biopsy if abnormal or change in periods and >40 years. Consider magnetic resonance imaging. Full blood count, urea and electrolytes, abdominal and chest computed tomography, glucose, electrocardiogram
Staging	Staging is surgico-pathological 1 Uterus only: 1A: <½ myometrial invasion; 1B: >½ myometrial invasion 2 Cervix also 3 Pelvic/para-aortic lymph nodes 4 Bowel and bladder or distant spread
Treatment	Usually total laparoscopic hysterectomy and bilateral salpingo-oophorectomy Radiotherapy if lymph nodes positive/likely to be positive
Prognosis	Dependent on clinical stage, histology, grade, patient's fitness Overall 75% 5-year survival

CHAPTER 4
The cervix and its disorders

Anatomy and function of the cervix

Anatomy

The cervix is a tubular structure, continuous with the uterus, 2–3 cm long and made up predominantly of elastic connective tissue. It connects the uterus and vagina, allowing sperm in and menstrual flow out. In pregnancy it holds the fetus in the uterus and then dilates in labour to allow delivery. It is attached posteriorly to the sacrum by the uterosacral ligaments and laterally to the pelvic side wall by the cardinal ligaments. Lateral to the cervix is the parametrium, containing connective tissue, uterine vessels and the ureters.

Histology and the transformation zone

The endocervix (canal) is lined by columnar (glandular) epithelium. The ectocervix, continuous with the vagina, is covered in squamous epithelium. The two types of cell meet at the 'squamocolumnar junction' (Fig. 4.1). During puberty and pregnancy, partial eversion of the cervix occurs. The lower pH of the vagina causes the now exposed area of columnar epithelium to undergo metaplasia to squamous epithelium, producing a 'transformation zone' at the squamocolumnar junction (see Fig. 4.1). Cells undergoing metaplasia are vulnerable to agents that induce neoplastic change, and it is from this area that cervical carcinoma commonly originates.

Blood supply and lymph drainage

The blood supply is from upper vaginal branches and the uterine artery. Lymph drains to the obturator and internal and external iliac nodes, and thence to the common iliac and para-aortic nodes. Cervical carcinoma characteristically spreads in the lymph and locally by direct invasion into the uterus, vagina, bladder and rectum.

Benign conditions of the cervix

Cervical ectropion (previously called erosion) is when the columnar epithelium of the endocervix is visible as a red area around the os on the surface of the cervix (Fig. 4.2a). This is due to eversion and is a normal finding in younger women, particularly those who are pregnant or taking the 'pill'. Normally asymptomatic, ectropions occasionally cause vaginal discharge or postcoital bleeding (PCB). This can be treated by freezing (cryotherapy) without anaesthetic, but only after a smear and, ideally, colposcopy have excluded a carcinoma. Exposed columnar epithelium is also prone to infection.

Acute cervicitis is rare but often results from sexually transmitted disease. Ulceration and infection are occasionally found in severe degrees of prolapse when the cervix protrudes or is held back with a pessary.

Obstetrics & Gynaecology, Fifth Edition. Lawrence Impey, Tim Child.
© 2017 John Wiley & Sons, Ltd. Published 2017 by John Wiley & Sons, Ltd.

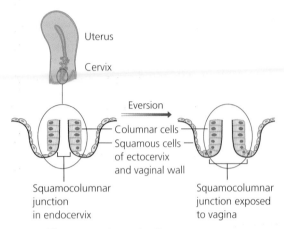

Fig. 4.1 The squamocolumnar junction.

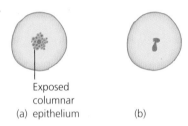

Fig. 4.2 (a) Cervical ectropion, (b) cervical polyp.

Chronic cervicitis is chronic inflammation or infection, often of an ectropion. It is a common cause of vaginal discharge and may cause 'inflammatory' smears. Cryotherapy is used, with or without antibiotics, depending upon bacterial culture.

Cervical polyps are benign tumours of the endocervical epithelium (Fig. 4.2b). They are most common in women above the age of 40 years and are seldom larger than 1 cm. They may be asymptomatic or cause intermenstrual bleeding (IMB) or PCB. Small polyps are avulsed without anaesthetic and examined histologically, but bleeding abnormalities must still be investigated.

Nabothian follicles occur where squamous epithelium has formed by metaplasia over endocervical cells. The columnar cell secretions are trapped and form retention cysts, which appear as white or opaque swellings on the ectocervix. Treatment is not required unless symptomatic (rare).

In *congenital malformations* the uterus and cervix may be absent or varying degrees of duplication may occur.

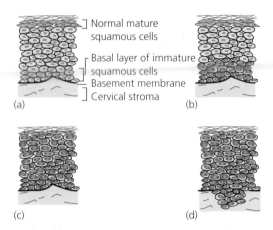

Fig. 4.3 The cervical epithelium and cervical intraepithelial neoplasia (CIN). (a) Normal cervical epithelium; proliferation in basal layer only with small nuclei. (b) CIN I–II: abnormal cells with larger nuclei proliferating in the lower one-third to two-thirds of the epithelium. (c) CIN III: abnormal cells occupying the entire epithelium. (d) Microinvasion: abnormal cells have penetrated the basement membrane.

Premalignant conditions of the cervix: cervical intraepithelial neoplasia

Definitions

Cervical intraepithelial neoplasia (CIN), or cervical dysplasia, is the presence of atypical cells within the squamous epithelium. These atypical cells are dyskaryotic, exhibiting larger nuclei with frequent mitoses. The severity of CIN is graded I–III and is dependent on the extent to which these cells are found in the epithelium (Fig. 4.3). CIN is therefore a *histological* diagnosis.

- *CIN I (mild dysplasia)*: Atypical cells are found only in the lower third of the epithelium.
- *CIN II (moderate dysplasia)*: Atypical cells are found in the lower two-thirds of the epithelium.
- *CIN III (severe dysplasia)*: Atypical cells occupy the full thickness of the epithelium. This is carcinoma *in situ*; the cells are similar in appearance to those in malignant lesions, but there is no invasion. Malignancy ensues if these abnormal cells invade through the basement membrane.

If untreated, about one-third of women with CIN II/III will develop cervical cancer over the next 10 years.

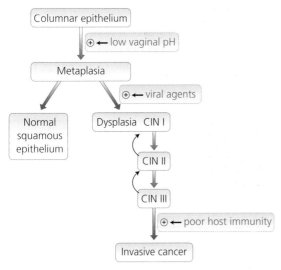

Fig. 4.4 Natural history of cervical intraepithelial neoplasia (CIN).

CIN I has the least malignant potential: it can progress to CIN II/III, but commonly regresses spontaneously (Fig. 4.4).

Epidemiology

Cervical intraepithelial neoplasia is becoming more common. Ninety per cent of cases of CIN III are in women under 45 years, with peak incidence in those 25–29 years of age.

Aetiology

Human papilloma virus (HPV): The most important factor is the number of sexual contacts, particularly at an early age; CIN is almost unknown in virgins. This is because infection with a HPV is sexually transmitted. Of over 130 different HPV strains, types 16, 18, 31 and 33 are most frequently associated with cervical cancer, though around 13 are considered 'high risk'.

Vaccination against individual viruses reduces the incidence of precancerous cervical lesions and therefore, potentially, cervical cancer. The vaccine is given before first sexual contact (i.e. to children/young adolescents) as it has a prophylactic effect, and does not help to treat established CIN. A UK national vaccination programme for adolescent girls began in 2008. The vaccine targets HPV types 16 and 18, which are responsible for 75% of cervical cancer cases in the UK. Because cervical cancer affects adult women, it will be many years before the full impact of immunization is seen. The vaccination of adolescent boys as part of the UK programme is under consideration. This would reduce the rate of penile cancer (mostly HPV related) and reduce the HPV transmission rate to unvaccinated women.

Other factors: Oral contraceptive usage and smoking are associated with a slightly increased risk of CIN. Immunocompromised patients (e.g. human immunodeficiency virus (HIV), those on long-term steroids) are also at increased risk of early progression to malignancy.

Pathology

As the columnar epithelium undergoes metaplasia to squamous epithelium in the transformation zone, exposure to certain HPV results in incorporation of viral deoxyribonucleic acid (DNA) into cell DNA. Viral proteins inactivate key cell tumour suppressor gene products and push the cell into a cell cycle. Over time, other mutations accumulate and can lead to carcinoma. Viruses also cause changes to hide the infected cell from the immune system. Failure of the immune system to detect and destroy such cells, either because of these cell changes or because of immunosuppression (transplant patient or acquired immunodeficiency syndrome (AIDS)), can result in malignancy.

Diagnosis: screening for cervical cancer

Cervical intraepithelial neoplasia causes no symptoms and is not visible on the cervix. However, the diagnosis identifies women at high risk of developing carcinoma of the cervix who could be treated before the disease develops. Identification of CIN is therefore the principal step in screening for cervical cancer.

Cervical smears

Screening is performed with cervical smears. These should be performed in all women from the age of 25 years, or after first intercourse if later, and then repeated every 3 years until the age of 49. Between 50 and 64 years of age smears are performed every 5 years. From the age of 65, only those who have not been screened since age 50 or have had recent abnormal tests are screened. The abnormal smear identifies women

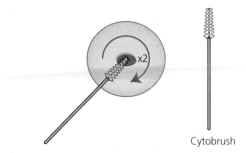

Cytobrush

Fig. 4.5 Taking a cervical smear.

likely to have CIN and therefore at risk of subsequent development of invasive cancer. Women younger than 25 years often have abnormal cervical changes but the risk of cervical cancer is very low. Commencing screening at 25 reduces the number of unnecessary recalls and colposcopies. The number of women diagnosed with cervical cancer in the UK has halved since the NHS screening programme was introduced in 1988 and screening now prevents around 5000 deaths per year. Around 80% of eligible women undergo screening.

Method

Using a Cusco's speculum, a brush is gently scraped around the external os of the cervix to pick up loose cells over the transformation zone (Fig. 4.5). The brush tip is broken into preservative fluid and transported to the laboratory, then the fluid is centrifuged and spread on a slide for microscopy (liquid-based cytology or LBC). LBC has replaced the use of a wooden spatula followed by direct smearing on a slide. The move to LBC as a method of cervical screening has reduced the number of inadequate samples and test recalls from 9% to 2.5%. LBC also allows testing for HPV within the same sample, with subsequent management dependent on the presence or absence of high-risk HPV types ('HPV triage').

Results

Smears identify cellular, not histological, abnormalities as only superficial cells are sampled. Cellular abnormalities are called *dyskaryosis* and classified as borderline, low or high grade. Dyskaryosis suggests the presence of CIN, and the grade partly reflects the severity of CIN. Smears are therefore often reported in histological terms; if high =0grade dyskaryosis is seen, for instance, the report may read 'CIN III'. This does not mean that CIN III is present, merely that a biopsy would be likely to find it.

Women with borderline or low-grade cellular abnormalities previously were invited back for a repeat smear after 6 months. If the abnormality remained then colposcopy was undertaken. From 2011, using HPV triage, women with borderline or low-grade dyskaryosis have their sample tested for HPV and if a high-risk HPV type is present then colposcopy is arranged. If the sample is negative for a high-risk HPV then the woman is returned to routine 3–5-yearly recall.

Human papilloma virus testing is also used as a 'test of cure'. Previously, women with CIN who underwent colposcopy treatment were recalled for annual smears for up to 10 years. Now, however, if follow-up smears show normal cells and the absence of high-risk HPV, then they can be entered back into the routine call and recall system. The use of combined cytological and HPV testing therefore reduces the number of repeat tests, colposcopy treatments and patient anxiety.

Occasionally, abnormal columnar cells are visible (cervical glandular intraepithelial neoplasia (CGIN)). Adenocarcinoma of the cervix or endometrium should then be excluded, using both colposcopy and endocervical curettage (sampling cells within the cervical canal) or with cone biopsy. Hysteroscopy is used if the cause of the abnormal cells is still unclear.

Colposcopy

The cervix is inspected via a speculum using an operating microscope with magnification 10–20-fold. Grades of CIN have characteristic appearances when stained with 5% acetic acid, although the diagnosis is only confirmed histologically and therefore biopsy is usual.

Management of the abnormal smear (with HPV triage)	
Smear result	*Action*
Normal	Repeat every 3 years (5 years if over age 50)
Borderline or low-grade dyskaryosis	If HPV negative: back to routine recall
	If HPV positive: colposcopy
High-grade dyskaryosis	Colposcopy
Cervical glandular intraepithelial neoplasia (any grade)	Colposcopy; if abnormality not found then hysteroscopy

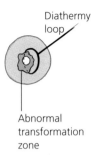

Diathermy
loop

Abnormal
transformation
zone

Fig. 4.6 Large loop excision of transformation zone (LLETZ).

Prevention of cervical cancer
Human papilloma virus vaccination Prevention of CIN : sexual and (barrier) contraceptive education Identification and treatment of CIN: cervical smear programmes

Treatment: prevention of invasive cervical cancer

If CIN II or III is present, the transformation zone is excised with cutting diathermy under local anaesthetic. This is called large loop excision of transformation zone (LLETZ) (Fig. 4.6), also sometimes called diathermy loop excision (DLE). The specimen is examined histologically. Occasionally an unsuspected malignancy is detected. LLETZ enables diagnosis and treatment to be achieved at the same time ('see and treat') and has replaced laser or diathermy ablation treatment. Alternatively, a small biopsy of the abnormal area can be taken colposcopically and confirmatory results awaited before performing LLETZ. The only major complication of LLETZ, postoperative haemorrhage, is uncommon but the risk of subsequent preterm delivery is increased in proportion to the depth of excision (*BMJ* 2014; **349**: g6233).

Results and problems with screening for cervical cancer

Cervical screening by 3–5-yearly smear can prevent around 45% of cervical cancer cases in women in their 30s, rising with age to 75% in women in their 50s and 60s who attend regularly. Screening prevents around 5000 deaths in the UK each year. Most women with cervical carcinoma have never had a smear, and those who

have tend to be identified at an earlier stage. Nevertheless, there is a significant false-negative rate with cervical smears, dependent on both sampling and interpretation techniques. Furthermore, the distinctions between grades of dyskaryosis and CIN are blurred and spontaneous regression of CIN can occur. Some women do not have cervical smears through fear or lack of awareness.

Psychological aspects of cervical screening

The woman with an abnormal smear must be handled sensitively. Many will assume they have cancer so an explanation of the 'early warning cells' found will allay fears. Discussion of sexual history and the papilloma virus is usually inappropriate because of feelings of guilt and recrimination. If CIN III is found then the woman can be advised that *without treatment*, she has around a 30% chance of developing cancer over 8–15 years. However, colposcopic treatment is straightforward and successful.

Malignant disease of the cervix

Epidemiology

Cervical cancer is the third most common gynaecological cancer after uterine and ovarian. In the UK there are around 3000 new cases diagnosed and 1000 deaths per year. It is the most common cancer in females under the age of 35 in the UK. Whilst the UK incidence decreased by nearly 50% between the late 1980s (when the NHS cervical screening programme was introduced) and the early 2000s, the last decade has seen an increase in rates in young women. The disease can occur at any age after first intercourse, but has two peaks of incidence: during a woman's 30s and her 80s. The majority of cases occur in women aged 25–49 years. Cervical cancer mortality rates decreased overall in the UK by 70% between 1972 and 2012.

Pathology

Ninety per cent of cervical malignancies are squamous cell carcinomas. Ten per cent are adenocarcinomas originating from the columnar epithelium; these have a worse prognosis and are increasing in proportion as the smear programme prevents proportionally more squamous carcinomas.

Aetiology

Cervical intraepithelial neoplasia is the preinvasive stage; causative factors are therefore the same. HPV is found in all cervical cancers; vaccination is likely to prevent many cases in the future. Cervical cancer is more common when screening has been inadequate. Immunosuppression (e.g. HIV or steroids) accelerates the process of invasion from CIN. Cervical cancer is not familial.

Clinical features

Occult carcinoma

This is when there are no symptoms, but the diagnosis is made by biopsy or LLETZ.

Clinical carcinoma

History: Postcoital bleeding, an offensive vaginal discharge and IMB or postmenopausal bleeding (PMB) are common. Pain is not an early feature. In the later stages of the disease, involvement of ureters, bladder, rectum and nerves causes uraemia, haematuria, rectal bleeding and pain, respectively. Smears have often been missed.

Examination: An ulcer or mass may be visible (Fig. 4.7) or palpable on the cervix. With early disease, the cervix may appear normal to the naked eye.

Spread and staging

The tumour spreads locally to the parametrium and vagina and then to the pelvic side wall. Lymphatic spread to the pelvic nodes is an early feature. Ovarian spread is rare with squamous carcinomas. Blood-borne spread occurs late. The International Federation of Gynaecology and Obstetrics (FIGO) classification is clinical (from examination), although divisions of stage 1 are histological (from local excision). It is limited as a predictor of survival because it does not include whether or not there is lymph node (LN) involvement. LN involvement is, however, more likely with advanced stages.

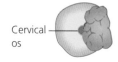

Fig. 4.7 Cervical carcinoma.

Spread and staging for cervical carcinoma	
Stage 1	*Lesions confined to the cervix*
1a(i)	Diagnosed only by microscope, invasion <3 mm in depth and lateral spread <7 mm
1a(ii)	Diagnosed with microscope, invasion >3 mm and <5 mm with lateral spread <7 mm
1b(i)	Clinically visible lesion or greater than 1a(ii), <4 cm in greatest dimension
1b(ii)	Clinically visible lesion, >4 cm in greatest dimension
Stage 2	*Invasion is into vagina, but not the pelvic side wall*
2a(i)	Involvement of upper two-thirds vagina, without parametrial invasion, <4 cm in greatest dimension
2a(ii)	>4 cm in greatest dimension
2b	Invasion of parametrium
Stage 3	*Invasion of lower vagina or pelvic wall, or causing ureteric obstruction*
Stage 4	*Invasion of bladder or rectal mucosa, or beyond the true pelvis*

Investigations

To confirm the diagnosis, the tumour is biopsied.

To stage the disease, vaginal and rectal examination is used to assess the size of the lesion and parametrial or rectal invasion. Unless it is clearly small, examination under anaesthetic (EUA) is performed. Cystoscopy detects bladder involvement and magnetic resonance imaging (MRI) detects tumour size, spread and LN involvement.

To assess the patient's fitness for surgery, a chest X-ray, full blood count (FBC) and urea and electrolytes (U&E) are checked. These may be abnormal with advanced disease. Blood is cross-matched before surgery.

Treatment of cervical malignancies

Microinvasive disease

Stage 1a(i) can be treated with cone biopsy (Fig. 4.8), as the risk of LN spread is only 0.5%. Postoperative haemorrhage and preterm labour in subsequent pregnancies are the main complications. Simple hysterectomy is preferred in older women.

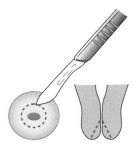

Fig. 4.8 Cone biopsy.

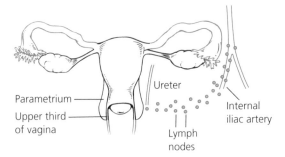

Parametrium

Upper third
of vagina

Ureter

Internal
iliac artery

Lymph
nodes

Fig. 4.9 Wertheim's hysterectomy.

All other stage 1 and stage 2a

The choice is between surgery and chemo-radiotherapy. If the LNs are involved, the latter is preferred; treatment is as for beyond stage 2a. LN involvement can be established at MRI, but LN sampling is still required if apparently negative, as MRI is not sensitive enough.
Radical hysterectomy (Wertheim's hysterectomy) involves pelvic node clearance, hysterectomy and removal of the parametrium and upper third of the vagina (Fig. 4.9). The ovaries are left only in the young woman with squamous carcinoma. Specific complications include haemorrhage, ureteric and bladder damage and fistulae, voiding problems and accumulation of lymph (lymphocyst). Increasingly, radical hysterectomy is undertaken using a minimal access approach.
Radical trachelectomy is a less invasive procedure for women who wish to conserve fertility. Laparoscopic pelvic lymphadenectomy is first performed. If nodes are positive then chemo-radiotherapy is used instead of surgery. If nodes are negative then radical trachelectomy is an option and involves removal of 80% of the cervix and the upper vagina (*Gynecol Oncol* 2011; **121**: 290). It is appropriate within stage 1a(ii)–1b(i) provided

the tumour is <20 mm in diameter. A cervical suture is inserted to help prevent preterm delivery. If the excision margins are incomplete then chemo-radiotherapy is required.

Proceeding straight to chemo-radiotherapy, particularly in older or medically unfit women, remains an alternative even if the nodes are negative, and survival rates are actually similar to surgery.

Stage 2b and worse or positive lymph nodes

These should be treated with radiotherapy and chemotherapy, e.g. platinum agents, the use of which reduces recurrence and increases survival. Palliative radiotherapy is used for bone pain or haemorrhage.

Recurrent tumours

Chemo-radiotherapy is given if it has not been used before. If it has, pelvic exenteration can be considered if the disease is central. Preoperative MRI and positron emission tomography (PET) scans are used to look for metastases. Pelvic exenteration involves removal of the vagina (the uterus and cervix if not already removed), the bladder and/or rectum, and is tried in the young, fit woman with a central recurrence. There is about a 30% cure rate in carefully selected patients.

Stages of cervical carcinoma and treatment	
Stage	*Treatment*
1a(i)	Cone biopsy or simple hysterectomy
1a(ii)–1b(i)	Laparoscopic lymphadenectomy and radical trachelectomy
1a(ii)–2a	Radical hysterectomy (if lymph nodes negative) or chemo-radiotherapy
2b and above or lymph nodes positive	Chemo-radiotherapy alone

Indications for chemo-radiotherapy for cervical carcinoma
Lymph nodes positive on magnetic resonance imaging or after lymphadenectomy
If lymph nodes negative as an alternative to hysterectomy
Surgical resection margins not clear
Palliation for bone pain or haemorrhage (radiotherapy)

Prognosis of cervical carcinoma	
Indicator	*Five-year survival (%)*
Stage Ia	95
Stage 1b	80
Stage 2	60
Stage 3–4	10–30
Lymph nodes involved	40
Lymph nodes clear	80
Overall	65

Prognosis

Patients are reviewed at 3 and 6 months and then every 6 months for 5 years. Recurrent disease is commonly central. Poor prognostic indicators are LN involvement, advanced clinical stage, large primary tumour, a poorly differentiated tumour and early recurrence. Death is commonly from uraemia due to ureteric obstruction.

Further reading

Crosbie EJ, Einstein MH, Franceschi S, Kitchener HC. Human papillomavirus and cervical cancer. *Lancet* 2013; **382**: 889–899.
NHS Cervical Screening: Programme Overview. Available at: www.cancerscreening.nhs.uk/cervical/ (accessed 7 July 2016).

Carcinoma of the cervix at a glance

Epidemiology	Becoming less common in the UK, deaths reducing
Pathology	90% squamous, also adenocarcinomas
Aetiology	Human papilloma virus (HPV), which is sexually transmitted, causing cervical intraepithelial neoplasia (CIN). HPV vaccine (types 16/18) given to all girls. Smoking, combined oral contraceptive, immunosuppression
Clinical features	None if occult. Postcoital (PCB) or intermenstrual bleeding (IMB), offensive discharge. Cervix initially appears normal, then ulcerated, then replaced by irregular mass
Screening	Routine use. Liquid-based cytology (LBC). HPV triage. Three-yearly cervical smears age 25–49; 5-yearly ages 50–64, colposcopy if abnormal
Investigations	Biopsy. Unless early, examination under anaesthetic (EUA) + cystoscopy and magnetic resonance imaging (MRI) to stage. Chest X-ray, urea and electrolytes (U&E), full blood count (FBC)
Staging	**1** Cervix and uterus: 1a(i) <3 mm depth, <7 mm across; 1a(ii) <5 mm depth, <7 mm across; 1b rest **2** Upper vagina also: 2a not parametrium; 2b in parametrium **3** Lower vagina or pelvic wall, or ureteric obstruction **4** Into bladder or rectum, or beyond pelvis

Treatment	Depends on clinical stage:	
	1a(i): Cone biopsy or simple hysterectomy	Cone biopsy or simple hysterectomy
	1a(ii)–1b(i): Laparoscopic lymphadenectomy and radical trachelectomy	Laparoscopic lymphadenectomy (to confirm negative LNs) and radical trachelectomy to preserve fertility
	1a(ii)–2a: Radical hysterectomy (if lymph nodes (LNs) negative) or chemo-radiotherapy	LNs negative: Wertheim's hysterectomy or chemo-radiotherapy LNs positive: Chemo-radiotherapy without surgery
	2b–4: Chemo-radiotherapy alone	Chemo-radiotherapy without surgery
Prognosis	Depends on LN involvement, clinical stage and histological grade Overall 65% 5-year survival	

Cervical intraepithelial neoplasia (CIN) at a glance

Definitions	Histological abnormality of the cervix in which abnormal epithelial cells occupy varying degrees of the squamous epithelium	
	CIN I/mild dysplasia: Atypical cells in the lower third of the epithelium	Atypical cells in lower third
	CIN II/moderate dysplasia: Atypical cells in the lower two-thirds of the epithelium	Atypical cells in lower two-thirds
	CIN III/severe dysplasia: Atypical cells occupy the full thickness of the epithelium	Atypical cells in full thickness (carcinoma *in situ*)
	Dyskaryosis: cellular abnormalities; borderline, low or high grade	Describes cellular (nuclear) abnormality only from cervical smear. Suggests presence of CIN
Epidemiology	Becoming more common, vaccination may reduce	
Prevention	Vaccination against HPV 16 and 18	
Aetiology	As for cervical carcinoma	
Diagnosis	No clinical features. Cervical smear abnormality and colposcopic abnormality suggests presence. Diagnosis confirmed histologically	
Treatment	Rationale: to prevent progression to invasion	
	CIN I usually observed; CIN II and III removed with large loop excision of transformation zone (LLETZ)	

CHAPTER 5
The ovary and its disorders

Anatomy and function of the ovaries

The normal ovaries occupy the ovarian fossa on the lateral pelvic wall overlying the ureter, but are attached to the broad ligament by the mesovarium, to the pelvic side wall by the infundibulopelvic ligament and to the uterus by the ovarian ligament. Blood supply is from the ovarian artery, but there is an anastomosis with branches of the uterine artery in the broad ligament (Fig. 5.1).

The ovaries have an outer cortex covered by 'germinal' epithelium (the most common carcinoma derives from this layer). The inner medulla contains connective tissue and blood vessels. The cortex contains the follicles and theca cells. Oestrogen is secreted by granulosa cells in the growing follicles and also by theca cells. The rare tumours of these cells secrete oestrogens. A few follicles start to enlarge every month under the influence of pituitary follicle-stimulating hormone (FSH), but only one will reach about 20 mm in size and rupture in response to the mid-cycle surge of pituitary luteinizing hormone (LH) to release its oocyte (see Fig. 2.3). After ovulation, the collapsed follicle becomes a corpus luteum, which continues to produce oestrogen and progesterone to support the endometrium whilst awaiting fertilization and implantation. If none occurs then the corpus luteum involutes, hormone levels decline and menstruation begins. If fertilization and implantation occur then human chorionic gonadotrophin (hCG) produced from trophoblasts maintains corpus luteum function and hormone production until 7–9 weeks' gestation when the fetoplacental unit takes over. Follicular and lutein cysts result from persistence of these structures in non-pregnant women.

Ovarian symptoms

Ovarian masses are often silent and detected either when they are very large and cause abdominal distension or on ultrasound scan. Acute presentation is associated with 'accidents'.

Ovarian cyst 'accidents'

Rupture of the contents of an ovarian cyst into the peritoneal cavity causes intense pain, particularly with an endometrioma or dermoid cyst (Fig. 5.2a). *Haemorrhage* into a cyst (Fig. 5.2b) or the peritoneal cavity often causes pain. Peritoneal cavity haemorrhage is occasionally so severe as to cause hypovolaemic shock. *Torsion* of the pedicle (bulky due to the cyst) causes infarction of the ovary ± tube and severe pain (Fig. 5.2c). Urgent surgery and detorsion are required if the ovary is to be saved.

Disorders of ovarian function

Polycystic ovary syndrome (PCOS) is a common disorder that causes oligomenorrhoea, hirsutism and subfertility. The 'cysts' are actually small, multiple, poorly developed follicles.

Premature menopause is when the last period is reached before the age of 40 years.

Problems of gonadal development include the gonadal dysgeneses, the most common of which is Turner's syndrome.

Obstetrics & Gynaecology, Fifth Edition. Lawrence Impey, Tim Child.
© 2017 John Wiley & Sons, Ltd. Published 2017 by John Wiley & Sons, Ltd.

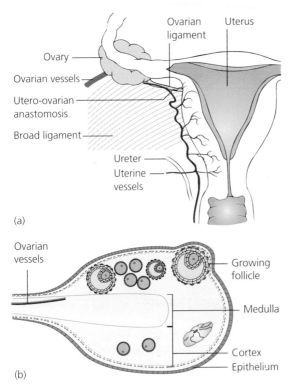

(a)

(b)

Fig. 5.1 Anatomy of the normal ovary. (a) Relations of the ovary. (b) Transverse section of the normal ovary.

Classification of ovarian tumours

Primary neoplasms

These can be benign or malignant. They are classified together because a benign cyst may undergo malignant change. They fall into three main groups.

Epithelial tumours

These are most common in postmenopausal women and are derived from the epithelium covering the ovary or, particularly for high-grade serous adenocarcinomas, the fallopian tube. Uniquely, histology may demonstrate 'borderline' malignancy, when malignant histological features are present but invasion is not. Such tumours may become frankly malignant: surgery is advised but their optimum management is disputed. In younger women with a borderline cyst, close observation may be offered following removal only of the cyst or affected ovary to retain fertility. Recurrence, as a borderline or invasive tumour, can occur up to 20 years later.

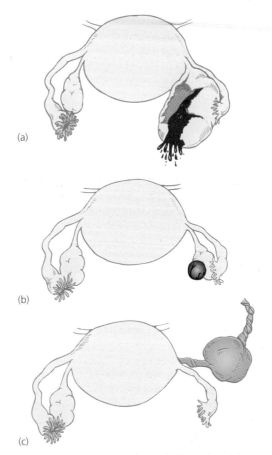

(a)

(b)

(c)

Fig. 5.2 (a) Rupture of an ovarian cyst. (b) Haemorrhage into an ovarian cyst (view from the abdomen). (c) Cyst twisting on its blood supply.

Serous cystadenoma or adenocarcinoma: The malignant variety is the most common malignant ovarian neoplasm and is classed as high grade (70% of ovarian malignancies) or low grade (<5% of malignancies). Benign and 'borderline' forms also exist.
Endometrioid carcinoma: This malignant variant accounts for 10% of ovarian malignancies. It is similar histologically to endometrial carcinoma, with which it is associated in 20% of cases.
Clear cell carcinoma is a malignant variant that accounts for 10% of ovarian malignancies and has a particularly poor prognosis.
Mucinous cystadenoma or adenocarcinoma can become very large. Mucinous adenocarcinoma accounts for 3% of ovarian malignancies. A rare 'borderline' variant is pseudomyxoma peritonei, in which the abdominal

cavity fills with gelatinous mucin secretions. An appendiceal primary tumour is more commonly the cause. *Brenner tumours* are rare and usually small and benign.

Germ cell tumours

These originate from the undifferentiated primordial germ cells of the gonad and account for 3% of ovarian malignancies.

Teratoma or dermoid cyst is a common benign tumour usually arising in young premenopausal women. It may contain fully differentiated tissue of all cell lines, commonly hair and teeth. It is commonly bilateral, seldom large and often asymptomatic. However, rupture is very painful. A malignant form, the solid teratoma, also occurs in this age group but is very rare.

Yolk sac tumours are highly malignant and present in children or young women.

Dysgerminoma is the female equivalent of the seminoma. Although rare, it is the most common ovarian malignancy in younger women. It is sensitive to radiotherapy.

Sex cord tumours

These originate from the stroma of the gonad and account for <2% of ovarian malignancies.

Granulosa cell tumours are usually malignant but slow growing. They are rare and are usually found in postmenopausal women. They secrete high levels of oestrogens and inhibin; stimulation of the endometrium can cause bleeding, endometrial hyperplasia, endometrial malignancy and, rarely, in young girls, precocious puberty. Serum inhibin levels are used as tumour markers to monitor for recurrence.

Thecomas are very rare, usually benign, and can secrete oestrogens and/or androgens.

Fibromas are rare and benign. They can cause Meigs' syndrome, whereby ascites and a (usually) right pleural effusion are found in conjunction with the small ovarian mass. The effusion is benign and cured by removal of the mass.

Common ovarian masses	
Premenopausal	Follicular/ lutein cysts
	Dermoid cysts
	Endometriomas
	Benign epithelial tumour
Postmenopausal	Benign epithelial tumour
	Malignancy

Secondary malignancies

The ovary is a common site for metastases, particularly from the breast and gastrointestinal tract. Secondaries account for 10% of malignant ovarian masses. A few contain 'signet ring' cells and if from the gut are called Krukenberg tumours. The primary malignancy may be difficult to detect and the prognosis is very poor.

Tumour-like conditions

The word 'cyst' can include anything from the malignant to the physiological, but is often interpreted as cancer by patients.

Endometriotic cysts: Endometriosis commonly causes altered blood to accumulate in 'chocolate cysts'. In the ovary, such cysts are called *endometriomas*. Rupture is very painful though uncommon.

Functional cysts: Follicular cysts and lutein cysts are persistently enlarged follicles and corpora lutea, respectively. They are therefore only found in premenopausal women. The combined pill protects against functional cysts by inhibiting ovulation. Lutein cysts tend to cause more symptoms. If symptoms are absent, treatment is not required and the cyst is observed using serial ultrasound scans. However, because of the remote possibility of malignancy, if an apparently functional cyst >5 cm persists beyond 2 months, the serum cancer antigen 125 (CA 125) level is measured and a laparoscopy considered to remove or drain the cyst (Fig. 5.3).

Ovarian cancer

The silent nature of this malignancy causes it to present late, meaning that the disease is widely metastatic within the abdomen. The 10-year survival rate is therefore 40–50%.

Epidemiology

There are 7000 new cases per year in the UK, causing 4200 deaths. The lifetime risk of developing ovarian cancer in the UK is 1 in 60. Rates increase with age and the median age of diagnosis in the general population is 63 years. There is marked geographical variation. After decades of increasing incidence, a steady slow fall has been noted in the UK and many other European countries since the early 2000s. This may be due

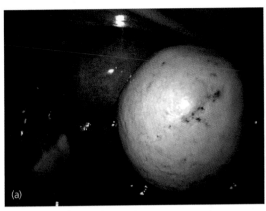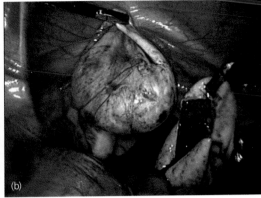

Fig. 5.3 (a) Laparoscopic photograph of a right ovarian benign epithelial cyst. (b) The cyst stripped and taken from within the ovary. The ovary returns to normal size within weeks of the operation.

to widespread use of the oral contraceptive pill (OCP), which reduces risk.

Histological types of primary ovarian malignancy	
Serous adenocarcinoma (high and low grades)	75%
Endometrioid carcinoma	10%
Clear cell carcinoma	10%
Mucinous adenocarcinoma	3%
Other (non-epithelial: germ cell and sex cord)	<5%

Pathology (see classification of ovarian tumours)

Ninety-five per cent overall are epithelial carcinomas and the management outlined applies largely to this group. The 'grade' of malignancy includes borderline, low and high grade. Germ cell tumours are the most common in the rare event of a woman under the age of 30 years being affected. Primary peritoneal cancer and fallopian tube cancer are rare malignancies but share many similarities with ovarian cancer. These three cancers are managed in a similar manner.

Aetiology

Benign cysts can undergo malignant change, but a pre-malignant phase is not normally recognized. The risk factors relate to the number of ovulations. Therefore, an early menarche, late menopause and nulliparity are risk factors, whilst pregnancy, lactation and use of the pill are protective. Ovarian carcinoma may also be

familial (5%) via the *BRCA1*, *BRCA2* (*Genet Med* 2010; **12**: 245–259) or *HNPCC* gene mutations. If two relatives are affected, the lifetime risk is 13%. If the *BRCA1* mutation is present, the risk approaches 50%. *BRCA1* and *BRCA2* gene mutations, with an overall prevalence of around 1:600, are also associated with breast cancer whilst *HNPCC* (also called Lynch's syndrome) is also associated with an increased risk of bowel (80% lifetime risk) and endometrial cancer. There is increasing recognition that the majority of high-grade serous adenocarcinomas, the most common type of ovarian cancer, actually originate in the fallopian tube.

Screening for ovarian cancer

There is currently no UK national screening programme for ovarian cancer. Unlike cervical cancer, screening is generally for early malignant rather than premalignant disease. Ovarian carcinoma presents late and, whilst the prognosis is much better for early disease, the recent results of a large trial (UKCTOCS) involving over 200 000 postmenopausal women randomized to annual transvaginal ultrasound scan, CA 125 checks or just observation showed no clear benefit of screening (*Lancet* 2016; **387**: 945–956). Women with a family history can be offered counselling and testing for genetic mutations in *BRCA1* and *BRCA2* genes. Those with the mutations are offered prophylactic salpingo-oophorectomy.

Clinical features

History. Symptoms are often initially vague and/or absent and 70% of patients present with stage 3–4 disease.

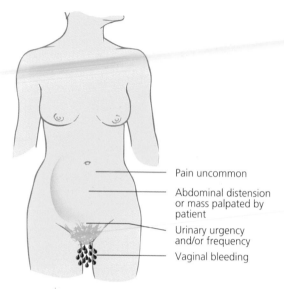

Pain uncommon

Abdominal distension or mass palpated by patient

Urinary urgency and/or frequency

Vaginal bleeding

Fig. 5.4 Ovarian cancer presents late as it is commonly asymptomatic.

Spread and staging for ovarian cancer (FIGO 2013)

Stage 1	*Disease macroscopically confined to the ovaries*
1a	One ovary is affected, capsule is intact
1b	Both ovaries are affected, capsule is intact
1c	1a or 1b with tumour on the surface, ruptured capsule, cytologically positive ascites, or positive peritoneal washings
Stage 2	*Disease extending to the pelvis* e.g. uterus, fallopian tubes or other pelvic tissues
Stage 3	*Abdominal disease and/or affected lymph nodes* The omentum, small bowel and peritoneum are frequently involved
Stage 4	*Disease is beyond the abdomen, e.g. in the lungs or liver parenchyma*

The histological type, including degree of differentiation or 'grade', is also reported

---

Increased awareness amongst women and GPs of warning symptoms and signs is vital to achieve earlier diagnosis, e.g. persistent abdominal distension ('bloating'), feeling full (early satiety) and/or loss of appetite, pelvic or abdominal pain, or increased urinary urgency and/or frequency (Fig. 5.4). Many of the symptoms are similar to those of irritable bowel syndrome (IBS) but since this rarely presents for the first time in older women, ovarian cancer must be excluded. It is important to ask about breast and gastrointestinal symptoms because a mass may be metastatic from these sites.

Examination: Examination may reveal cachexia, an abdominal or pelvic mass and ascites. Very large masses are less likely to be malignant. The breasts should be palpated.

Is the ovarian mass malignant?

More likely if:
Rapid growth, >5 cm
Ascites
Advanced age
Bilateral masses
Solid or septate nature on ultrasound scan
Increased vascularity

Spread and staging

Ovarian adenocarcinoma spreads directly within the pelvis and abdomen (called transcoelomic spread). Lymphatic and, more rarely, blood-borne spread also occur. Staging is surgical and histological.

Investigations

Initial detection (primary care)

CA 125 levels should be measured in women over 50 with many abdominal symptoms. These symptoms include persistent or frequent abdominal pain or distension ('bloating'), loss of appetite, weight loss and fatigue, change in bowel habit, urinary frequency and/or urgency, or with symptoms similar to IBS. If the CA 125 level is raised (>35 IU/mL), an ultrasound of the abdomen and pelvis is arranged (Fig. 5.5). If ultrasound or physical examination identifies ascites and/or a pelvic or abdominal mass, urgent referral to secondary care is undertaken.

Establishing the diagnosis (secondary care)

If not already performed, the CA 125 is measured and an ultrasound is arranged. In women under 40, levels of alpha fetoprotein (AFP) and hCG are measured to

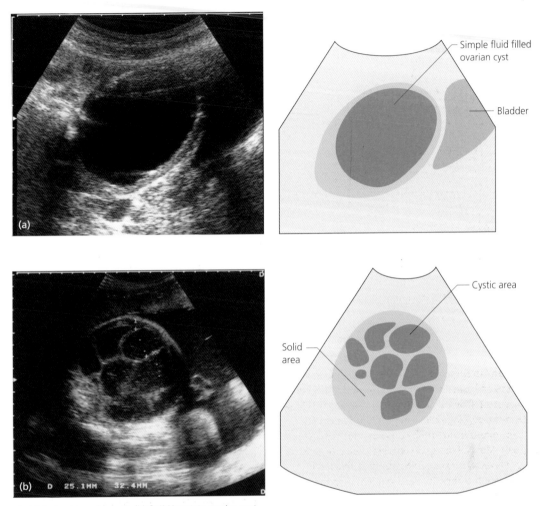

Fig. 5.5 (a) A simple ovarian cyst. (b) Solid/ septate ovarian cyst.

identify women who may not have epithelial ovarian cancer, levels being raised in germ cell tumours.

The *risk of malignancy index* (RMI) is calculated from the product of the ultrasound scan score (U), menopausal status (M) and serum CA 125 level, i.e. RMI = U × M × CA125. The ultrasound result is scored 1 point for each of the following characteristics: multilocular cysts, solid areas, metastases, ascites, bilateral lesions. U = 0 for an ultrasound score of 0 points, U = 1 for an ultrasound score of 1 point, and U = 3 for an ultrasound score of 2–5 points. Menopausal status is scored as 1 = premenopausal and 3 = postmenopausal. All women with a RMI ≥250 are referred to a specialist multidisciplinary team (MDT).

A computed tomography (CT) scan of the pelvis and abdomen (and thorax if clinically indicated) is performed to establish the extent of disease, but further staging is usually performed using surgery.

Management of ovarian cancer

Assessment of fitness for surgery may be extensive as many affected women are elderly. Blood is cross-matched before surgery.

Surgical

A mid-line laparotomy (Fig. 5.6) allows thorough assessment of the abdomen and pelvis (*Cochrane* 2013;

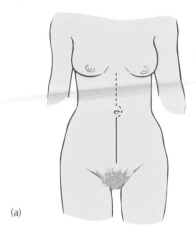

(a)

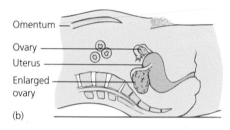

Omentum

Ovary

Uterus

Enlarged ovary

(b)

Fig. 5.6 (a) Site of incision for suspected ovarian cancer (dotted line is potential extension if abdominal disease). (b) Laparotomy for ovarian cancer. The uterus, ovaries, omentum and as much of the affected tissue as possible are removed.

CD005344). A total hysterectomy, bilateral salpingo-oophorectomy and partial omentectomy is performed, with biopsies of any peritoneal deposits, random biopsies of the peritoneum and retroperitoneal lymph node assessment. In women with suspected stage 1 ovarian cancer (disease confined to the ovaries), the retroperitoneal lymph nodes are sampled; in stage 2 or greater, they are removed through block dissection if enlarged. For advanced tumours, the prognosis relates to the effectiveness of the initial debulking procedure. Patients who have complete debulking have a better prognosis. So-called 'ultraradical' surgery is increasingly being performed which may include bowel resection, splenectomy and peritoneal stripping to achieve complete cytoreduction. In young women wishing to preserve fertility, where disease appears early or is 'borderline', the uterus and unaffected ovary may be preserved but meticulous further staging and follow-up are required.

Chemotherapy

A confirmed tissue diagnosis is required before offering chemotherapy. If surgery has not been performed then tissue for histology can be obtained through percutaneous image-guided biopsy or laparoscopy. If tissue for histology cannot be gained then cytology from paracentesis of ascites can be performed. CA 125 levels, if initially elevated, can be used to monitor the response to chemotherapy.

Very early (low-grade histology, stage 1a and 1b): Chemotherapy is not usually given (*Cochrane* 2012; CD004706). *Other stage 1* (high grade, stage 1c): six cycles of the platinum agent carboplatin are used.

Stage 2–4: Carboplatin (or cisplatin) alone or in combination with paclitaxel is used.

Two-thirds of women whose tumours initially respond to first-line chemotherapy relapse within 2 years of completing treatment. Many women now receive neoadjuvant chemotherapy, i.e. they do not have surgery initially but receive chemotherapy and have surgery halfway through the course of chemotherapy. This causes less morbidity although current evidence suggests there is no difference in survival with this approach.

Early-stage malignant germ cell tumours can often be adequately treated with removal of the adnexa alone, allowing preservation of fertility. Higher risk and more advanced germ cell tumours are usually treated with chemotherapy and are generally highly sensitive. Whilst dysgerminomas are sensitive to radiotherapy, chemotherapy is more effective and so preferred.

Follow-up and prognosis

Levels of CA 125 are useful after as well as during chemotherapy. CT scanning aids detection of residual disease or relapse. Interval debulking of residual tissue, if not all could be removed at first surgery, may be beneficial, but routine 'second-look' laparoscopy or laparotomy to monitor the response is not. Chemotherapy prolongs short-term survival and improves quality of life. Poor prognostic indicators are advanced stage, poorly differentiated tumours, clear cell tumours and slow or poor response to chemotherapy. Death is commonly from bowel obstruction or perforation. The prognosis of ovarian cancer is improving, but largely for the minority of women with early-stage disease.

Support: Women must be offered support and written information, including regarding psychosocial and psychosexual issues and genetic aspects, throughout the process of investigation, diagnosis and treatment. This should be appropriate to them and their disease stage.

Prognosis of ovarian cancer	
Stage	*Five-year survival (%)*
1a/b	85+
1c	80
2	70
3 (most patients)	40
4	10
Overall	<50

Palliative care

Only 30% of women are cured of their gynaecological carcinoma. Ovarian cancer causes the most deaths, but the principles outlined are applicable to all terminal disease.

Definition and aims

Palliative care is 'the active total care of the patient whose disease is incurable'. The aim is to increase quality of life for the patient and her family. This involves addressing symptoms such as pain, nausea, bleeding and symptoms of intestinal obstruction, as well as meeting the patient's social, psychological and spiritual needs. Care therefore needs to be individualized. Important issues include the problems of prolongation of poor-quality life, euthanasia, symptom control versus drug side effects, making the transition from curative to palliative care, and resource allocation.

Organization of palliative care

Three levels of care are involved, usually working together: the general practitioner, specialist practitioners such as Macmillan nurses, and specialist hospices or gynaecology units.

Symptom control

Pain: The 'analgesic ladder' (Fig. 5.7) describes the differing analgesic strengths of drugs. Co-analgesics such as antidepressants, steroids and cytotoxics may also be used. Accurate appreciation of pain and drug side effects is important. Opioid analgesia can be 'patient controlled' and is normally accompanied by antiemetics. Alternative therapies such as acupuncture or behavioural techniques may allow greater patient control.

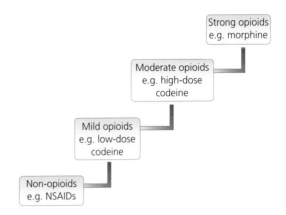

Fig. 5.7 The analgesic ladder. NSAIDs, non-steroidal anti-inflammatory drugs.

Nausea and vomiting affects 60% of patients with advanced carcinoma. It may be due to opiates, metabolic causes (e.g. uraemia), vagal stimulation (e.g. bowel distension) or psychological factors, all of which should be addressed. Antiemetics include anticholinergics, antihistamines, dopamine antagonists or 5HT-3 antagonists (e.g. ondansetron).

Heavy vaginal bleeding may occur with advanced cervical and endometrial carcinomas. High-dose progestogens may be helpful; radiotherapy is often used if it has not been used before.

Ascites and bowel obstruction are particular features of advanced ovarian carcinoma. Ascites is best drained slowly by repeated paracentesis. Obstruction is ideally managed at home.

Spontaneous resolution occurs in up to one-third of patients. If obstruction is partial, metoclopramide is used (pro-motility and antiemetic) and stool softeners, with enemas for constipation and a trial of dexamethasone to reduce tissue oedema. For complete obstruction, cyclizine and ondansetron are used for nausea and vomiting, with hyoscine for spasm. The patient is encouraged to eat and drink small amounts as she feels able. Some may be managed for many months like this. Surgical palliation is indicated with acute, single-site obstruction; stents may also be inserted low in the sigmoid colon or rectum.

Terminal distress: The last 24 hours are often the memories the relatives will retain. The terminal stage should be managed sensitively with time for the patient and relatives in a quiet environment. Good symptom control with anxiolytics and analgesics without overly sedating can allow valuable time with the family.

Further reading

Patient support website: www.ovacome.org.uk (accessed 7 July 2016).

Gynaecological cancers information: www.oncolink. com (accessed 7 July 2016).

Jacobs J, Menon U, Ryan A, *et al*. Ovarian cancer screening and mortality in the UK Collaborative Trial of Ovarian Cancer Screening (UKCTOCS):

a randomised controlled trial. *Lancet* 2016; **387**: 945–956.

Jayson GC, Kohn EC, Kitchener HC, Lederman JA. Ovarian cancer. *Lancet* 2014; **384**: 1376–1388.

National Institute for Health and Care Excellence. *Ovarian Cancer: The Recognition and Initial Management of Ovarian Cancer*. Available at: www.nice.org. uk/guidance/cg122 (accessed 7 July 2016).

Classification of ovarian tumours at a glance

Tumour-like conditions	Endometriotic cysts, follicular and lutein cysts	
Primary tumours	Benign, borderline and malignant types	
	Epithelial tumours	Serous cystadenomas (benign or malignant)
		Mucinous cystadenomas (benign or malignant)
		Endometrioid carcinoma (malignant)
		Clear cell carcinoma (malignant)
		Brenner tumour (benign)
	Germ cell tumours	Dermoid cyst (benign)
		Solid teratoma (malignant)
		Dysgerminoma (malignant)
	Sex cord tumours	Granulosa cell tumours (benign or malignant)
		Thecomas (usually benign)
		Fibromas (benign)
Secondary malignancies	Usually from breast or bowel	

Carcinoma of the ovary at a glance

Epidemiology	Causes most gynaecological cancer deaths; postmenopausal, more common in the West
Pathology	Epithelial 90%, germ cell tumour if <30 years
Aetiology	Family history, nulliparity, early menarche, late menopause
Clinical features	Silent in early stage: 75% present in stages 3–4, usually with abdominal bloating, distension or mass, pain or vaginal bleeding
Screening	Not routine and limited use. Ultrasound scan (USS), CA 125 and family history/gene testing
Investigations	USS, CA 125, risk of malignancy index, CT, surgery
Staging	1 Ovaries only; 1c with capsule breached or malignant cells in abdomen 2 Pelvis only 3 Abdomen and pelvis 4 Distant, including liver
Treatment	Surgery: total abdominal hysterectomy (TAH), bilateral salpingo-oophorectomy (BSO), omentectomy, at staging laparotomy. Lymph node biopsy/removal Debulk all advanced tumours Possible laparoscopy and oophorectomy alone for young women wanting fertility (very close monitoring) Then chemotherapy unless 'borderline' or low-risk stage 1a/b
Prognosis	Poor (<50% 5-year survival) because of late presentation

CHAPTER 6
Disorders of the vulva and vagina

Anatomy

The vulva is the area of skin that stretches from the labia majora laterally to the mons pubis anteriorly and the perineum posteriorly. It overlaps with the vestibule, the area between the labia minora and the hymen, which surrounds the urethral and vaginal orifices. The vagina is 7–10 cm long. It is lined by squamous epithelium. Anteriorly lie the bladder and urethra. Posterior to the upper third is the pouch of Douglas (peritoneal cavity). The lower posterior wall is close to the rectum. Most lymph drainage occurs via the inguinal lymph nodes, which drain to the femoral and thence to the external iliac nodes of the pelvis (Fig. 6.1). This is a route for metastatic spread of carcinoma of the vulva.

Vulval symptoms

The most common vulval symptoms are *pruritus* (itching), *soreness*, *burning* and *superficial dyspareunia* (pain on sexual penetration). Symptoms can be due to local problems including infection, dermatological disease, malignant and premalignant disease and the vulval pain syndromes. Skin disease affects the vulva but rarely in isolation. Systemic disease may predispose to certain vulval conditions (e.g. candidiasis with diabetes mellitus).

Causes of pruritus vulvae

Infections
Candidiasis (± vaginal discharge)
Vulval warts (condylomata acuminata)
Pubic lice, scabies

Dermatological disease
Any condition but especially eczema, psoriasis, lichen simplex, lichen sclerosus, lichen planus, contact dermatitis

Neoplasia
Carcinoma
Premalignant disease (vulval intraepithelial neoplasia, VIN)

Miscellaneous benign disorders of the vulva and vagina

Lichen simplex (or chronic vulval dermatitis) (Fig. 6.2)

Women with sensitive skin, dermatitis or eczema can present with vulval symptoms, which can result in lichen simplex, a chronic inflammatory skin condition. This presents with severe intractable pruritus, especially at night. The area, typically the labia majora, is inflamed and thickened with hyper- and hypopigmentation.

Obstetrics & Gynaecology, Fifth Edition. Lawrence Impey, Tim Child.
© 2017 John Wiley & Sons, Ltd. Published 2017 by John Wiley & Sons, Ltd.

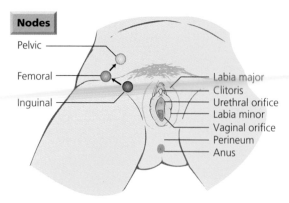

Fig. 6.1 Anatomy and lymph drainage of the vulva.

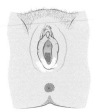

Fig. 6.2 Lichen simplex.

The symptoms can be exacerbated by chemical or contact dermatitis and are sometimes linked to stress or low body iron stores. Vulval biopsy is indicated if the diagnosis is in doubt. Irritants such as soap should be avoided; emollients, moderately potent steroid creams and antihistamines are used with the aim of breaking the itch–scratch cycle.

Lichen planus

A common disease which may affect skin anywhere on the body, but particularly mucosal surfaces such as in the mouth and genital region. Lichen planus presents with flat, papular, purplish lesions. In the mouth and genital region, it can be erosive and is more commonly associated with pain than with pruritus. The aetiology is unknown but may be autoimmune related. It can affect all ages and is not linked to hormonal status. Treatment is with high-potency steroid creams; surgery should be avoided.

Lichen sclerosus

The vulval epithelium is thin with loss of collagen. This may have an autoimmune basis and thyroid disease and

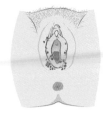

Fig. 6.3 Extensive vulval warts.

vitiligo may coexist. Around 40% of women have or go on to develop another autoimmune condition. The typical patient is postmenopausal but much younger women are occasionally affected. It causes severe pruritus, which may be worse at night. Uncontrollable scratching may cause trauma with bleeding and skin splitting and symptoms of discomfort, pain and dyspareunia. The appearance is of pink-white papules, which coalesce to form parchment-like skin with fissures. Inflammatory adhesions can form, potentially causing fusion of the labia and narrowing of the introitus. Vulval carcinoma can develop in 5% of cases. Biopsy is important to exclude carcinoma and to confirm the diagnosis. Treatment is with ultra-potent topical steroids.

Vulvar dysaesthesia (vulvodynia) or the vulval pain syndromes

These are diagnoses of exclusion, with no evidence of organic vulval disease. They are divided into provoked or spontaneous vulvar dysaesthesia and subdivided according to site: local (e.g. vestibular) or generalized. They are associated with many factors including a history of genital tract infections, former use of oral contraceptives and psychosexual disorders. Spontaneous generalized vulvar dysaesthesia (formerly essential vulvodynia) describes a burning pain that is more common in older patients. Vulvar dysaesthesia of the vestibule causes superficial dyspareunia or pain using tampons and is more common in younger women, in whom introital damage must be excluded. For both conditions, topical agents are seldom helpful and oral drugs such as amitriptyline or gabapentin are sometimes used.

Infections of the vulva and vestibule

Herpes simplex, vulval warts (condylomata acuminata) (Fig. 6.3), syphilis and donovanosis may all affect the vulva.

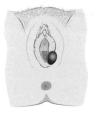

Fig. 6.4 Bartholin's abscess.

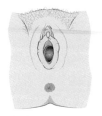

Fig. 6.5 Congenital vaginal cyst.

Candidiasis may affect the vulva if there has been prolonged exposure to moisture. Candidiasis is more common in diabetics, the obese, in pregnancy, when antibiotics have been used or when immunity is compromised, and tends to present with irritation and soreness of the vulva and anus rather than discharge. Prolonged topical or oral antifungal therapy may be necessary.

Bartholin's gland cyst and abscess

The two glands behind the labia minora secrete lubricating mucus for coitus. Blockage of the duct causes cyst formation. If infection occurs, commonly with *Staphylococcus* or *Escherichia coli*, an abscess forms (Fig. 6.4). This is acutely painful and a large tender red swelling is evident. Treatment is with incision and drainage, and marsupialization, whereby the incision is sutured open to reduce the risk of re-formation.

Introital damage

This commonly follows childbirth. Overtightening, incorrect apposition at perineal repair or extensive scar tissue commonly present with superficial dyspareunia. Symptoms often resolve with time. If the introitus is too tight, vaginal dilators or surgery (Fenton's repair) are used.

Vaginal cysts

Congenital cysts commonly arise in the vagina (Fig. 6.5). They have a smooth white appearance, can be as large as a golf ball, and are often mistaken for a prolapse. They seldom cause symptoms, but if there is dyspareunia they should be excised.

Vaginal adenosis

When columnar epithelium is found in the normally squamous epithelium of the vagina, it is called vaginal adenosis. It commonly occurs in women whose mothers received diethylstilboestrol (DES) in pregnancy, when it is associated with genital tract anomalies. Spontaneous resolution is usual, but it very occasionally turns malignant (clear cell carcinoma of the vagina). Women with DES exposure *in utero* are screened annually by colposcopy. It may also occur secondarily to trauma.

Vaginal wall prolapse and vaginal discharge are discussed in Chapters 7 and 10, respectively.

Premalignant disease of the vulva: vulval intraepithelial neoplasia

Vulval intraepithelial neoplasia (VIN) is the presence of atypical cells in the vulval epithelium. VIN is divided into two types depending on its histopathological characteristics.

Usual type VIN: Nearly all VIN is of usual type, can be warty, basaloid or mixed, and is more common in women aged 35–55. It is associated with HPV (especially HPV-16), cervical intraepithelial neoplasia (CIN), cigarette smoking and chronic immunosuppression. Clinically it may be multifocal and appearances vary widely: red, white or pigmented; plaques, papules or patches; erosions, nodules, warty or hyperkeratosis. Usual type VIN is associated with warty or basaloid squamous cell carcinoma.

Differentiated type VIN: This is rarer than usual type, can be associated with lichen sclerosis, and is seen in older women. The lesion is usually unifocal in the form of an ulcer or plaque and is linked to keratinizing squamous cell carcinomas of the vulva. The risk of progression to cancer is higher than for usual type VIN.

Pruritus or pain is common with VIN. Emollients or a mild topical steroid may help. The gold standard for VIN is local surgical excision to relieve symptoms, confirm histology and exclude invasive disease. Fifteen per cent of women having excision have unrecognized invasive disease, so if conservative or medical treatment is used, adequate biopsies must be taken.

Carcinoma of the vulva

Epidemiology

Carcinoma of the vulva accounts for 5% of genital tract cancers, with up to 1200 new cases each year in the UK and 400 deaths. It is most common after the age of 60 years.

Pathology

Ninety-five per cent of vulval malignancies are squamous cell carcinomas. Melanomas, basal cell carcinomas, adenocarcinomas and a variety of others, including sarcomas, account for the rest.

Aetiology

Although VIN is a premalignant stage of squamous carcinoma, carcinoma often arises *de novo*. It is also associated with lichen sclerosis, immunosuppression, smoking and Paget's disease of the vulva.

Clinical features

History: The patient experiences pruritus, bleeding or a discharge, or may find a mass, but malignancy often presents late as lesions go unnoticed or cause embarrassment.

Examination: This will reveal an ulcer or mass, most commonly on the labia majora or clitoris (Fig. 6.6). The inguinal lymph nodes may be enlarged, hard and immobile.

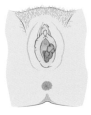

Fig. 6.6 Vulval carcinoma.

Spread and staging

Fifty per cent of patients present with stage 1 disease. Vulval carcinoma spreads locally and via the lymph drainage of the vulva. Spread is to the superficial and then to the deep inguinal nodes, and thence to the femoral and subsequently external iliac nodes (see Fig. 6.1). Contralateral spread may occur. Staging is surgical and histological (i.e. after surgery).

Spread and staging for carcinoma of the vulva	
Stage 1a	Tumour confined to vulva/perineum; ≤2 cm in size with stromal invasion ≤1 mm; negative nodes
Stage 1b	Tumour confined to vulva/perineum; >2 cm in size or with stromal invasion >1 mm; negative nodes
Stage 2	Tumour of any size with adjacent spread (lower urethra/vagina or anus); negative nodes
Stage 3	Tumour of any size with positive inguinofemoral nodes
Stage 4	Tumour invades upper urethra/vagina, rectum, bladder, bone (4a); or distant metastases (4b)

Investigations

To establish the diagnosis and histological type, a biopsy is taken.

To assess fitness for surgery, a chest X-ray, electrocardiogram (ECG), full blood count (FBC) and urea and electrolytes (U&E) are required, as these patients are usually elderly. Blood is cross-matched.

Treatment

For Stage 1a disease, wide local excision is adequate, without inguinal lymphadenectomy, as the risk of spread is negligible.

For other stages: For women with unifocal squamous cancers of <4 cm dimension, with no clinical or radiological suspicion of lymph node metastasis, increasing use is being made of sentinel lymph node biopsy (SLNB). A radioactive isotope and/or blue dye are

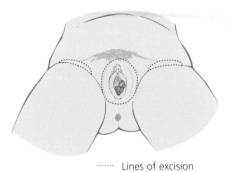

······ Lines of excision

Fig. 6.7 Skin-sparing and separate incisions for a vulvectomy.

injected around the tumour site and any sentinel node identified is biopsied to assess the presence of metastasis. If no sentinel node is present then complete inguinofemoral lymphadenectomy is considered. The use of SLNB appears to reduce morbidity without affecting the accuracy of diagnosis or outcomes in terms of relapse, although trials are ongoing.

If SLNB is not indicated or available, or if the sentinel node is positive, then wide local excision and groin lymphadenectomy is performed through separate 'skin-sparing' incisions (Fig. 6.7) – so-called triple incision radical vulvectomy. If the tumour does not extend to within 2 cm of the mid-line, unilateral excision and lymphadenectomy only are used. This approach has largely replaced the traditional radical vulvectomy through a 'butterfly incision', which dissected the entire vulva and groins *en bloc*. Complications include wound breakdown, infection, leg lymphoedema, lymphocyst formation and sexual and body image problems. *Radiotherapy* may be used to shrink large tumours prior to surgery, postoperatively if groin lymph nodes are positive, or palliatively to treat severe symptoms. Reconstructive surgery involving a plastic surgeon is considered where a major resection is planned.

Prognosis

Many of these patients die from other diseases related to their age. Survival at 5 years in stage 1 is >90%; in stages 3–4 the figure is 40%.

Malignancies of the vagina

Secondary vaginal carcinoma is common and arises from local infiltration from cervix, endometrium or vulva, or from metastatic spread from cervix, endometrium or gastrointestinal tumours.

Primary carcinoma of the vagina accounts for 2% of genital tract malignancies, affects older women and is usually squamous. Presentation is with bleeding or discharge and a mass or ulcer is evident. Treatment is with intravaginal radiotherapy or, occasionally, radical surgery. The average survival at 5 years is 50%.

Clear cell adenocarcinoma of the vagina: Most are a rare complication affecting the daughters of women prescribed DES during pregnancy to try to prevent miscarriage, during the 1950s to early 1970s. With radical surgery and radiotherapy, survival rates are good.

Further reading

Cancer statistics: http://info.cancerresearchuk.org/cancerstats/types/vulva/ (accessed 8 July 2016).

Royal College of Obstetricians and Gynaecologists. *Guidelines for the Diagnosis and Management of Vulval Carcinoma.* Available at: www.rcog.org.uk/globalassets/documents/guidelines/vulvalcancer-guideline.pdf (accessed 8 July 2016).

Royal College of Obstetricians and Gynaecologists. *The Management of Vulval Skin Disorders. Green-top Guideline* 58. Available at: www.rcog.org.uk/globalassets/documents/guidelines/gtg_58.pdf (accessed 8 July 2016).

Carcinoma of the vulva at a glance

Epidemiology	1200 cases per year in UK. Age >60 years
Aetiology	Vulvar intraepithelial neoplasia (VIN) and oncogenic human papilloma viruses (HPVs), lichen sclerosis
Pathology	95% squamous cell carcinomas
Features	Pruritus, bleeding, discharge, mass
Spread	Local and lymph
Staging	1 Confined to vulva/perineum and no nodes: 1a <2 cm size and stromal invasion <1 mm; 1b >2 cm size or stromal invasion >1 mm
	2 Any size with local spread, no nodes
	3 Any size with positive nodes
	4 In upper urethra/vagina, rectum/bone/bladder or distant metastases
Treatment	Tumour biopsy, possible sentinel lymph node biopsy, then wide local excision with separate groin node dissection, bilateral unless tumour >2 cm from mid-line
	Radiotherapy if lymph nodes involved
Prognosis	>90% 5-year survival in stage 1; 40% in stages 3–4

CHAPTER 7

Prolapse of the uterus and vagina

Prolapse is descent of the uterus and/or vaginal walls beyond normal anatomical confines. It occurs as a result of weakness in the supporting structures. Behind the vaginal walls, the bladder, urethra, rectum and small bowel descend and produce a form of herniation. Prolapse is extremely common and is present to variable degrees in most older parous women.

Anatomy and physiology of the pelvic supports

The pelvic floor consists of muscular and fascial structures that provide support to the pelvic viscera and the external openings of the vagina, urethra and rectum. The uterus and vagina are suspended from the pelvic side walls by endopelvic fascial attachments that support the vagina at three levels.

Level 1: The cervix and upper third of the vagina are supported by the cardinal (transverse cervical) and uterosacral ligaments (Fig. 7.1). These are attached to the cervix and suspend the uterus from the pelvic side wall and sacrum, respectively.

Level 2: The mid-portion of the vagina is attached by endofascial condensation (endopelvic fascia) laterally to the pelvic side walls.

Level 3: The lower third of the vagina is supported by the levator ani muscles and the perineal body. The levator ani muscles form the floor of the pelvis from attachments on the bony pelvic walls and incorporate the perineal body in the perineum. The levator ani, together with its associated fascia, is termed the pelvic diaphragm.

Prolapse

Types of prolapse

Types of uterovaginal prolapse are classified anatomically according to the site of the defect and the pelvic viscera that are involved (Fig. 7.2).

Urethrocoele is prolapse of the lower anterior vaginal wall, involving the urethra only.

Cystocoele is prolapse of the upper anterior vaginal wall, involving the bladder. Often there is an associated prolapse of the urethra, in which case the term *cystourethrocoele* is used (Fig. 7.2c).

Apical prolapse is the term used to describe prolapse of the uterus, cervix and upper vagina (Fig. 7.2b). If the uterus has been removed, the vault or top of the vagina, where the uterus used to be, can itself prolapse.

Enterocoele is prolapse of the upper posterior wall of the vagina (Fig. 7.2e). The resulting pouch usually contains loops of small bowel.

Rectocoele is prolapse of the lower posterior wall of the vagina, involving the anterior wall of the rectum (Fig. 7.2d).

Grading of prolapse

There are many grading systems. None is perfect and some are complex, impractical and only of interest to specialist urogynaecologists. For all measurements, the condition of the examination must be specified, i.e. position of the patient, at rest or straining and whether traction is employed. One of the simpler measurement

Obstetrics & Gynaecology, Fifth Edition. Lawrence Impey, Tim Child.
© 2017 John Wiley & Sons, Ltd. Published 2017 by John Wiley & Sons, Ltd.

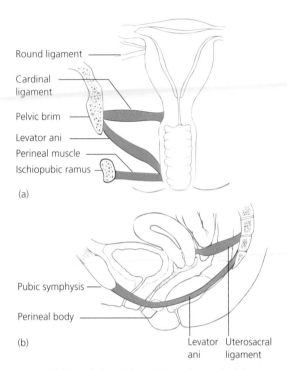

Fig. 7.1 (a) Coronal view of the pelvis showing cardinal ligaments and the levator ani. (b) Lateral view of the pelvis showing the uterosacral ligaments and levator ani.

systems grades prolapse as 1–4 in severity: this is the Baden–Walker classification.

Baden–Walker classification	
0	No descent of pelvic organs during straining
1	Leading surface of prolapse does not descend below 1 cm above the hymenal ring
2	Leading edge of prolapse extends from 1 cm above to 1 cm below the hymenal ring
3	Prolapse extends 1 cm or more below the hymenal ring but without complete vaginal eversion
4	Vagina completely everted (complete procidentia)

Female genital prolapse	
Anterior wall	Bladder (cystocoele) and/or urethra (urethrocoele)
Apical	Uterus, cervix and upper vagina; vaginal vault if previous hysterectomy
Posterior wall	Rectum (rectocoele) and/or pouch of Douglas (enterocoele)

Epidemiology

Half of all parous women have some degree of prolapse and 10–20% seek medical attention.

Aetiology of prolapse

Attenuation of the vaginal support mechanisms may occur as a result of one of the following causes.

Vaginal delivery and pregnancy: Prolapse is uncommon in nulliparous women. Vaginal delivery may cause mechanical injuries and denervation of the pelvic floor, which contribute to subsequent prolapse. These risks are increased with large infants, prolonged second stage and instrumental delivery.

Congenital factors: Abnormal collagen metabolism, e.g. Ehlers–Danlos syndrome, can predispose to prolapse.

Menopause: The incidence of prolapse increases with age. It is thought that this is due to the deterioration of collagenous connective tissue that occurs following oestrogen withdrawal.

Chronic predisposing factors: Prolapse is aggravated by any chronic increase in intra-abdominal pressure, resulting from factors such as obesity, chronic cough, constipation, heavy lifting or pelvic mass.

Iatrogenic factors: Pelvic surgery may also influence the occurrence of urogenital prolapse. For example, hysterectomy incises the uterosacral ligaments and can be associated with subsequent vaginal vault prolapse. Continence procedures, whilst elevating the bladder neck, may lead to defects in other pelvic compartments.

Causes of prolapse
Vaginal delivery and pregnancy
Congenital collagen deficiency
Menopause
Chronic elevated abdominal pressure
Pelvic surgery

Clinical features

History: Symptoms are often absent, but a dragging sensation or the sensation of a lump is common, usually worse at the end of the day or when standing up. Back pain is unusual. Severe prolapse interferes with intercourse, may ulcerate and cause bleeding

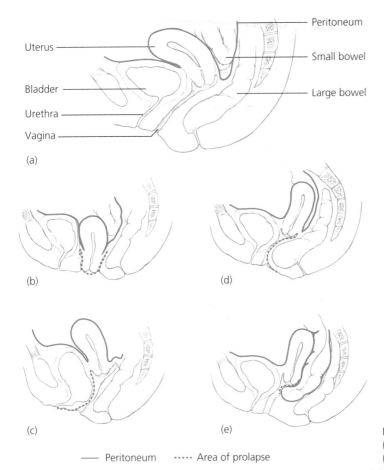

Uterus

Bladder

Urethra

Vagina

(a)

Peritoneum

Small bowel

Large bowel

(b)

(d)

(c)

(e)

—— Peritoneum   ····· Area of prolapse

Fig. 7.2 Types of prolapse. (a) Normal pelvis, (b) uterine prolapse, (c) cystocoele, (d) rectocoele, (e) enterocoele.

or discharge. A cystourethrocoele can cause urinary frequency and incomplete bladder emptying. Stress incontinence is common, but it may be incidental. A rectocoele often causes no symptoms, but occasionally causes difficulty in defaecating. Some women have to reduce the prolapse with their fingers to enable the passing of urine or stool.

Examination: This should include abdominal examination to exclude pelvic masses. A large prolapse is visible from the outside (Fig. 7.3), but a smaller prolapse requires speculum examination. A Sims' speculum allows separate inspection of the anterior and posterior vaginal walls: the patient is asked to bear down to demonstrate prolapse. An enterocoele may be mistaken for a rectocoele, but a finger in the rectum will be seen to bulge into a rectocoele but not into an enterocoele, which does not contain rectum. Large polyps and vaginal cysts may be mistaken for a prolapse. Stress incontinence should be sought with the prolapse temporarily reduced by asking the patient to strain/cough.

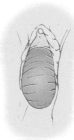

Fig. 7.3 Appearance of cystocoele.

Symptoms of prolapse	
Often asymptomatic	
General	Dragging sensation, vaginal lump
Cystourethrocoele	Urinary frequency, incontinence
Rectocoele	Occasional difficulty in defaecating

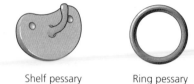

Shelf pessary   Ring pessary

Fig. 7.4 Pessaries for uterovaginal prolapse. (a) Shelf pessary, (b) ring pessary.

Investigations

Usually no investigations are required; the diagnosis is a clinical one. Consider a pelvic ultrasound if a pelvic mass is suspected. Urodynamic testing is required if urinary incontinence is the principal complaint.

To assess fitness for surgery (if appropriate), an electrocardiogram (ECG), chest X-ray, full blood count (FBC) and renal function may be required, as the women are often elderly.

Prevention

Prevention involves recognition of obstructed labour and the avoidance of an excessively long second stage. Pelvic floor exercises after childbirth are encouraged.

Management

Prolapse can be an incidental finding (e.g. noted at the time of a routine cervical smear). If asymptomatic, women should be reassured and advised to avoid treatment. Prolapse should only be treated if symptoms are impacting significantly on quality of life.

Weight reduction is often appropriate. Smoking is discouraged. *Physiotherapy* may help mild-to-moderate degrees of prolapse and reduce the stress incontinence that can be associated, although evidence is limited (*Cochrane* 2006; CD003882).

Pessaries

These are used in the woman who is unwilling or unfit for surgery. They act like an artificial pelvic floor, placed in the vagina to stay behind the symphysis pubis and in front of the sacrum. The most commonly used is the ring pessary, but the shelf pessary is more effective for severe forms of prolapse (Fig. 7.4). They are changed every 6–9 months; postmenopausal women may require oestrogen replacement, either topical oestrogen alone or as standard hormone replacement therapy (HRT), to prevent vaginal ulceration. Occasionally,

pessaries cause pain, urinary retention or infection, or fall out.

Surgical treatment

Prolapse may kink the urethra, masking stress incontinence. As repair could precipitate incontinence, concomitant surgery for stress incontinence may be required. Synthetic meshes are used for sacrocolpopexy, hysteropexy and some vaginal operations. Meshes reinforce weak connective tissue, reducing recurrent prolapse risk. They can, however, be associated with complications, particularly when inserted through a vaginal incision. In particular, there is a risk of mesh extrusion or erosion (where the mesh protrudes through the vagina); careful discussion of risks and benefits is required before their use.

Uterine prolapse

Vaginal hysterectomy has been the traditional surgical treatment for uterovaginal prolapse but, alone, often fails to address the underlying deficiencies in pelvic support that cause uterovaginal prolapse. Indeed, up to 40% of women undergoing hysterectomy subsequently present with vaginal vault prolapse.

Hysteropexy, open or laparoscopic, is an effective procedure for correcting uterine prolapse without recourse to hysterectomy. The uterus and cervix are attached to the sacrum using a bifurcated non-absorbable mesh. It is effective because it restores the length of the vagina without compromising its calibre (*BJOG* 2010; **117**: 62–68).

Vaginal vault prolapse

Sacrocolpopexy, which can be laparoscopic or open, fixes the vault to the sacrum using a mesh. Complications include mesh erosion and haemorrhage.

Sacrospinous fixation is performed vaginally and suspends the vault to the sacrospinous ligament. Complications include nerve or vessel injury, infection and buttock pain. It is less effective but recovery is faster.

Vaginal wall prolapse

Anterior and *posterior 'repairs'* are used for the relevant prolapse but, as several prolapses may occur in one patient, these operations are often combined.

Surgery for urodynamic stress incontinence

If this is present, the tension-free vaginal tape (TVT), transobturator tape (TOT) procedures, or *Burch*

colposuspension may be performed at the same time as prolapse repair.

Further reading

Maher C, Feiner B, Baessler K, Schmid C. Surgical management of pelvic organ prolapse in women. *Cochrane Database of Systematic Reviews*. Available at: www.cochrane.org/CD004014/INCONT_surgical-management-of-pelvic-organ-prolapse-in-women (accessed 8 July 2016).

Genital prolapse at a glance

Definition	Descent of the uterus and/or vaginal walls beyond normal anatomical confines	
Types	Anterior wall (bladder and/or urethra) is a cystourethrocoele Posterior wall is a rectocoele (rectum) or enterocoele (pouch of Douglas) Uterovaginal prolapse graded 1–4, depending on descent Vault prolapse after hysterectomy	
Epidemiology	Very common; older multiparous women	
Aetiology	Pregnancy and vaginal delivery, oestrogen deficiency, obesity, chronic cough, pelvic masses, surgery, iatrogenic (vault)	
Features	Often asymptomatic. Dragging sensation or feeling of lump coming down Bulge of vaginal wall visible from outside or with Sims' speculum	
Prevention	Pelvic floor exercise, improved management of labour	
Treatment	General	Lose weight, treat chest problems including smoking
	Pessaries	Ring or shelf, if frail. Change 6–9 monthly
	Surgery	Hysteropexy or vaginal hysterectomy for uterine prolapse Anterior repair for cystocoele, posterior repair for rectocoele Sacrospinous fixation or sacrocolpopexy for vault prolapse Consider surgery for stress incontinence

CHAPTER 8
Disorders of the urinary tract

Anatomy and function of the female lower urinary tract system

Voluntary control of urine release is achieved by the bladder and urethra. During the filling phase of the cycle, normal lower urinary tract function depends upon adequate bladder capacity and a competent urethral sphincter. The voiding phase is dependent upon detrusor contractility and co-ordinated urethral relaxation.

The bladder has a smooth muscle wall (detrusor muscle) and can normally 'store' about 500 mL of urine, although the normal first urge to void is at about 200 mL. It is drained by the urethra, which is about 4 cm long and has a muscular wall and an external orifice in the vestibule just above the vaginal introitus.

Neural control of the bladder and urethra

Parasympathetic nerves aid voiding; sympathetic nerves prevent it. The voiding reflex consists of afferent fibres, which respond to distension of the bladder wall and pass to the spinal cord. Efferent parasympathetic fibres pass back to the detrusor muscle and cause contraction. They also enable opening of the bladder neck. Meanwhile, efferent sympathetic fibres to the detrusor muscle are inhibited. This 'micturition reflex' is controlled at the level of the pons. The cerebral cortex modifies the reflex and can relax or contract the pelvic floor and the striated muscle of the urethra.

Continence

Continence is dependent on the pressure in the urethra being greater than that in the bladder (Fig. 8.1). Bladder pressure is influenced by detrusor pressure and external (intra-abdominal) pressure. Urethral pressure is influenced by the inherent urethral muscle tone and also by external pressure, namely the pelvic floor and, normally, intra-abdominal pressure. The detrusor muscle is expandable: as the bladder fills, there is no increase in pressure. Increases in abdominal pressure such as coughing will be transmitted equally to the bladder and upper urethra because both lie within the abdomen. Normally, therefore, coughing does not alter the pressure difference and does not lead to incontinence.

Micturition

Micturition results when bladder pressure exceeds urethral pressure. This is achieved voluntarily by a simultaneous drop in urethral pressure (partly due to pelvic floor relaxation) and an increase in bladder pressure due to a detrusor muscle contraction.

Incontinence

Essentially there are two main causes of female incontinence.
Uncontrolled increases in detrusor pressure increasing bladder pressure beyond that of the normal urethra.

Obstetrics & Gynaecology, Fifth Edition. Lawrence Impey, Tim Child.
© 2017 John Wiley & Sons, Ltd. Published 2017 by John Wiley & Sons, Ltd.

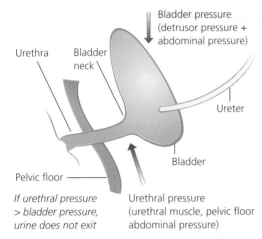

Fig. 8.1 Anatomy of the lower urinary tract and contributors to bladder and urethral pressure.

'Overactive bladder' (OAB) or 'urinary urge incontinence', previously called 'detrusor instability', is the most common cause of this mechanism.

Increased intra-abdominal pressure transmitted to bladder but not urethra, because the upper urethra neck has slipped from the abdomen. Bladder pressure therefore exceeds urethral pressure when intra-abdominal pressure is raised, for example when coughing. 'Urinary stress incontinence' is the most common cause of this mechanism.

Rarer causes include urine bypassing the sphincter through a fistula or the pressure of urine overwhelming the sphincter due to overfilling of the bladder due to neurogenic causes or outlet obstruction: 'overflow incontinence'.

Common urinary symptoms

Urinary incontinence is involuntary urinary leakage, which can be divided, broadly, into stress incontinence and urge incontinence.

Daytime frequency is the number of times a woman voids during her waking hours. This should normally be between 4 and 7 voids per day. Increased daytime frequency is defined as occurring when a patient perceives that she voids too often by day.

Nocturia is waking at night one or more times to void. Up to the age of 70 years, more than a single void is considered abnormal.

Nocturnal enuresis is urinary incontinence occurring during sleep.

Urgency is the sudden compelling desire to pass urine, which is difficult to defer. Urgency is most frequently secondary to detrusor overactivity, although inflammatory bladder conditions such as interstitial cystitis may also present with this.

Bladder pain is felt suprapubically or retropubically. Typically, pain occurs with bladder filling and is relieved by emptying it. Pain is indicative of an intravesical pathology, such as interstitial cystitis or malignancy, and warrants further investigation.

Urethral pain is pain felt in the urethra.

Dysuria is pain experienced in the bladder or urethra on passing urine, frequently associated with urinary tract infections.

Haematuria is the presence of blood in the urine. This can be microscopic or macroscopic (frank). It is always significant and always warrants further investigation.

Investigation of the urinary tract

Urine dipstick tests: Urine dipstick testing for blood, glucose, protein leucocytes and nitrites is essential whenever a patient presents with urinary symptoms. Nitrites suggest the presence of infection: if positive, a urine sample is sent for microscopy and culture to confirm infection and the type and antibiotic sensitivity of the organism(s). Glycosuria suggests diabetes; haematuria suggests bladder carcinoma or calculi.

Urinary diary: The patient keeps a record for a week of the time and volume of fluid intake and micturition. This gives invaluable information about drinking habits, frequency and bladder capacity.

Postmicturition ultrasound or catheterization: These exclude chronic retention of urine.

Urodynamic studies, cystometry: These are necessary prior to surgery for stress incontinence or for women whose overactive bladder symptoms do not respond to medical therapy. Urodynamics may be performed with or without video imaging. Cystometry directly measures, via a catheter, the pressure in the bladder (vesical pressure) whilst the bladder is filled and provoked with coughing. A pressure transducer is also placed in the rectum (or vagina) to measure abdominal pressure (Fig. 8.2). The true detrusor pressure (i.e. the pressure generated by true contraction of the detrusor muscle) can be automatically calculated by subtracting the abdominal pressure from the vesical pressure. The detrusor pressure does not normally alter with filling or provocation (raised intra-abdominal pressure).

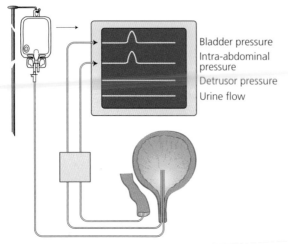

Bladder pressure

Intra-abdominal pressure

Detrusor pressure

Urine flow

Fig. 8.2 Diagram of cystometry set-up.

If leaking occurs with coughing, in the absence of a detrusor contraction, then the problem is likely to be 'urodynamic stress incontinence' (USI). If an involuntary detrusor contraction occurs, 'detrusor overactivity' is diagnosed. Initially, the patient experiences urgency and then incontinence if bladder pressure is increased beyond that of the urethra. Cystometry is widely used to investigate symptoms of urinary incontinence as both USI and detrusor overactivity can cause leakage with exertion, but their treatments are very different.

Ultrasonography: Excludes incomplete bladder emptying, checks for congenital abnormalities, calculi and tumours, and detects cortical scarring of the kidneys.

Abdominal X-ray diagnoses conditions such as foreign bodies and calculi.

Computed tomography (CT) urogram: With the use of contrast, the integrity and route of the ureter are examined.

Methylene dye test: Blue dye is instilled into the bladder. Leakage from places other than the urethra, i.e. fistulae, can be seen.

Cystoscopy: Inspection of the bladder cavity is useful to exclude tumours, stones, fistulae and interstitial cystitis but gives little indication of bladder performance.

Urinary stress incontinence

Definition

Urinary stress incontinence is a complaint of involuntary leakage of urine on effort or exertion, or on sneezing or coughing. When confirmed on urodynamic studies, it is called urodynamic stress incontinence (USI). The diagnosis can only be made with certainty after excluding an overactive bladder using cystometry (Fig. 8.3).

Epidemiology

Stress incontinence accounts for almost 50% of causes of incontinence in the female and occurs to varying degrees in more than 10% of all women.

Aetiology

Important causes of stress incontinence include pregnancy and vaginal delivery, particularly prolonged labour and forceps delivery, obesity and age (particularly postmenopausal). Prolapse commonly coexists but is not always related. Previous hysterectomy (not for prolapse or urine symptoms) may predispose to USI (*Lancet* 2007; **370**: 1494).

Mechanism of incontinence

When there is an increase in intra-abdominal pressure ('stress'), the bladder is compressed and its pressure rises. In the normal woman, the bladder neck is equally compressed so that the pressure difference is unchanged. However, if the bladder neck has slipped below the pelvic floor because its supports are weak, it will not be compressed and its pressure remains unchanged (Fig. 8.4). If the rest of the urethra and the pelvic floor are unable to compensate, the bladder pressure exceeds urethral pressure and incontinence results.

Clinical features

History: This must assess the degree to which the patient's life is disrupted. Stress incontinence predominates, but many patients also complain of frequency, urgency or urge incontinence. It is important to have the patient prioritize her symptoms as the treatment for USI differs from that for the overactive bladder. Faecal incontinence, also due to childbirth injury, may coexist.

Examination with a Sims' speculum often, but not invariably, reveals a cystocoele or urethrocoele. Leakage of urine with coughing may be seen. The abdomen is palpated to exclude a distended bladder.

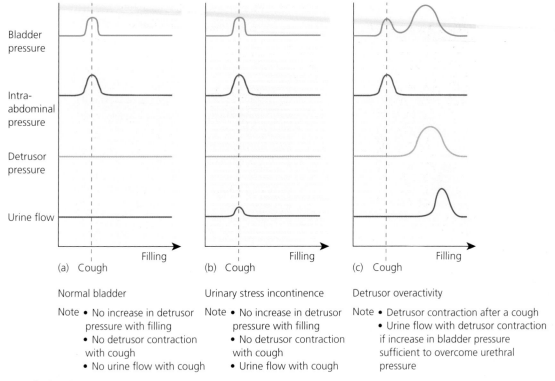

Bladder pressure

Intra-abdominal pressure

Detrusor pressure

Urine flow

(a) Cough   Filling

(b) Cough   Filling

(c) Cough   Filling

Normal bladder

Note
- No increase in detrusor pressure with filling
- No detrusor contraction with cough
- No urine flow with cough

Urinary stress incontinence

Note
- No increase in detrusor pressure with filling
- No detrusor contraction with cough
- Urine flow with cough

Detrusor overactivity

Note
- Detrusor contraction after a cough
- Urine flow with detrusor contraction if increase in bladder pressure sufficient to overcome urethral pressure

Fig. 8.3 Cystometry.

Investigations

Urine dipstick is important to exclude infection. Cystometry (see Fig. 8.3b) is required to exclude OAB if surgery is considered or if OAB symptoms fail to respond to medical treatment.

Management

If obese, the patient is encouraged to lose weight. Causes of a chronic cough (e.g. smoking) are addressed. She should reduce excessive fluid intake.

Conservative

Conservative treatment is aimed at strengthening the pelvic floor. Pelvic floor muscle training (PFMT) is a first-line treatment for at least 3 months and is taught by a physiotherapist. The strength of pelvic floor muscle contraction should be digitally assessed before treatment. PFMT should consist of at least eight contractions, three times per day. If PFMT is beneficial then continue an exercise programme. Vaginal 'cones' or sponges are used to alleviate incontinence adequately in more than half of patients. The 'cones' are inserted into the vagina and held in position by voluntary muscle contraction. Increasing sizes are used as muscle strength increases.

Drugs

Duloxetine is the only drug licensed for the treatment of moderate-to-severe USI. It is a serotonin and noradrenaline reuptake inhibitor (SNRI) that enhances urethral striated sphincter activity via a centrally mediated pathway. Duloxetine is associated with significant and dose-dependent decreases in frequency of incontinence episodes. Nausea is the most frequently reported side effect (up to 25%). Other side effects, including dyspepsia, dry mouth, dizziness, insomnia or drowsiness, can limit its use. Consequently it is not recommended by NICE for routine use.

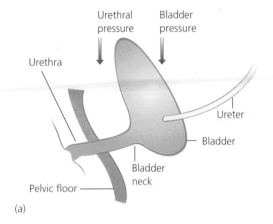

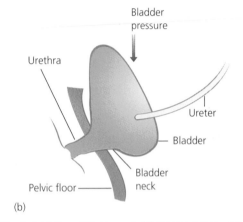

Fig. 8.4 (a) Normal bladder neck. (b) Bladder neck in urodynamic stress incontinence (USI).

Surgery

Surgery for stress urinary incontinence can be considered when conservative measures have failed and the woman's quality of life is compromised. It is important to be clear about the underlying cause of the incontinence, as the effects of surgery are largely irreversible.

Currently, 'mid-urethral sling' procedures such as the tension-free vaginal tape (TVT) and the transobturator tape (TOT) are the usual first-line surgical options, with cure rates of up to 90%. They are less invasive and therefore have largely replaced the traditional Burch colposuspension. Complications include bladder perforation, postoperative voiding difficulty, bleeding, infection, *de novo* detrusor overactivity and suture or mesh erosion (in 'sling' procedures).

Tension-free vaginal tape (TVT): A synthetic polypropylene tape is placed in a U-shape under the midurethra via a small vaginal anterior wall incision, using local, regional or general anaesthesia. The tension is then adjusted to prevent leakage as the woman coughs. Cystourethroscopy is performed to ensure that there has been no damage to the bladder or urethra. The procedure is minimally invasive and most women can return to normal activity within a few weeks.

Transobturator tape (TOT) is similar to the TVT although a different insertion technique is used. The polypropylene tape is passed via the transobturator foramen, through the transobturator and puborectalis muscles. Unlike the TVT, therefore, the retropubic space is not entered and so bladder perforation is rare. Early data suggest that this approach has a success rate similar to that of TVT.

Injectable periurethral bulking agents have a lower immediate success rate of 40–60%. Cure rates are low (less than 20%) and there is also a long-term continued decline in continence. However, the procedure has low morbidity and injections can be performed under local anaesthesia. Injections can be particularly appropriate in women who have not yet completed childbirth, in the frail elderly and if previous surgery has failed.

Other operations. There are other surgical procedures available, such as colposuspension and rectus fascial slings. They are more invasive and were largely abandoned after the 1990s, when polypropylene synthetic TVT/TOT slings were introduced. Recently, there has been adverse publicity regarding synthetic mesh implants. The majority view among urogynaecology specialists is that minimally invasive synthetic mesh TVT-type surgery remains the 'gold standard' operation for the majority of patients.

Distinction between urodynamic stress incontinence and stress incontinence

- Urodynamic stress incontinence (USI) is a *disorder* diagnosed only after cystometry, of which stress incontinence is the major symptom.
- Stress incontinence is a *symptom*: 'I leak when I cough'. It can be due to USI, but it may also be the result of overactive bladder or overflow incontinence.

Overactive bladder

Definition

The overactive bladder (OAB) is defined as urgency, with or without urge incontinence, usually with frequency or nocturia, in the absence of proven infection. The symptom combinations are suggestive of detrusor overactivity but can be due to other forms of urinary tract dysfunction.

Detrusor overactivity is a urodynamic diagnosis characterized by involuntary detrusor contractions during the filling phase which may be spontaneous or provoked by, for instance, coughing (see Fig. 8.3c).

These definitions recognize that not all women with symptoms of OAB will have detrusor overactivity, and not all women with detrusor overactivity will have symptoms of overactive bladder. This reflects the non-physiological nature of urodynamic studies.

Epidemiology

Overactive bladder causes 35% of cases of female incontinence.

Aetiology

It is most commonly idiopathic. The condition can follow operations for USI and is then probably the result of bladder neck obstruction. Occasionally, OAB is due to involuntary detrusor contractions (detrusor overactivity), occurring in the presence of underlying neuropathy such as multiple sclerosis or spinal cord injury.

Mechanism of incontinence

The detrusor contraction is normally felt as urgency. If strong enough, it causes the bladder pressure to overcome the urethral pressure and the patient leaks: urge incontinence. This can occur spontaneously or with provocation, for example, with a rise in intra-abdominal pressure or a running tap. Coughing may therefore lead to urine loss and be confused with stress incontinence.

Clinical features

History: Urgency and urge incontinence, frequency and nocturia are usual. Stress incontinence is common. Some patients leak at night or at orgasm. A history of childhood enuresis is common, as is faecal urgency.

Examination is often normal, but an incidental cystocoele may be present.

Investigations

The urinary diary will show frequent passage of small volumes of urine, particularly at night, and may show high intake of caffeine-containing drinks such as tea/coffee or colas. With detrusor overactivity, cystometry demonstrates contractions on filling or provocation (see Fig. 8.3c). Occasionally, the bladder pressure merely rises steadily with filling. However, cystometry is generally not indicated until either there has been failure of lifestyle changes and drug management of OAB symptoms, or if surgery for stress incontinence is considered.

Management

Conservative

Simple advice is tried first. Reducing fluid intake, if the urinary diary suggests this is excessive, or avoiding caffeinated products can have a dramatic effect. Drugs that alter bladder function, such as diuretics and antipsychotics, should be reviewed.

Bladder training consists of (i) education, (ii) timed voiding with systematic delay in voiding, and (iii) positive reinforcement. The woman is asked to resist the sensation of urgency, and void according to a timetable. This should be used for at least 6 weeks, often in combination with anticholinergic therapy.

Drugs

Anticholinergics (antimuscarinics) suppress detrusor overactivity and are the most widely used treatment. These block the muscarinic receptors that mediate detrusor smooth muscle contraction, relaxing the detrusor muscle. Different drugs vary in their selectivity for various muscarinic receptors and some have additional actions, such as direct smooth muscle effects. These drugs are safe, but side effects include a dry mouth. Recently, an association with dementia following long-term use has been reported, though this has yet to be proven.

Sympathomimetics (e.g. Mirabegron) have recently been licensed as bladder antispasmodics and have no anticholinergic side effects. They should be considered if anticholinergic drugs are poorly tolerated. There is an association with hypertension so blood pressure monitoring is required.

Referral to a specialist clinic is indicated if oral bladder relaxants fail to improve symptoms after 1–2 months.

Oestrogens: Many women develop bladder-filling symptoms after the menopause. Oestrogen treatment in postmenopausal women improves symptoms of vaginal atrophy, such as vaginal dryness and irritation. Vaginal oestrogen administration reduces symptoms of urgency, urge incontinence, frequency and nocturia.

Botulinum toxin A (BTX) blocks neuromuscular transmission, causing the affected muscle to become weak. The toxin is injected cystoscopically under local or general anaesthesia into the detrusor muscle in 10–30 different locations, while sparing the trigonum. Results suggest cure or improvement rates of 60–90% at 3 weeks to 12 months follow-up, with a duration of, on average, 6 months after one dose. The most common complication reported is voiding dysfunction and urinary retention (5–20%), which usually resolves as the effect of treatment declines. BTX is suitable if anticholinergics fail.

Other treatments

Neuromodulation and sacral nerve stimulation provide continuous stimulation of the S3 nerve root via an implanted electrical pulse generator and improve the ability to suppress detrusor contractions. This treatment is appropriate for refractory detrusor overactivity, and has a 30–50% clinical success rate.

Surgery (clam augmentation ileocystoplasty) is used only for very severe and resistant symptoms.

Causes of incontinence	
Stress incontinence (USI)	50%
Overactive bladder	35.0%
Mixed	10.0%
Overflow incontinence	1.0%
Fistulae	0.3%
Unknown	4.0%

Causes of urgency and frequency
Urinary infection
Bladder pathology
Pelvic mass compressing the bladder
Overactive bladder
Urodynamic stress incontinence (USI)

Other urinary disorders

'Mixed' USI and overactive bladder

This accounts for 10% of all cases of incontinence. The diagnosis is made at cystometry. The most bothersome symptom is treated first.

Acute urinary retention

The patient is unable to pass urine for 12 hours or more, catheterization producing as much or more urine than the normal bladder capacity. It is painful, except when due to epidural anaesthesia or failure of the afferent pathways. Causes include childbirth (particularly with an epidural), vulval or perineal pain (e.g. herpes simplex), surgery (hence the need to monitor bladder function postoperatively before discharge from hospital), drugs such as anticholinergics, the retroverted gravid uterus, pelvic masses and neurological disease (e.g. multiple sclerosis or cerebrovascular accident). Catheterization is maintained for 48 hours whilst the cause is treated.

Chronic retention and urinary overflow

This accounts for only 1% of cases of incontinence. Leaking occurs because bladder overdistension eventually causes overflow. It can be due to either urethral obstruction or detrusor inactivity. Pelvic masses and incontinence surgery are common causes of urethral obstruction. Autonomic neuropathies (e.g. diabetes) and previous overdistension of the bladder (e.g. unrecognized acute retention after epidural anaesthesia) cause detrusor inactivity. Presentation may mimic stress incontinence or urinary loss may be continuous. Examination reveals a distended non-tender bladder. The diagnosis is confirmed by ultrasound or catheterization after micturition. Intermittent self-catheterization is commonly required.

Painful bladder syndrome and interstitial cystitis

Painful bladder syndrome (PBS) is a condition in which a patient experiences suprapubic pain related to bladder filling, accompanied by other symptoms such as frequency, in the absence of urinary tract infection (UTI) or other obvious pathology. The diagnosis of interstitial cystitis is confined to patients with painful bladder symptoms who have characteristic cystoscopic and histological features. The aetiology is unknown. Treatments include dietary changes, bladder training, tricyclic antidepressants, analgesics and intravesical infusion of various drugs.

Fistulae

These are abnormal connections between the urinary tract and other organs (Fig. 8.5). The most common are the vesicovaginal and urethrovaginal fistulae. In the developing world, they are common as a result of obstructed labour: in the West they are rare and usually due to surgery, radiotherapy or malignancy. Investigation is with a CT urogram or cystoscopy. Whilst small fistulae may resolve spontaneously, surgery is usually required, the timing depending on the site and the cause.

Further reading

www.bladderandbowelfoundation.org (accessed 11 July 2016).

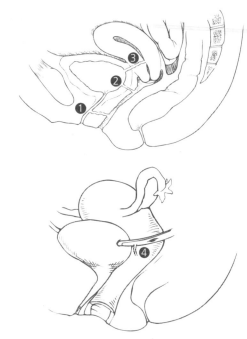

Fig. 8.5 Urinary fistulae: 1, urethrovaginal; 2, vesicovaginal; 3, vesicouterine; 4, ureterovaginal.

Garely A, Noor N. Diagnosis and surgical treatment of stress urinary incontinence. *Obstetrics and Gynecology* 2014; **124**(5):1011–1027.

Gormley EA, Lightner D, Burgio K, *et al.* Diagnosis and treatment of overactive bladder (non-neurogenic) in adults: AUA/SUFU guideline. *Journal of Urology* 2012; **188**: 2455–2463.

Urinary stress incontinence at a glance

Definition	The complaint of involuntary leakage of urine on effort or exertion, or on sneezing or coughing, and confirmed on urodynamic testing	
Epidemiology	10% of women, varying severity. More common with age	
Aetiology	Childbirth and the menopause	
Clinical features	Stress incontinence, also frequency and urgency. Prolapse common	
Investigations	Urine dipstick; diary; cystometry before surgery to confirm diagnosis	
Treatment	Conservative	Physiotherapy
	Medical	Duloxetine
	Surgical	Tension-free vaginal tape (TVT) or transobturator tape (TOT). Colposuspension if these fail

CHAPTER 9
Endometriosis and chronic pelvic pain

Endometriosis

Definition and epidemiology

Endometriosis is the presence and growth of tissue similar to endometrium outside the uterus. Some 1–2% of women are diagnosed as having endometriosis, particularly between the ages of 30 and 45 years, although endometriotic lesions may occur in 1–20% of all women, albeit asymptomatically. It is more common in nulliparous women.

Pathology

Endometriosis, like normal endometrium, is oestrogen dependent: it regresses after the menopause and during pregnancy. It can occur throughout the pelvis, particularly in the uterosacral ligaments, and on or behind the ovaries (Fig. 9.1). Occasionally it affects the umbilicus or abdominal wound scars, the vagina, bladder, rectum and even the lungs. Accumulated altered blood is dark brown and can form a 'chocolate cyst' or endometrioma in the ovaries.

Endometriosis causes inflammation, with progressive fibrosis and adhesions. In its most severe form, the entire pelvis is 'frozen', the pelvic organs rendered immobile by adhesions.

Aetiology

Endometriosis in the pelvis is probably a result of retrograde menstruation ('Sampson's theory'; *Am J Pathol* 1927; **3**: 93–110). More distant foci may result from mechanical, lymphatic or blood-borne spread. As retrograde menstruation is common, but is not always associated with endometriosis, unknown individual factors appear to determine whether the retrograde menstrual endometrium implants and grows. Affected women have an impaired immune system and endometriosis deposits show evidence of both neuro- and angiogenic activity, leading to increased density of adjacent nerve fibres and hence pain (*Hum Reprod Update* 2014; **20**: 717–736). Genetic linkage studies suggest a degree of inherited predisposition (*Nat Genet* 2011; **43**: 51–54). A currently less popular theory is that endometriosis is the result of metaplasia of coelomic cells. It is also not understood why symptoms correlate poorly with the extent of the disease.

Clinical features

History: Symptoms are often absent, but endometriosis is an important cause of chronic pelvic pain. This is usually cyclical. Presenting complaints include dysmenorrhoea before the onset of menstruation, deep dyspareunia, subfertility, pain on passing stool (dyschezia) during menses, and, occasionally, menstrual problems. Rupture of endometriosis ovarian cysts is uncommon but the associated pain may be the first symptom. Cyclical haematuria, rectal bleeding or bleeding from the umbilicus are uncommon and suggest severe disease.

Examination: Common findings on vaginal examination are tenderness and/or thickening behind the uterus or in the adnexa. In advanced cases, the uterus is retroverted and immobile (due to adhesions) and a rectovaginal nodule of endometriosis may be

Obstetrics & Gynaecology, Fifth Edition. Lawrence Impey, Tim Child.
© 2017 John Wiley & Sons, Ltd. Published 2017 by John Wiley & Sons, Ltd.

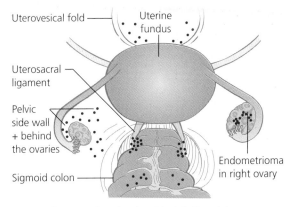

Fig. 9.1 Common sites of endometriosis in the pelvis.

apparent on digital examination and even visible on speculum examination posterior to the cervix if full thickness vaginally. With mild endometriosis, the pelvis often feels normal.

Investigations

Laparoscopy: The diagnosis is only made with certainty after visualization ± biopsy, usually at laparoscopy. Active lesions are red vesicles or punctate marks on the peritoneum. White scars or brown spots ('powder burn') represent less active endometriosis (Figs 9.2, 9.3), while extensive adhesions and ovarian endometriomas (endometriosis cysts) indicate severe disease.

Transvaginal ultrasound is useful to make and to exclude the diagnosis of an ovarian endometrioma (Fig. 9.4)

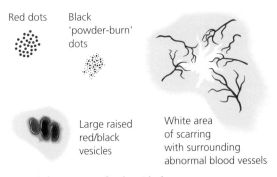

Fig. 9.2 Appearances of endometriosis.

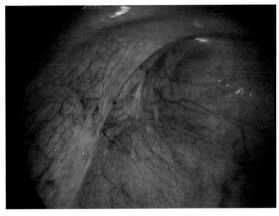

Fig. 9.3 Laparoscopic view of peritoneal endometriosis: scarring with surrounding abnormal blood vessels.

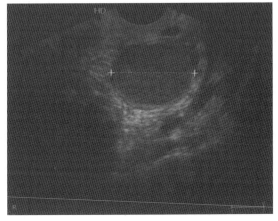

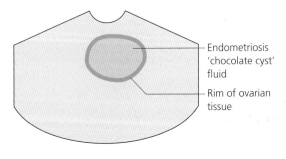

Fig. 9.4 Transvaginal ultrasound photograph of an ovarian endometrioma. The 'ground glass' appearance of the altered blood is typical.

and may also suggest the presence of adenomyosis (although magnetic resonance imaging (MRI) is a better investigation if adenomyosis is suspected).

Other: Peritoneal endometriosis will not be visualized on ultrasound scan but may be on MRI. If there is clinical evidence of deeply infiltrating endometriosis, ureteric, bladder and bowel involvement should be assessed with an MRI ± intravenous pyelogram (IVP) and barium studies. Serum cancer antigen 125 (CA 125) levels are sometimes raised but have little diagnostic value. It is likely that the non-invasive diagnosis of endometriosis using blood or endometrial (from an outpatient uterine cavity biopsy) markers will soon become reality (*Hum Reprod Update* 2014; **20**: 717–736).

The revised American Fertility Society (rev-AFS) grading system is used. At laparoscopy, points are scored dependent on the presence and position of endometriosis deposits and adhesions. The sum of the points allocates the disease extent to one of four grades: grade 1 (minimal); grade 2 (mild); grade 3 (moderate) or grade 4 (severe). The relationship between disease severity (grade) and symptoms such as pain or infertility is limited. It also takes time to undertake scoring during surgery. Consequently, many gynaecologists do not use the system during routine clinical practice, reserving it for research studies.

Symptoms of endometriosis
None
Dysmenorrhoea
Chronic pelvic pain
Deep dyspareunia
Subfertility
Cyclical bowel or bladder symptoms including pain and/or bleeding
Dyschezia (pain on defaecation)
Dysuria

Differential diagnosis of endometriosis
Adenomyosis
Chronic pelvic inflammatory disease
Chronic pelvic pain
Other causes of pelvic masses
Irritable bowel syndrome

Management

Endometriosis is a common incidental finding at laparoscopy. In more than 50% of women, the disease regresses or does not progress. Asymptomatic endometriosis does not require treatment although consideration should be given to removing endometriomas in view of the (very low) risk of misdiagnosing ovarian cancer. Symptoms should be ascribed to endometriosis with caution and the diagnosis reviewed if treatment does not relieve the patient's symptoms. Pain that is suggestive of endometriosis can be treated with a therapeutic 'trial' of a hormonal drug to suppress ovarian activity and is appropriate without a definitive diagnosis.

Medical

Some women prefer to avoid hormonal therapy and can manage pain symptoms effectively with *analgesia* (e.g. non-steroidal anti-inflammatory drugs (NSAIDs)). These can be combined with paracetamol and opiates.

Hormonal treatment is used based upon the observations that symptoms regress during pregnancy, in the postmenopausal period and under the influence of androgens. Treatment therefore mimics pregnancy (e.g. the 'pill' or progestogens) or the menopause (e.g. gonadotrophin-releasing hormone (GnRH) analogues) or is androgenic (e.g. danazol). Suppression of ovarian function with these hormonal drugs reduces endometriosis-associated pain. The hormonal drugs are equally effective but differ in their adverse effect and cost profiles. Symptom recurrence is common following medical treatment. The treatments are contraceptive so are not suitable for women who are trying to conceive.

The combined oral contraceptive is widely used and has high acceptability. It is not suitable for older women and/or smokers. It is often used in a back-to-back or a 'tricycling' regime when two or three pill packets are taken without a break to reduce the frequency of painful withdrawal bleeds.

Progestogen preparations are used on a cyclical or continuous basis. Although generally well tolerated, the side effects of fluid retention, weight gain, erratic bleeding and premenstrual syndrome-like symptoms are severe in a few patients.

GnRH analogues act by inducing a temporary menopausal state: overstimulation of the pituitary leads to downregulation of its GnRH receptors (Fig. 9.5). Pituitary gonadotrophin and therefore ovarian hormone production are inhibited. Side effects mimic the menopause: reversible bone demineralization limits therapy to 6 months, although it can be extended for up to 2 years or more using 'add-back' hormone replacement therapy (HRT), which prevents bone loss and reduces menopausal side effects.

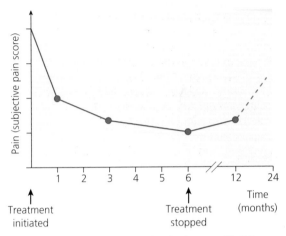

Fig. 9.5 Effect of gonadotrophin-releasing hormone (GnRH) analogue on pain score in patients with endometriosis.

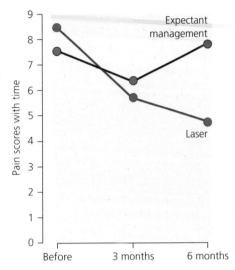

Fig. 9.6 Pain scores over time following laparoscopic removal or observation of minimal to moderate endometriosis. Source: Sutton CJ *et al. Fertil Steril* 1994; **62**: 696–700. Reproduced with permission of Elsevier.

Danazol and *gestrinone*, synthetic compounds with androgenic effects, are seldom used now because of their severe side effects.

Intrauterine system (IUS): An alternative to systemic hormone treatment is a progestogen IUS that reduces pain, especially dysmenorrhoea, with symptom control maintained over 3–5 years dependent on IUS type.

Surgical

Scissors, laser or *bipolar diathermy* can be used laparoscopically at the time of diagnosis to destroy endometriotic lesions ('see and treat') (Fig. 9.6). Surgery may also improve conception rates so is preferable to medical treatment for women with endometriosis-related pain and infertility.

   More radical surgery involves dissection of adhesions and removal of ovarian endometriomas, or even a hysterectomy with bilateral salpingo-oophorectomy (BSO). When treating ovarian endometriotic cysts, the first step is to open and then drain the 'chocolate' fluid within. The cyst wall can either then be stripped away from the ovarian stroma using grasping forceps and removed for pathological analysis, or an attempt made to ablate the cyst wall within the ovary using laser or diathermy. Stripping of the cyst wall is associated with a lower cyst recurrence rate and higher spontaneous conception rate though there may be more chance of causing ovarian damage compared with ablation.

   Surgery can be very difficult due to the severity of adhesions and anatomical distortion; there are risks of damaging bowel, bladder, blood vessels and the ureters. In expert hands, symptomatic improvement is seen in 70% of patients: this may be longer term than with medical therapy. Hysterectomy should be considered a 'last resort'; it is only appropriate in the woman whose family is complete. HRT will be required if the ovaries are removed, and only exceptionally causes a reactivation. However, if endometriosis remains then, when prescribing HRT, consideration is given to using a combined (oestrogen and progestogen) preparation to avoid prolonged unopposed oestrogen stimulation that has been linked to the development of malignant change in ectopic endometrium.

Treatment of endometriosis	
Medical	Analgesia
	Combined oral contraceptives
	Progestogens
	Gonadotrophin-releasing hormone (GnRH) analogues ± hormone replacement therapy (HRT)
	Intrauterine system (IUS)
Surgical	Laparoscopic laser ablation/ diathermy/ scissors ± adhesiolysis
	Hysterectomy and bilateral salpingo-oophorectomy (BSO)

Endometriosis and fertility

Endometriosis is found in 25% of laparoscopies for investigation of subfertility. The more severe the endometriosis, the greater the chance of subfertility. If the fallopian tubes are unaffected, medical treatment will not increase fertility, but laparoscopic excision or ablation of deposits may (*Cochrane* 2014; CD011031). Drainage and stripping of ovarian endometrioma cysts improves fertility compared to drainage and cyst wall ablation. With severe disease affecting the fallopian tubes, surgery has limited benefit and *in vitro* fertilization (IVF) is the best option.

Chronic pelvic pain

Definition

Chronic pelvic pain (CPP) is defined as intermittent or constant pain in the lower abdomen or pelvis of at least 6 months' duration, not occurring exclusively with menstruation or intercourse. CPP presents in primary care as often as migraine or low back pain and affects about 15% of adult women. It carries a heavy social and economic price.

Assessment and investigation

This needs time. The woman's own ideas on the cause of the pain need to be elicited and discussed. There is frequently more than one component to the pain. A full history will prevent non-gynaecological diagnoses being missed. Psychological evaluation is helpful with some patients. It is obvious, but essential to remember, that just because no cause can be found for pain, this does not mean that it does not exist. Possible investigations include transvaginal ultrasound, MRI or laparoscopy as appropriate.

Possible causes of pain

Pelvic pain that varies considerably over the menstrual cycle may be due to hormonally driven gynaecological conditions including *endometriosis* or *adenomyosis*. Oestrogen activity appears to be important as postmenopausal pain is rare (and more likely to be due to malignancy) and suppression of ovarian activity cures two-thirds of cases. There may be gynaecological or pelvic adhesions, although these may be incidental findings and evidence for pain benefit of dividing adhesions is lacking. However, ovarian tissue can become trapped within adhesions (e.g. following previous surgery such as hysterectomy or ovarian cystectomy) and cause cyclical pain treated by oophorectomy or adhesiolysis.

Symptoms suggestive of *irritable bowel syndrome* or *interstitial cystitis* are often present in women with CPP. These conditions may be a primary cause or a component of the pain. *Psychological factors* are important. Depression and sleep disorders are common. A substantial number give a history of childhood and/or ongoing sexual or physical abuse. Other possible theories include the 'pelvic congestion syndrome', in which venous congestion in the pelvis is said to cause chronic pain, and the 'myofascial syndrome', in which, it is said, the pain originates in muscle trigger points or trapped nerves.

Management

If symptoms are suggestive of irritable bowel syndrome then dietary change and a trial of antispasmodics should be tried first. Appropriate analgesia should be arranged for the pain. Women with cyclical pain should be offered a therapeutic trial using the *combined oral contraceptive* pill or a GnRH analogue with add-back HRT for a period of 3–6 months before having a diagnostic laparoscopy if the pain is unresolved. The *progestogen IUS* could also be considered.

Laparoscopy may have a role in developing a woman's beliefs about her pain, even if the findings are normal, but further invasive investigation is usually counterproductive. Counselling and psychotherapy are useful and pain management programmes involve relaxation techniques, sex therapy, diet and exercise. Even if no explanation for the pain can be found, attempts should be made to treat the pain empirically and to develop a management plan in partnership with the woman. Drugs such as amitriptyline or gabapentin may be used to manage the pain.

Further reading

Cochrane Collaboration. *Endometriosis: An Overview of Cochrane Reviews.* Available at: www.cochrane.org/CD009590/MENSTR_endometriosis-an-overview-of-cochrane-reviews (accessed 11 July 2016).

Endometriosis.org: http://endometriosis.org/support/ (accessed 11 July 2016).

European Society of Human Reproduction and Embryology. *Guideline on the Management of Women with Endometriosis.* Available at: www.eshre.eu/Guidelines-and-Legal/Guidelines/Endometriosis-guideline.aspx (accessed 11 July 2016).

Royal College of Obstetricians and Gynaecologists. *Chronic Pelvic Pain, Initial Management.* Green-top Guideline No. 41. Available at: www.rcog.org.uk/en/guidelines-research-services/guidelines/gtg41/ (accessed 11 July 2016).

Endometriosis at a glance

Definition	Endometrium outside the uterus
Epidemiology	Common (1–20%). More prevalent in nulliparous women, diagnosed at 35–40 years
Aetiology	Poorly understood. Probably retrograde menstruation that implants. Genetic susceptibility
Pathology	Peritoneal inflammation causes fibrosis, adhesions, endometriomas ('chocolate cysts')
Clinical features	Pelvic pain, dysmenorrhoea, dyspareunia, dyschezia, dysuria, subfertility
Investigations	Laparoscopy, biopsy. Transvaginal ultrasound, MRI
Medical treatment	Ovarian suppression (combined pill, progestogens, gonadotrophin-releasing hormone (GnRH) analogues ± hormone replacement therapy (HRT)). Progestogen-releasing intrauterine system (IUS) Medical treatment does not improve fertility
Surgical treatment	Laparoscopic ablation ± adhesiolysis. May improve symptoms and fertility. Ovarian cystectomy. Hysterectomy and bilateral salpingo-oophorectomy (BSO) if severe in older woman
Prognosis	Disease usually recurs after cessation of medical treatment

In women of reproductive age, the vagina is lined by squamous epithelium. It is richly colonized by bacterial flora, predominantly lactobacilli, and has an acidic pH (<4.5). This normal flora has a significant role in defence against infection by pathogens. In prepubertal girls and postmenopausal women, lack of oestrogen results in a thinner epithelium, a higher pH (6.5–7.5) and reduced resistance to infection.

The healthy vagina		
Prepubertal	*Pubertal*	*Postmenopausal*
Simple cuboidal epithelium	Stratified squamous epithelium	Atrophic changes
Colonized by organisms similar to skin commensals	Lactobacilli dominant	Flora similar to skin commensals
Alkaline pH	pH 3.5–4.5	Alkaline pH

Genital infections, several of which are sexually transmitted, are a common cause of gynaecological symptoms, but may also be asymptomatic. In recent years, the incidence of most sexually transmitted infections (STIs) has risen in the UK as a result of changes in sexual behaviour, particularly frequent partner change, among young people.

Infections of the vulva and vagina

Three common infections are associated with vaginal discharge: bacterial vaginosis (BV), trichomoniasis and candidiasis, of which trichomoniasis is a STI.

Non-sexually transmitted infections

Bacterial vaginosis (formerly Gardnerella or anaerobic vaginosis)

This is the most common cause of vaginal discharge in women of reproductive age. It is associated with a loss of lactobacilli and increase of anaerobic and highly specific fastidious BV-associated bacteria in the vagina. These produce proteolytic enzymes, which break down vaginal peptides into volatile, malodorous amines. The rise in pH facilitates adherence of *G. vaginalis* (90%) and *Atopobium vaginae* to exfoliating epithelial cells and development of a biofilm which adheres to the epithelium. A grey-white discharge is present with a characteristic fishy odour, but no vulvovaginitis. The diagnosis is established by a raised vaginal pH, the typical discharge, a positive 'whiff' test (fishy odour when 10% potassium hydroxide (KOH) is added to the secretions) and the presence of 'clue cells' (epithelial cells studded with Gram-variable coccobacilli) on microscopy. Treatment of symptomatic women is with metronidazole or clindamycin cream. These bacteria can cause secondary infection in pelvic inflammatory disease (PID). There is also an association with preterm labour.

Candidiasis (thrush)

Candida spp, a yeast-like fungus (Fig. 10.1), is identified in the lower genital tract in:
- 10–20% of healthy women in the reproductive age group
- 6–7% of menopausal women (higher if taking hormone replacement therapy (HRT))
- 3–6% of prepubertal girls.

Obstetrics & Gynaecology, Fifth Edition. Lawrence Impey, Tim Child.
© 2017 John Wiley & Sons, Ltd. Published 2017 by John Wiley & Sons, Ltd.

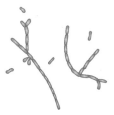

Fig. 10.1 *Candida albicans* showing budding hyphae and oval spores.

Symptomatic candidiasis is due to a hypersensitivity response to the commensal and up to half of all women report at least one symptomatic lifetime episode. Most are due to *C. albicans*. Pregnancy, diabetes and the use of antibiotics are risk factors. Recurrent candidiasis is more common in the immunocompromised, and in patients with uncontrolled diabetes. The classic symptoms are 'cottage cheese' discharge with vulval irritation and itching. Superficial dyspareunia and dysuria may occur. The vagina and/or vulva can be inflamed and red. The diagnosis is established by culture and treatment is with topical imidazoles (e.g. clotrimazole pessary) or oral fluconazole.

Other non-STIs

Toxic shock syndrome usually occurs as a rare complication of the retained, particularly hyperabsorbable, tampon. A toxin-producing *Staphylococcus aureus* is responsible; a high fever, hypotension and multisystem failure can occur. Treatment is with antibiotics and intensive care.

Sexually transmitted infections (STIs)

Risk factors for acquisition of STIs

- *Number of partners*: 2+ partners in last 6 months, new partner in the last 3 months or concurrent partners.
- *Non-use of condoms*: condoms greatly reduce the risk of blood-borne viruses, gonorrhoea and chlamydia, but are less effective against warts and herpes.
- *Other STIs*, including STI (or symptoms) in partner and previous STI.
- *Young age*: under 20 years is a strong risk factor.
- *Sexual preference*: men who have sex with men (MSM).

Principles in the management of STIs

Screening for concurrent infections is important because more than one STI may be present.

Partner notification (contact tracing) involves identification and contacting recent sexual contacts, for screening and treatment. This is to reduce the risk of complications in partners and to reduce onward transmission of infection.

Confidentiality is pivotal to the doctor–patient relationship within any consultation, but particularly in the setting of sexual health due to the sensitive content. The doctor is breaching confidentiality if he/she informs sexual contacts of his/her patient of the diagnosis without their permission. The diagnosis of an STI is emotive and patients need to be handled sensitively and with adequate explanation. Sexually transmitted infections can occur within monogamous relationships (e.g. genital herpes following orogenital sex).

Education: Concerns about an STI offer the opportunity to deliver health promotion to reduce the risk of reinfection and to avoid onward transmission of infection.

Chlamydia

Chlamydia trachomatis is a small bacterium (Fig. 10.2) and is now the most common sexually transmitted bacterial organism in the developed world; 3.0% of 18–24 year olds in the UK have chlamydia at any one time. More than 70% of infected women with chlamydia do not have any genital symptoms. The most common symptoms in women are altered vaginal discharge, intermenstrual and/or postcoital bleeding and low abdominal pain and dyspareunia. The principal complication is pelvic infection, which may also be silent. This can cause tubal damage leading to subfertility and/or chronic pelvic pain. Chlamydia infection may precipitate sexually acquired reactive arthritis (SARA),

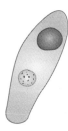

Fig. 10.2 *Chlamydia trachomatis*.

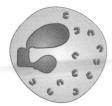

Fig. 10.3 Gram-negative *Neisseria gonorrhoeae* in pairs in a human neutrophil.

characterized by a triad of urethritis, conjunctivitis and arthritis. Nucleic acid amplification tests (NAATs) are best and can be used on urine for screening purposes. Treatment is with azithromycin or doxycycline.

Gonorrhoea

This is caused by *Neisseria gonorrhoeae*, a Gram-negative diplococcus (Fig. 10.3). It is common, particularly in the developing world. Men usually develop urethritis but it is commonly asymptomatic in women, although vaginal discharge, urethritis, bartholinitis, cervicitis and pelvic infection can occur. Systemic complications are rare and include bacteraemia and acute, usually monoarticular, septic arthritis. Diagnosis is from NAATs of endocervical or vulvovaginal swabs, which should always be confirmed on a second platform. Positive NAATs should be followed by culture to check antibiotic sensitivities. Antibiotic resistance is increasing, including to quinolones, azithromycin, and cefixime. IM ceftriaxone is usually required in combination.

Genital warts (condylomata acuminata)

There are more than 80 types of human papilloma virus (HPV). HPV is passed through close physical (skin to skin) contact, almost always genital for genital warts. Many people have subclinical infection so have no obvious warts but may transmit the virus to partners. External genital warts are most commonly caused by HPV 6 and 11, which are rarely associated with severe dysplasia and do not cause genital or anal cancers. Certain oncogenic types (mostly 16 and 18) are associated with the development of cervical intraepithelial neoplasia (CIN). The vulva, perianus, cervix and vagina (less frequently) are common sites for warts in women which may be hard or soft, range from solitary to multiple, and may be pigmented. They may itch. The diagnosis is usually clinical.

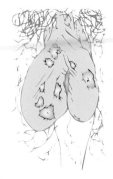

Fig. 10.4 Genital herpes.

It is not currently possible to eradicate the virus. No treatment is an option, as warts may regress spontaneously. It is important to explain that patients may remain infectious even in the absence of visible warts. Options include chemical applications with podophyllin, podophyllotoxin, trichloroacetic acid solution, or imiquimod and/or physical ablation with cryotherapy. There is a high recurrence rate (up to 25%). A vaccine against HPV is now administered to adolescent girls for the purpose of preventing cervical neoplasia.

Genital herpes

Both herpes simplex viruses (HSV), HSV-1 and HSV-2 can affect the genitals and anal area (genital herpes) (Fig. 10.4). HSV-1 causes cold sores and with an increase in oral sex, now commonly causes genital herpes. Most people will have no visible signs or symptoms. About one in three people will experience a primary infection within 4–14 days of becoming infected. They may feel generally unwell with flu-like symptoms such as fever, tiredness and headache. This is often followed by stinging or itching in the genital or anal area. Small vesicles then occur, which burst within a day or two and will then crust over and heal. Local lymphadenopathy and dysuria are common; secondary bacterial infection, aseptic meningitis or acute urinary retention are rarer. The virus then lies dormant in the dorsal root ganglia and reactivations may occur. Typically, a patient diagnosed with HSV-2 will have 4–6 recurrences each year. People with HSV-1 will have infrequent recurrences – on average this will be less than once per year. Recurrences are usually much milder and clear more quickly than the first outbreak. There is often a tingling sensation or mild flu-like illness before an outbreak. Aciclovir (also valaciclovir or famciclovir) is used in severe infections and will also reduce the duration of symptoms if started early in a reactivation. Neonatal herpes has a high mortality and can be prevented.

Syphilis

Infection by the spirochaete *Treponema pallidum* (Fig. 10.5) is common in the developing world, and while uncommon in the UK, the incidence is rising, primarily in MSM. Sexual transmission occurs in the first 2 years of untreated infection, although transmission to the fetus may occur up to 10 years after the primary infection. Primary or secondary syphilis during pregnancy carries a high risk of *congenital infection.*

Many patients who acquire syphilis are unaware and only diagnosed when positive serology is noted some years later. *Primary syphilis* is characterized by a solitary painless genital ulcer (chancre). Untreated, *secondary syphilis* may develop weeks later, often with a rash, influenza-like symptoms and warty genital or perioral growths (condylomata lata). There is a systemic vasculitis and any organ can be involved with manifestations, including hepatitis, uveitis and alopecia. The symptoms resolve without treatment and *latent syphilis* follows. *Tertiary syphilis* is now very rare. It develops many years later and virtually any organ can be affected. Aortic regurgitation, dementia, tabes dorsalis and gummata in skin and bone are the best known complications. A variety of diagnostic tests are used (including the enzyme immunoassay (syphilis EIA) and Venereal Disease Research Laboratories (VDRL) tests). Treatment of all stages is with parenteral (usually intramuscular) penicillin.

Trichomoniasis

Trichomonas vaginalis is a flagellate protozoan (Fig. 10.6) that is very prevalent worldwide but relatively uncommon in the UK. Typical symptoms are an offensive grey-green discharge, vulval irritation, dysuria and superficial dyspareunia, but it is asymptomatic in up to 50% of women. The most common clinical finding is abnormal vaginal discharge in up to 70% of women. Diagnosis is by NAATs although motile trichomonads will be seen on wet film microscopy in about 60% of cases. Treatment is with systemic metronidazole.

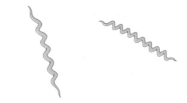

Fig. 10.5 *Treponema pallidum.*

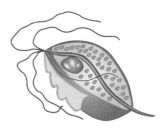

Fig. 10.6 *Trichomonas vaginalis.*

Other STIs causing genital ulcers

Other than herpes and syphilis, chancroid (*Haemophilus ducreyi*) and lymphogranuloma venereum (subtypes of *Chlamydia trachomatis*) may cause genital ulceration. They are rare in the UK but remain endemic in small areas in the tropics and are occasionally seen as 'imported' diseases.

Human immunodeficiency virus (HIV)/ acquired immunodeficiency syndrome (AIDS)

Infection with this retrovirus (Fig. 10.7) is the cause of the clinical syndrome acquired immune deficiency syndrome (AIDS). The overall prevalence in the UK in 2013 was 2.8 per 1000 population aged 15–59 years (1.9 per 1000 women and 3.7 per 1000 men). An estimated 59 500 people living with HIV in 2013 in the UK had acquired their infection through heterosexual contact. There has been a decline in the number of new HIV diagnoses in the UK reported among heterosexual men and women in recent years (from 4890 in 2004 to 2490 in 2013), due to fewer diagnoses among people born in sub-Saharan Africa. The HIV prevalence rate among black African heterosexuals is 56 per 1000 population aged 15–59 years (41 per 1000 men and 71 per 1000 women) (Fig. 10.8).

Seroconversion is often accompanied by an influenza-like illness with a rash and lymphadenopathy but most HIV-positive women are asymptomatically infected and can remain fit and well, albeit infectious, for many years. HIV infection causes a depletion of CD4 cells, which eventually puts patients at risk of certain opportunistic infections and tumours. Early deterioration may be associated with chronic skin problems, recurrent oral candida, fever and generalized lymphadenopathy. CIN is more common in HIV-infected women, affecting one-third. Yearly smears are recommended as progression to malignancy is more rapid. Genital infections, particularly candidiasis and menstrual disturbances, are more common. Vertical transmission to the fetus is virtually prevented by antiretroviral therapy, with or without elective caesarean and avoidance of breastfeeding. With current combination antiretroviral regimens, HIV is increasingly considered as a chronic controllable condition in a similar manner to diabetes.

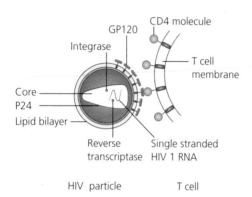

Fig. 10.7 Human immunodeficiency virus (HIV) particle attaching to a T lymphocyte.

Infections of the uterus and pelvis

Endometritis

This is infection confined to the cavity of the uterus alone. Untreated, spread of infection to the pelvis is common. Endometritis is often the result of instrumentation of the uterus or a complication of pregnancy, or both. Infecting organisms include chlamydia and gonorrhoea if these are present in the genital tract. However, anaerobes associated with bacterial vaginosis and organisms such as *Escherichia coli*, staphylococci and even clostridia may be implicated. It is common after caesarean section; it also occurs after miscarriage or

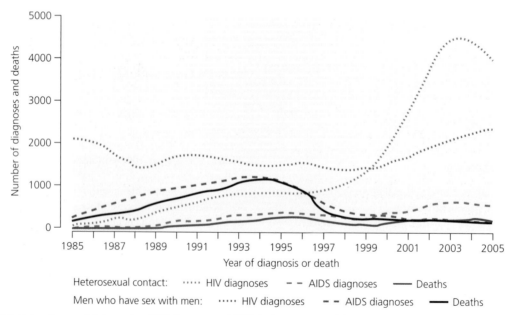

Fig. 10.8 Human immunodeficiency virus (HIV) diagnoses and AIDS deaths among men infected through same-sex contact or individuals infected through heterosexual contact, UK.

termination of pregnancy, particularly if some 'products of conception' are retained. Illegal terminations are now rare in the West but are particularly prone to sepsis. Endometritis presents with persistent and often heavy vaginal bleeding, usually accompanied by pain. The uterus is tender and the cervical os is commonly open. A fever may initially be absent but severe sepsis can ensue. Investigations include vaginal and cervical swabs and a full blood count (FBC); pelvic ultrasound is not reliable. Broad-spectrum antibiotics are given. An evacuation of retained products of conception (ERPC) is then performed if symptoms do not subside or if there are 'products' in the uterus at ultrasound examination.

Acute pelvic infection and pelvic inflammatory disease

Definition and epidemiology

Pelvic inflammatory disease (PID) or salpingitis traditionally describes sexually transmitted pelvic infection, but pelvic infection is best considered as a single entity. Endometritis usually coexists. The incidence is increasing: 2% of women will be affected during their lifetime. Pelvic infection is more common in women with STI risk factors, e.g. young age, multiple sexual partners, recent partner change and non-use of condoms. The combined oral contraceptive is partly protective, as is the intrauterine system (IUS). Younger, poorer, sexually active nulliparous women are at most risk. Pelvic infection almost never occurs in the presence of a viable pregnancy.

Aetiology

Ascending infection of bacteria in the vagina and cervix is most common, although descending infection from local organs such as the appendix can also occur. Spread of previously asymptomatic STIs to the pelvis is usually spontaneous but can be the result of uterine instrumentation (e.g. termination of pregnancy, ERPC, laparoscopy and dye test, and intrauterine devices) and/ or complications of childbirth and miscarriage. In these latter instances, infection is often due to introduction of non-sexually transmitted bacteria.

Pathology and bacteriology

Infection is frequently polymicrobial. Chlamydia (up to 60%) and gonorrhoea are the principal sexually transmitted organisms. Endometritis and a uni- or bilateral salpingitis and parametritis occur; the ovaries are rarely affected. Perihepatitis (Fitz-Hugh–Curtis syndrome) affects 10% and causes right upper quadrant pain due to adhesions, easily visible at laparoscopy, between the liver and the anterior abdominal wall.

Clinical features

Because of the difficulty of diagnosis and the potential for damage to the reproductive health of women (even by apparently mild or subclinical PID), clinicians should maintain a low threshold for the diagnosis and treatment of PID.

History: Many have no symptoms and present later with subfertility or menstrual problems. Bilateral lower abdominal pain with deep dyspareunia is the hallmark, usually with abnormal vaginal bleeding or discharge (Fig. 10.9).

Examination: In severe cases examination reveals a tachycardia and high fever, signs of lower abdominal peritonism with bilateral adnexal tenderness and cervical excitation (pain on moving the cervix). A mass (pelvic abscess) may be palpable vaginally. More frequently, the diagnosis is less clear and may be confused with appendicitis and ovarian cyst accidents (pain usually unilateral) or ectopic pregnancy (pregnancy test positive plus usually unilateral pain).

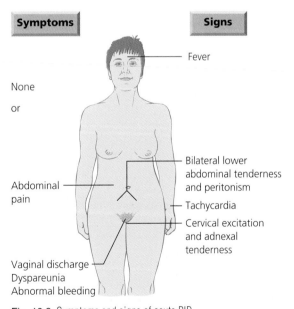

Fig. 10.9 Symptoms and signs of acute PID.

Investigations

Endocervical swabs should be taken for chlamydia and gonorrhoea, and blood cultures sent if there is a fever. The *white blood cell count* (WBC) and *C-reactive protein* (CRP) may be raised. *Pelvic ultrasound* helps to exclude an abscess or ovarian cyst. *Laparoscopy* with fimbrial biopsy and culture is the 'gold standard' although not commonly performed.

Treatment

Analgesics and either a parenteral cephalosporin, e.g. intramuscular ceftriaxone, followed by doxycycline and metronidazole, or ofloxacin with metronidazole are most effective. Febrile patients should be admitted for intravenous therapy. The diagnosis should be reviewed after 24 hours if there is no significant improvement and a laparoscopy performed. A pelvic abscess may not respond to antibiotic therapy and require drainage either under ultrasound guidance or laparoscopically. Rupture of a large pelvic abscess can be life-threatening. Sexual partners should be treated before the resumption of sexual activity.

Complications

The main early complication is the formation of an abscess or pyosalpinx. Later, many women develop tubal obstruction and subfertility, chronic pelvic infection or chronic pelvic pain. Ectopic pregnancy is six times more common after pelvic infection. The chance of tubal damage following one episode of acute PID is around 12%.

Chronic pelvic inflammatory disease

This is a persisting infection and is the result of non-treatment, inadequate treatment of acute PID, or reinfection following failure to treat sexual partners. Typically, there are dense pelvic adhesions and the fallopian tubes may be obstructed and dilated with fluid (hydrosalpinx) or pus (pyosalpinx) (Figs 10.10, 10.11). Common symptoms are chronic pelvic pain or dysmenorrhoea, deep dyspareunia, heavy and irregular menstruation, chronic vaginal discharge and subfertility. Examination may reveal features similar to endometriosis: abdominal and adnexal tenderness and a fixed retroverted uterus. Transvaginal ultrasound may reveal fluid collections within the fallopian tubes or surrounding adhesions. Laparoscopy is the best diagnostic tool; culture is often negative.

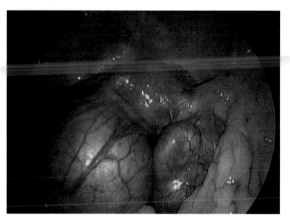

Fig. 10.10 Laparoscopic photograph of severe chronic PID.

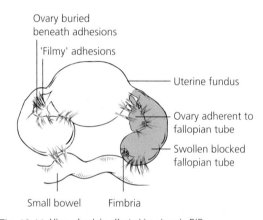

Ovary buried beneath adhesions

'Filmy' adhesions

Uterine fundus

Ovary adherent to fallopian tube

Swollen blocked fallopian tube

Small bowel   Fimbria

Fig. 10.11 View of pelvis affected by chronic PID.

Treatment is with analgesics and antibiotics if there is evidence of active infection. Severe cases occasionally respond to cutting of the adhesions (adhesiolysis), but sometimes removal of affected tubes (salpingectomy) is required.

Features of PID
Symptoms:
pelvic pain (may be unilateral), constant or intermittent
deep dyspareunia
vaginal discharge
irregular menses/intermenstrual or postcoital bleeding
Signs:
cervical motion pain (cervical excitation)
adnexal discomfort (commonly bilateral but may be unilateral)
fever (unusual in chronic infection)

Late complications of PID
Subfertility
Chronic pelvic pain
Ectopic pregnancy

Vaginal discharge: causes and treatment

Vaginal discharge is a common complaint and is often physiological. Normal discharge can range in appearance from mucoid, characteristically associated with ovulation, to opaque. It increases around ovulation, during pregnancy and in women taking the combined oral contraceptive. Exposure of columnar epithelium in cervical eversion and ectropion may cause discharge and can be treated by cryotherapy or diathermy once infection (cervicitis) has been excluded with swabs.

Abnormal discharge is associated with symptoms, which include malodour, itch and superficial dyspareunia. Some patients complaining of vaginal discharge may have a vulval problem. Three common infections are associated with vaginal discharge: BV, trichomoniasis (an STI) and candidiasis.

Vaginal discharge may be caused by a range of other physiological and pathological conditions, including cervicitis, aerobic vaginitis (AV), atrophic vaginitis and mucoid cervical ectopy. Psychosexual problems and depression can present with recurrent episodes of vaginal discharge. These need to be considered if tests for specific infections are negative. Many of the symptoms and signs are non-specific and a number of women may have other conditions, such as vulvar dermatoses or allergic and irritant reactions. Occasionally, cervical infection caused by chlamydia or gonorrhoea may result in vaginal discharge.

Further reading

British Association for Sexual Health and HIV. STI guidelines, regularly updated. *Available at*: www.bashh.org/guidelines *(accessed 11 July 2016).*

British HIV Association. HIV guidelines, regularly updated. *Available at*: www.bhiva.org/guidelines.aspx *(accessed 11 July 2016).*

British Association for Sexual Health and HIV and RCOG. *Management of Genital Herpes in Pregnancy.* Available at: www.rcog.org.uk/en/guidelines-research-services/guidelines/genital-herpes (accessed 11 July 2016).

Causes	*Features/clues in diagnosis*
Candidiasis	Itch, cottage cheese discharge ± vulvitis
Bacterial vaginosis	Malodour, worse with intercourse, not usually associated with vulvovaginitis
Trichomoniasis	Vulvovaginitis/cherry red cervix /(but 50% asymptomatic)
Gonorrhoea	Rare cause of discharge, but patients with gonorrhoea commonly have BV (30%)
Chlamydia	Rare cause of discharge, occasional mucopurulent cervicitis
Primary herpes simplex virus	Frank, vulvovaginitis with cervicitis and genital/cervical ulceration
Foreign body	Anaerobic/malodorous, will resolve with removal, antibiotics not usually required
Atrophic vaginitis	Due to oestrogen deficiency and common during lactation/ after the menopause
Ectropion/erosion	Pathogen-negative discharge often attributed to this finding but evidence is slender
Polyp	Rare cause of discharge
Cervical carcinoma	Rare but if causing symptoms, abnormal vaginal bleeding and discharge; should be clinically obvious

British Association for Sexual Health and HIV and FSRH. *Management of Vaginal Discharge in Non-Genitourinary Medicine Settings.* Available at: http://www.bashh.org/documents/4264.pdf (accessed 11 July 2016).

Sherrard J, Luzzi GA. Sexual history and examination. In: WarrellDA, CoxTM, FirthJD, eds. *Oxford Textbook of Medicine,* 5th edn. Oxford: Oxford University Press, 2010, pp. 1254–1255.

Acute pelvic inflammatory disease (PID) at a glance

Definition	Infection of the pelvis, usually sexually transmitted
Epidemiology	2% lifetime risk, younger, multiple partners
Aetiology	Ascending: sexually transmitted infections (STIs): chlamydia and gonorrhoea spontaneous or after childbirth/uterine instrumentation. Non-STIs: seldom spontaneous Descending: rarer; from other organs or blood
Clinical features	Chlamydial PID often silent. Bilateral abdominal pain, vaginal discharge, fever, erratic menstrual bleeding
Investigations	Swabs, full blood count (FBC), C-reactive protein (CRP). Laparoscopy if doubt or poor response to treatment. Pregnancy test
Treatment	Analgesia and antibiotics, e.g. metronidazole and ofloxacin
Complications	Pelvic abscess, chronic PID, chronic pelvic pain, subfertility, ectopic pregnancy

CHAPTER 11
Fertility and subfertility

Definitions

A couple are 'subfertile' if conception has not occurred after a year of regular unprotected intercourse. Fifteen per cent of couples are affected. Most couples do not have 'infertility' since they continue to have a monthly chance of conception, even though this may be lower than normal. Failure to conceive may be *primary*, meaning that the female partner has never conceived, or *secondary*, indicating that she has previously conceived, even if the pregnancy ended in miscarriage or termination.

Conditions for pregnancy

Four basic conditions are required for pregnancy.
1 An egg must be produced. Failure is 'anovulation' (30% of cases). Management of subfertility involves finding out if ovulation is occurring and, if not, why.
2 Adequate sperm must be released. 'Male factor' problems contribute to 25% of cases. The history, examination and investigations should involve the male, or at least examination of his semen.
3 The sperm must reach the egg. Most commonly, the fallopian tubes are damaged (25% of cases). Sexual (5%) and cervical (<5%) problems may also prevent fertilization.
4 The fertilized egg (embryo) must implant. The incidence of defective implantation is unknown. This may account for much of the 30% of couples with 'unexplained subfertility'.

Counselling and support for the subfertile couple

A trained counsellor should be available in every fertility clinic. Reproduction is a fundamental body function that these couples have not achieved and over which they have little control. One partner may feel responsible, or guilty about past pregnancy terminations or sexually transmitted disease. Many men feel disempowered and less 'male'. The relationship may suffer and intercourse becomes clinical. Counsellors allow couples to talk about these problems. They can also educate the couple and may even uncover a hidden (e.g. sexual) problem.

Contributors to subfertility	
Ovulatory problems	30%
Male problems	25%
Tubal problems	25%
Coital problems	5%
Cervical problems	<5%
Unexplained	30%
N.B. Because more than one cause may be present, the percentage total is more than 100%.	

Disorders of ovulation

Ovulatory dysfunction is a contributory cause in 30% of subfertile couples. Fertility declines with increasing female age due mainly to the reduced genetic 'quality' of remaining oocytes rather than ovulatory problems.

Physiology of ovulation

Anti-mullerian hormone (AMH) is produced from small (not large) ovarian follicles and reduces the release of oestrogen. At the beginning of each cycle, the *low* oestrogen levels exert a positive feedback to cause hypothalamic

Obstetrics & Gynaecology, Fifth Edition. Lawrence Impey, Tim Child.
© 2017 John Wiley & Sons, Ltd. Published 2017 by John Wiley & Sons, Ltd.

gonadotrophin-releasing hormone (GnRH) pulses to stimulate the anterior pituitary gland to produce gonadotrophins: follicle-stimulating hormone (FSH) and luteinizing hormone (LH) (Fig. 11.1). As a follicle grows, the production of AMH reduces and oestrogen levels consequently increase. The resulting *intermediate* oestradiol level has a negative feedback effect on the hypothalamus, such that less FSH and LH are produced. Therefore, the maturing follicles compete for less stimulating hormones. Usually only one (the *dominant follicle*) is large enough with sufficient gonadotrophin receptors to be able to survive and continue growth. The development

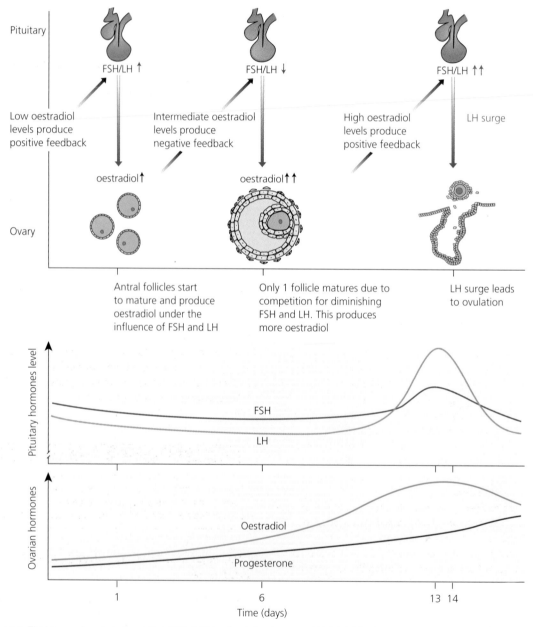

Fig. 11.1 The hormonal control of ovulation. FSH, follicle-stimulating hormone; LH, luteinizing hormone.

of this dominant follicle is also co-regulated by inhibin B, which also suppresses FSH. AMH therefore acts as the gatekeeper of follicular development (*Hum Reprod Update* 2014; **20**: 370–385).

As this follicle matures, its oestradiol output increases considerably. When a *high* 'threshold' level of oestradiol is attained, the negative feedback is reversed and positive feedback now causes LH and FSH levels to again increase and dramatically so: it is the peak of the former that ultimately leads to rupture of the now ripe follicle when it is around 2 cm diameter. This is ovulation and the egg spills onto the ovarian surface where it can be picked up by the fallopian tube. Following ovulation, the follicle becomes a corpus luteum and releases oestrogen and progesterone to maintain a secretory endometrium suitable for embryo implantation. If this does not occur, the corpus luteum involutes and hormone levels fall, leading to menstruation around 14 days after ovulation. If embryo implantation does occur, the human chorionic gonadotrophin (hCG) produced by the trophoblast tissue acts on the corpus luteum to maintain oestrogen and progesterone production until the fetoplacental unit takes over at 8–10 weeks' gestation.

Detection of ovulation

History: The vast majority of women with regular cycles are ovulatory. Some experience vaginal spotting or an increase in vaginal discharge or pelvic pain ('mittelschmerz') around the time of ovulation.

Examination: Cervical mucus preovulation is normally acellular, will 'fern' (form fern-like patterns) when on a dry slide (Fig. 11.2a) and will form 'spinnbarkeit' (elastic-like strings) of up to 15 cm (Fig. 11.2b). The body temperature normally drops some 0.2°C preovulation and then rises 0.5°C in the luteal phase. If the woman is asked to record her temperature every day, the pattern can be seen on a temperature chart (Fig. 11.2c). These examinations are generally not requested or performed.

Investigations are more reliable and are used more frequently. The only proof of ovulation is conception but positive investigations are strongly suggestive.

1 Elevated serum progesterone levels in the mid-luteal phase usually indicate that ovulation has occurred. The luteal phase (time from ovulation to subsequent menstruation) is constant at 14 days. Therefore a low progesterone result can only be interpreted as showing lack of ovulation if it was taken around 7 days before the

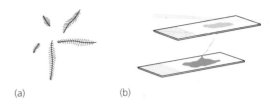
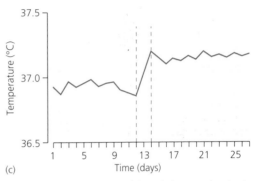

Fig. 11.2 Evidence of ovulation: (a) cervical mucus showing fern-like pattern; (b) spinnbarkeit formation of mucus between two glass slides; (c) temperature chart.

subsequent menstruation, i.e. day 21 of a 28-day cycle or day 28 of a 35-day cycle. For women with irregular cycles, repeat progesterone tests may be required until menstruation starts.

2 Ultrasound scans can serially monitor follicular growth and, after ovulation, demonstrate the fall in size and haemorrhagic nature of the corpus luteum. This is time-consuming and generally not performed.

3 Over-the-counter urine predictor kits will indicate if the LH surge has taken place. Ovulation should then follow.

Detection of ovulation

Mid-luteal phase serum progesterone (the standard test)
Ultrasound follicular tracking (time-consuming)
Temperature charts (not recommended)
Luteinizing hormone (LH) -based urine predictor kits

Causes of anovulation: polycystic ovary syndrome

Polycystic ovary syndrome (PCOS) is a diagnosis of exclusion. Other causes of irregular or absent periods need to be considered and investigated as appropriate.

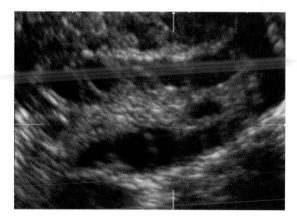

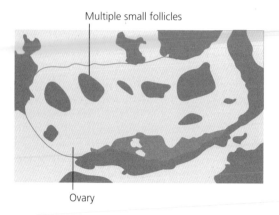

Multiple small follicles

Ovary

Fig. 11.3 Ultrasound of a polycystic ovary (PCO).

Definitions and epidemiology

Polycystic ovary (PCO) describes a characteristic transvaginal ultrasound appearance of multiple (12 or more) small (2–8 mm) follicles in an enlarged (>10 mL volume) ovary. PCO is found in about 20% of all women (Fig. 11.3), the majority of whom have regular ovulatory cycles. Women with PCO may develop other features of the full syndrome if they put on weight (see below).

Polycystic ovary syndrome: PCOS affects around 5% of women and causes over 80% of cases of anovulatory infertility. It is diagnosed when at least two out of the following three criteria are met: (i) PCO on ultrasound, (ii) irregular periods (>35 days apart) and (iii) hirsutism: clinical (acne or excess body hair) and/or biochemical (raised serum testosterone).

Pathology/aetiology

Susceptibility to PCO is mainly genetic. Affected women demonstrate disordered LH production and peripheral insulin resistance with compensatory raised insulin levels. The combination of raised levels of LH and insulin acting on the PCO leads to increased ovarian androgen production. Raised insulin levels also increase adrenal androgen production and reduce hepatic production of steroid hormone-binding globulin (SHBG) which leads to increased free androgen levels. Increased intraovarian androgens disrupt folliculogenesis, leading to excess small ovarian follicles (and the PCO picture) and irregular or absent ovulation. Raised peripheral androgens cause hirsutism (acne and/or excess body hair). Increasing body weight leads to increased insulin and

consequently androgen levels. Hence environmental factors (weight) can modify the phenotype of PCOS. Many women have a family history of type II diabetes.

Clinical features

PCO: Polycystic ovaries without the syndrome generally cause no symptoms.

PCOS: The stereotypical patient with the syndrome is obese, has acne, hirsutism and oligomenorrhoea or amenorrhoea; these may therefore be the presenting symptoms (Fig. 11.4). However, since only two out of the three criteria are necessary, presentation can vary. Although many women with severe PCOS have normal body weight,

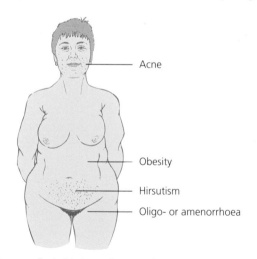

Acne

Obesity

Hirsutism

Oligo- or amenorrhoea

Fig. 11.4 Typical features of severe polycystic ovary syndrome (PCOS).

changes in weight over time will alter insulin levels and severity of the syndrome. Miscarriage is more common in PCOS and may be related to the increased levels of LH and/or insulin and also increased body weight.

Diagnosis of polycystic ovary syndrome

Two or more out of:
Ovaries with polycystic morphology on ultrasound
Irregular periods 5 weeks or more apart
Hirsutism (clinical and/or biochemical)

Investigations

Alternative causes for the symptoms need to be excluded.
Blood tests: Anovulation is investigated with FSH (raised in ovarian failure, low in hypothalamic disease, normal in PCOS), AMH (high in PCOS, low in ovarian failure), prolactin (to exclude a prolactinoma) and thyroid-stimulating hormone (TSH). Hirsutism is investigated with serum testosterone levels (possibility of androgen-secreting tumour or congenital adrenal hyperplasia if very raised). LH is measured (often raised in PCOS but not diagnostic).
Ultrasound: (Transvaginal scan) is used to look for polycystic ovaries (see Fig. 11.3).
Other: Screening for diabetes and abnormal lipids is also advised, particularly if the woman is obese or has a family history of diabetes, abnormal lipids or cardiovascular disease.

Clinical features of polycystic ovary syndrome (PCOS)

Subfertility
Oligomenorrhoea or amenorrhoea
Hirsutism and/or acne
Obesity
Miscarriage

Investigations for polycystic ovary syndrome (PCOS)

Transvaginal ultrasound scan
Follicle-stimulating hormone (FSH), luteinizing hormone (LH), anti-mullerian hormone (AMH), testosterone, prolactin, thyroid-stimulating hormone (TSH)
Fasting lipids and glucose to screen for complications

Complications of PCOS

Up to 50% of women with PCOS develop *type II diabetes* in later life; 30% develop *gestational diabetes* during pregnancy, a risk reduced by weight reduction. *Endometrial cancer* is more common in women with many years of amenorrhoea due to unopposed oestrogen action. In spite of a number of risk factors (weight, insulin resistance, diabetes, abnormal lipids), increased mortality rates have not been demonstrated in women with PCOS.

Treatment of symptoms other than infertility

Advice regarding diet and exercise is given. Normalization of weight should result in reduction in insulin levels and improvement in all PCOS symptoms. If fertility is not required, treatment with the combined oral contraceptive will regulate menstruation and treat hirsutism. At least three to four bleeds per year, whether spontaneous or induced, are necessary to protect the endometrium. The antiandrogens cyproterone acetate (also available combined as a contraceptive pill) or spironolactone are effective treatments for hirsutism but conception must be avoided. The insulin sensitizer metformin reduces insulin levels, and therefore androgens and hirsutism (and also promotes ovulation). Eflornithine is a topical antiandrogen used for facial hirsutism.

Other causes of anovulation

These may originate in the ovary, the pituitary or hypothalamus, or in other parts of the endocrine system (Fig. 11.5). Pregnancy causes amenorrhoea.

Hypothalamic causes

Hypothalamic hypogonadism: A reduction in hypothalamic GnRH release causes amenorrhoea, because reduced stimulation of the pituitary reduces FSH and LH levels, which in turn reduces oestradiol levels. This is usual with anorexia nervosa (Fig. 11.6) and common in women on diets, athletes and those under stress. Restoration of body weight, if appropriate, restores hypothalamic function. *Kallmann's syndrome* occurs when GnRH-secreting neurones fail to develop; in other patients, the cause is obscure. Exogenous

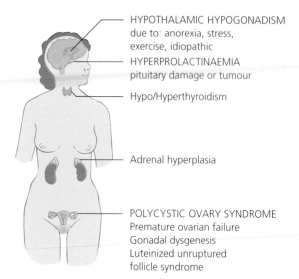

HYPOTHALAMIC HYPOGONADISM
due to: anorexia, stress,
exercise, idiopathic

HYPERPROLACTINAEMIA
pituitary damage or tumour

Hypo/Hyperthyroidism

Adrenal hyperplasia

POLYCYSTIC OVARY SYNDROME
Premature ovarian failure
Gonadal dysgenesis
Luteinized unruptured
follicle syndrome

Fig. 11.5 Causes of anovulation (common causes shown in capital letters).

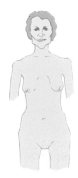

Fig. 11.6 Anorexia nervosa causes amenorrhoea and subfertility.

gonadotrophins or a GnRH pump will induce ovulation. Bone protection with the contraceptive pill or hormone replacement therapy (HRT) is required.

Pituitary causes

Hyperprolactinaemia is excess prolactin secretion, which reduces GnRH release. It is usually caused by benign tumours (adenomas) or hyperplasia of pituitary cells, but is also associated with PCOS, hypothyroidism and the use of psychotropic drugs. It accounts for 10% of anovulatory women, who commonly have oligomenorrhoea or amenorrhoea, galactorrhoea and, if a pituitary tumour is enlarging, headaches and a bitemporal hemianopia. Prolactin levels are elevated. Computed tomography (CT) imaging is indicated if neurological symptoms occur. Treatment with a dopamine agonist (bromocriptine or cabergoline) usually restores ovulation, because dopamine inhibits prolactin release. Surgery is needed if this fails or neurological symptoms warrant it.

Pituitary damage can reduce FSH and LH release. Production of GnRH is normal. This results from pressure from tumours or infarction following severe postpartum haemorrhage (Sheehan's syndrome).

Ovarian causes of anovulation (in addition to PCOS)

Premature ovarian insufficiency: As the ovary fails, oestradiol and inhibin levels are lowered, so reduced negative feedback on the pituitary causes FSH and LH levels to rise. The level of AMH, produced by the resting ovarian follicles, will be very low, as will the antral follicle count (AFC) on ultrasound scan. Exogenous gonadotrophins are of no use, since there are no ovarian follicles to respond, and donor eggs are required for pregnancy. Bone protection with HRT or the oral contraceptive pill is required.

Gonadal dysgenesis: These rare conditions usually present with primary amenorrhoea.

The luteinized unruptured follicle syndrome is present when a follicle develops but the egg is never released. It is unlikely to occur every month so does not cause persistent problems.

Other causes

Hypo- or *hyperthyroidism* reduces fertility. Menstrual disturbances are usual.

Androgen-secreting tumours cause amenorrhoea and virilization.

Common causes of anovulation
Polycystic ovary syndrome (PCOS)
Hypothalamic hypogonadism
Hyperprolactinaemia
Thyroid disease
Premature ovarian insufficiency

Induction of ovulation

Lifestyle changes and treatment of associated disease

Treatment of fertility involves health advice regarding pregnancy, the risks of multiple pregnancy with ovulation induction and the use of folic acid. Restoration of normal weight is advised: this alone may restore ovulation. Treatment of specific causes, such as a thyroid abnormality or hyperprolactinaemia, usually leads to restoration of ovulation. Smoking should cease.

Treatment of PCOS

Clomifene is the traditional first-line ovulation induction drug in PCOS. It is usually limited to 6 months' use and results in ovulation and live birth rates of around 70% and 40%, respectively. Clomifene is an antioestrogen, blocking oestrogen receptors in the hypothalamus and pituitary. As gonadotrophin release is normally inhibited by oestrogen, it increases the release of FSH and LH. Effectively, therefore, it 'fools' the pituitary into 'believing' there is no oestrogen. As it is only given at the start of the cycle, from days 2 to 6, it can initiate the process of follicular maturation which is thereafter self-perpetuating for that cycle. Clomifene cycles should be monitored by transvaginal ultrasound, at least in the first month, to assess ovarian response (both under and over) and endometrial thickness. If no follicles develop then the dose in subsequent cycles is increased. If three or more follicles develop, cycle cancellation is usually indicated to reduce the risk of multiple pregnancy (overall 10%). As clomifene is an antioestrogen, it has negative effects at the endometrium and, at higher doses, may cause a thin endometrium This might explain the low live birth rate (40%), despite the good ovulation rates (70%).

Metformin is an alternative first-line treatment. This oral, insulin-sensitizing drug is used to restore ovulation. It does not promote multiple ovulation so there is no increase in multiple pregnancies (and no need for scan monitoring). Unlike clomifene, it needs to be taken every day through the cycle in multiple doses; gastrointestinal side effects are common. For women with a body mass index (BMI) <30, metformin is more efficacious than clomifene and vice versa for BMI >30 (NICE Fertility Guidelines 2013). Metformin increases the effectiveness of clomifene in clomifene-resistant women so can be used jointly as a second-line treatment. It treats hirsutism so may be a suitable first-line fertility treatment for anovulatory women who want hirsutism treated and to avoid multiple pregnancy. Additional benefits, when metformin is continued during pregnancy, may include a reduction in both early miscarriage and the development of gestational diabetes, which are more common with PCOS.

Oral aromatase inhibitors such as *letrozole* can be used to induce ovulation, resulting in a higher live birth rate than clomifene (*NEJM* 2014; **371**: 1462–1464). This may be due to reduced negative effects at the endometrium. Aromatase inhibitors are not licensed for fertility treatment and are not yet currently widely used.

If ovulation does not occur with the above first-line treatments then second-line options include the following.

Laparoscopic ovarian diathermy is as effective as gonadotrophins (*Cochrane* 2012; CD001122) and with a lower multiple pregnancy rate. Each ovary is monopolar diathermied at a few points for a few seconds. During the same operation, tubal patency can be tested using methylene blue insufflation and any comorbidities such as endometriosis or adhesions treated. If successful then regular ovulations can continue for years. Patients are warned of the risks of surgery, including periovarian adhesion formation and, rarely, ovarian failure.

Clomifene + metformin can be used as dual therapy; *gonadotrophins* (see below) are also used.

Gonadotrophin induction of ovulation

This is used when first-line treatments have failed, but also in hypothalamic hypogonadism if the weight is normal. Recombinant or purified urinary FSH ± LH acts as a substitute for the normal pituitary production and is given by daily subcutaneous injection to stimulate follicular growth. The result is often maturation of more than one follicle. For PCOS patients, a 'low-dose step-up' regimen is used in which the gonadotrophin dose is increased in small increments every 5–7 days until the ovaries begin to respond. This reduces the multiple pregnancy rate to <10%. Follicular development is monitored with ultrasound. Once a follicle is of a size adequate for ovulation (about 17 mm), the process can be artificially stimulated by injection of hCG (which is structurally similar to LH) or recombinant LH. As an alternative to gonadotrophin induction of ovulation, women with hypothalamic hypogonadism can use a continuous subcutaneous GnRH pump. This stimulates FSH and LH production from the pituitary in a physiological manner and achieves normal pregnancy and multiple pregnancy rates. However, the need to wear the pump continuously limits the method's acceptability.

Inducing ovulation	
If polycystic ovary syndrome (PCOS)	Weight loss and lifestyle changes. If inappropriate/ fails . . . Clomifene or metformin (or letrozole). If fails… Clomifene + metformin Gonadotrophins Ovarian diathermy. If fails . . . *In vitro* fertilization (IVF)
If hypothalamic hypogonadism	Restore weight Gonadotrophins if weight normal
If hyperprolactinaemia	Bromocriptine or cabergoline
If ovulation or pregnancy does not occur following second-line treatments then IVF is the next step.	

Side effects of ovulation induction

Multiple pregnancy is more likely with clomifene, letrozole and particularly gonadotrophins (but not metformin) as more than one follicle may mature. Multiple pregnancy increases perinatal complication rates. High order multiple pregnancies now more commonly follow ovulation induction alone than IVF, since with the latter only one or two embryos are replaced in the majority of women, and in the former follicular growth and ovulation are less controlled.

Ovarian hyperstimulation syndrome (OHSS): Gonadotrophin stimulation 'overstimulates' the follicles, which get very large and painful. It is more common during IVF (severe in approximately 1% of cycles) than standard ovulation induction. The risk factors for OHSS include gonadotrophin stimulation, age <35 years, previous OHSS, and ovaries of polycystic morphology on ultrasound scan. Prevention involves use of the lowest effective gonadotrophin doses, ultrasound monitoring of follicular growth and, if this is excessive, 'coasting'

(withdrawing gonadotrophins for a few days) or cancellation of IVF cycle (withholding hCG injection). During IVF, the 'short antagonist protocol' significantly reduces OHSS rates in PCOS women. The risk is reduced further still by replacing the final hCG injection trigger with a GnRH agonist (*Cochrane* 2014; CD008046). In severe cases, hypovolaemia, electrolyte disturbances, ascites, thromboembolism and pulmonary oedema may develop; OHSS can be fatal. Hospitalization is required in such cases for restoration of intravascular volume, electrolyte monitoring and correction, analgesia and thromboprophylaxis. Drainage of ascitic fluid is occasionally necessary to increase comfort and, by reducing splinting of the diaphragm, ease breathing.

Ovarian and breast carcinoma: The evidence is conflicting but generally reassuring (*Hum Reprod Update* 2014; **20**: 106–123).

Male subfertility

Male factors contribute in 25% of subfertile couples.

Physiology of sperm production

Spermatogenesis in the testis is dependent on pituitary LH and FSH, the former largely acting via testosterone production in the Leydig cells of the testis. FSH and testosterone control Sertoli cells, which are involved in synthesis and transport of sperm. Testosterone and other steroids inhibit the release of LH, completing a negative feedback control mechanism with the hypothalamic–pituitary axis. It takes about 70 days for sperm to develop fully.

Detection of adequate sperm production: semen analysis

A normal semen analysis result virtually excludes a male cause for infertility. The sample should be produced by masturbation with the last ejaculation having occurred 2–7 days previously. The sample must be analysed within 1–2 hours of production. An abnormal analysis result must be repeated after 12 weeks (no delay if azoospermia). If persistently abnormal, examination and investigation of the male must follow (Fig. 11.7). The World Health Organization changed the normal reference values in 2010 (*Hum Reprod Update* 2010; **16**: 231).

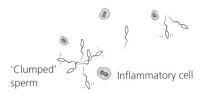

'Clumped' sperp   Inflammatory cell

Fig. 11.7 Semen analysis. Antisperm antibodies causing clumping.

Normal semen analysis	
Volume	>1.5mL
Sperm count	>15 million/mL
Progressive motility	>32%

Definitions of terms describing abnormal semen	
Azoospermia	No sperm present
Oligospermia	<15 million/mL
Severe oligospermia	<5 million/mL
Asthenospermia	Absent or low motility

Common causes of abnormal semen analysis
Unknown
Smoking/alcohol/drugs/chemicals/inadequate local cooling
Genetic factors
Antisperm antibodies

Male factor investigations and treatment
Semen analysis

If abnormal repeat and:
  Examine the scrotum
  Optimize lifestyle factors

If oligospermic then: Intrauterine insemination
If moderate-to-severe oligospermia then: *In vitro* fertilization (IVF) ± intracytoplasmic sperm injection (ICSI)

If azoospermic then:
  Examine for presence of vas deferens
  Check karyotype, cystic fibrosis, hormone profile
  Surgical sperm retrieval then IVF + ICSI or donor insemination

Common causes of abnormal/absent sperm release

Idiopathic oligospermia and *asthenozoospermia* are common. Sperm numbers and/or motility are low but not absent.

Drug exposure: Alcohol, smoking, drugs (e.g. sulfasalazine or anabolic steroids ('body builders'), and exposure to industrial chemicals, particularly solvents, can impair male fertility.

Varicocoele: This refers to varicosities of the pampiniform venous plexus and usually occurs on the left side. It is present in about 25% of infertile men (but 15% of all men). It is not fully understood how it impairs fertility and its surgical treatment does not improve conception.

Antisperm antibodies are present in about 5% of infertile men and are common after vasectomy reversal. Poor motility and 'clumping' together of the sperm are evident on the semen analysis.

Other causes include infections (e.g. epididymitis), mumps orchitis, testicular abnormalities (e.g. in Klinefelter's syndrome XXY), obstruction to delivery (e.g. congenital absence of the vas usually associated with cystic fibrosis), hypothalamic problems and Kallmann's syndrome (hypogonadotrophic hypogonadism), hyperprolactinaemia and retrograde ejaculation (ejaculation into the bladder, e.g. due to neurological disease secondary to diabetes, or transurethral resection of prostate gland (TURP)).

Investigations

All male partners should have a semen analysis, repeated 12 weeks later if abnormal or immediately if azoospermic.

If azoospermia is diagnosed, then a blood test for FSH, LH, testosterone, prolactin and TSH will find treatable causes (e.g. hypogonadotropic hypogonadism (very low FSH, LH and testosterone), hyperprolactinaemia or thyroid dysfunction) though these are not common. High levels of FSH and LH and low testosterone suggest primary testicular failure, which may be associated with cryptorchidism (failure of testes to have descended by birth) or due to surgery or radiochemotherapy, though the cause is often not found. A serum karyotype will also demonstrate genetic causes of azoospermia including Klinefelter's syndrome (XXY) or chromosomal translocations. Men with azoospermia and absent vas deferens should have a blood test for cystic fibrosis.

Management of male factor subfertility

General advice: Lifestyle changes and drug exposures are addressed. The testicles should be below body temperature: advice on wearing loose clothing and testicular cooling is given.

Specific measures: Ligation of a varicocoele does not significantly improve fertility so is not recommended. Hypogonadotrophic hypogonadism may be treated with thrice-weekly subcutaneous injections of FSH and LH (± hCG) for 6–12 months. Spermatogenesis and testicular androgen production should return towards normal.

Assisted conception techniques: Intrauterine insemination (IUI) may help if there is mild-to-moderate sperm dysfunction though success rate data are conflicting. If more severe oligospermia is present then *IVF* is used; if this is very severe then *intracytoplasmic sperm injection* (ICSI) is used as part of an IVF cycle. If there is azoospermia, sperm can be extracted direct from the testis (surgical sperm retrieval (SSR)) in 50–80% of men and then used for ICSI-IVF (*Fertil Steril* 2007; **88**: 374). Or donor sperm may be used, after appropriate counselling; this is called donor insemination (DI). Frozen-thawed sperm is injected into the uterus during a natural menstrual or mildly stimulated cycle at the time of ovulation. Children born from current sperm, oocyte or embryo donations in the UK can contact the donor from the age of 18, contributing to a critical national shortage of gamete and embryo donors.

Disorders of fertilization

The egg and sperm are unable to meet in 30% of subfertile couples.

Physiology of fertilization

At ovulation, the fallopian tube moves so that the fimbrial end collects the oocyte from the ovary. The tube must have adequate mobility to move onto the ovary to achieve this. Peristaltic contractions and cilia in the tube help sweep the oocyte along toward the sperm. Blockage or ciliary damage will impair this. At ejaculation, millions of sperm enter the vagina. The cervical mucus helps them get through the cervix.

Why the sperm might not meet the egg	
Tubal damage	Infection
	Endometriosis
	Surgery/adhesions
Cervical problems	
Sexual problems	

Causes of failure to fertilize: tubal damage

This contributes in 25% of subfertile couples.

Infection

Pelvic inflammatory disease (PID), particularly due to sexually transmitted infections (e.g. chlamydia), causes adhesion formation within and around the fallopian tubes (Fig. 11.8). It is the main cause of tubal damage and 12% of women will be infertile after one episode of infection. Infection at the time of insertion of intrauterine contraceptive devices or a ruptured appendix may also be responsible. Most women will have had no symptoms, but some give a previous history of pelvic pain, vaginal discharge or abnormal menstruation.

If there are peritubal adhesions or 'clubbed' and closed fimbrial ends of otherwise normal-looking tubes then laparoscopic adhesiolysis and salpingostomy can be performed. Ectopic pregnancy rates are increased. Success rates are very poor if the tube is damaged proximal to the fimbrial ends. Under these circumstances or if conception does not occur after surgery, IVF is indicated.

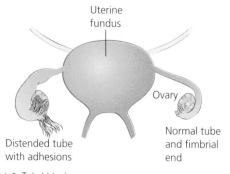

Fig. 11.8 Tubal blockage.

Endometriosis

This is found in 25% of subfertile women, but is probably contributory in fewer. Its role in subfertility is more than simply mechanical, but this is poorly understood. Laparoscopic surgery to remove endometriotic deposits improves fertility even in mild cases; medical treatment is not used since it suppresses ovulation. IVF is the next step if this fails.

Previous surgery/sterilization

Any pelvic surgery may cause adhesion formation. Treatment is as for infectious causes but IVF is often needed. If women have undergone tubal clip sterilization but now want pregnancy, the options are IVF or open microsurgical tubal reanastomosis (increased ectopic risk).

Other causes of failure to fertilize

Cervical problems

'Cervical factors' rarely contribute to subfertility. Cervical problems can be due to *antibody production* by the woman, whereby antibodies agglutinate or kill the sperm, *infection* in the vagina or cervix that prevents adequate mucus production or *cone biopsy* for microinvasive cervical carcinoma. IUI to bypass the cervix can be used.

Sexual problems

These occur in about 5% of subfertile couples. Impotence can be psychological or organic. Ignorance or discomfort can also prevent coitus. Counselling with a trained psychosexual counsellor is required, after exclusion of organic disease.

Detection of tubal damage

As pelvic infection and endometriosis are often symptomless, only limited information can be gained from the history and examination. One or other of the following tests is necessary for full assessment of subfertility. However, if severe male factor infertility is present, IVF ± ICSI will be required in any event and investigation of the tubes is not required.

Laparoscopy and dye test allows visualization and assessment of the fallopian tubes. Methylene blue dye is injected through the cervix from the outside. Whether it enters or spills from the tubes can then be seen, demonstrating whether the tubes are patent. *Hysteroscopy* is performed first to assess the uterine cavity for abnormalities.

Hysterosalpingogram (HSG): Without anaesthetic, radio-opaque contrast is injected through the cervix. Spillage from the fimbrial end (and filling defects) can be seen on X-ray. A variant of this test can be performed using transvaginal ultrasound and an ultrasound opaque liquid (HyCoSy). These tests are preferred in women with no risk factors for tubal disease and no symptoms or signs suggestive of endometriosis, as they are less invasive and safer than laparoscopy. However, both endometriosis and periovarian adhesions may not be diagnosed with HSG or HyCoSy unless they cause tubal damage, meaning that the possibility of surgical treatment of these pathologies to improve fertility is lost.

Assisted conception

Recent advances have greatly increased the success of fertility treatment. Over 1% of babies now born in the UK are conceived through assisted conception. The current methods are IUI, IVF with or without ICSI, frozen embryo replacement (FER), oocyte donation and preimplantation genetic diagnosis (PGD) and screening (PGS). They are often unavailable on the NHS. Success is best measured by the live birth rate; this declines after 35 years, and considerably after 40 years of age (Fig. 11.9). Sperm quality is important but ICSI has rendered this less significant.

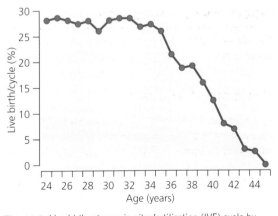

Fig. 11.9 Live birth rate per *in vitro* fertilization (IVF) cycle by female age.

Indications for assisted conception
When any/all other methods have failed
Unexplained subfertility
Male factor subfertility (intracytoplasmic sperm injection [ICSI])
Tubal blockage (standard in vitro fertilization [IVF])
Endometriosis
Genetic disorders

Intrauterine insemination (IUI)

Washed sperm are injected directly into the cavity of the uterus. IUI can be performed during a natural menstrual cycle ('natural cycle IUI'), using urinary LH testing for ovulation in order to time insemination or, more successfully, following gonadotrophin ovulation induction ('stimulated IUI').

This is suitable for couples with unexplained subfertility, cervical and sexual and some male factors, and is cheaper but much less successful than IVF. However, the tubes should be patent, as the oocyte(s) still need to travel from the ovary to the sperm. Cycles should be regular and ovulatory for natural cycle IUI. For stimulated IUI, the live birth rate is 5–10% per cycle with a 15% risk of multiple pregnancy.

In vitro fertilization (IVF)

The embryos are fertilized outside the uterus and transferred back. The live birth rate in women <36 years in good centres is about 35% per stimulated cycle; for women in their 40s, success rates are <10%. The fallopian tubes need not be patent. Normal 'ovarian reserve' is needed so that sufficient oocytes will be collected for fertilization and transfer, so IVF is not possible for women with ovarian failure. Ovarian reserve is best assessed using serum levels of AMH rather than FSH levels. Unlike FSH, AMH is produced in the ovary, so is a direct rather than indirect measure of reserve. An alternative is transvaginal ultrasound measurement of the number of resting small follicles in the ovaries (the 'antral follicle count' or AFC).

Stages of IVF

Multiple follicular development: This is a prerequisite for successful IVF and is achieved using 2 weeks of daily subcutaneous gonadotrophin injections (FSH ± LH). An additional drug must be used to prevent an endogenous LH surge and premature ovulation before oocyte collection. With 'long-protocol' IVF, daily GnRH analogue is started on day 21 of the menstrual cycle and continued for 2–3 weeks to eventually suppress pituitary FSH and LH production, which also leads to ovarian quiescence. Once suppression (or 'downregulation') is confirmed by a low serum oestradiol level or thin endometrium on scan, the gonadotrophin stimulation begins. The GnRH analogue is continued, along with gonadotrophin stimulation, until just before the egg collection. During 'short-protocol' IVF, pituitary suppression is not achieved before starting gonadotrophin stimulation. Instead, a daily GnRH antagonist is added from around day 5 of gonadotrophin stimulation and continued until just before the egg collection.

Ovulation and egg collection: Once an optimal number of mature size (15–20 mm diameter) ovarian follicles are confirmed with scan monitoring (Fig. 11.10), the gonadotrophins and GnRH analogue or antagonist are stopped. A single injection of hCG or LH is then given to switch on ('trigger') final oocyte maturation; 35–38 hours later the eggs are collected under intravenous sedation by aspirating follicles transvaginally under ultrasound control (Fig. 11.11).

Fertilization and culture: The eggs are incubated with washed sperm and transferred to a growth medium. The fertilized eggs (embryos) are cultured until the cleavage (day 2–3) or blastocyst (day 5–6) stage ready for transcervical uterine transfer. Spare, good-quality embryos can be frozen for future thawing and FER during a natural or HRT treatment cycle.

Embryo transfer: More embryos increase pregnancy rates, but miscarriage and preterm delivery rates are higher. Traditionally, two cleavage embryos were transferred, with a 25% twin pregnancy rate; no more than two is mandatory in women <40 years. As blastocysts have a higher implantation potential, single blastocyst transfer (elective single embryo transfer, eSET) may produce similar pregnancy rates, although are more prone to late division causing monochorionic twin pregnancies. Luteal phase support, using progesterone or hCG, is given until 4–8 weeks' gestation.

Intracytoplasmic sperm injection (ICSI)

This is the injection, with a very fine needle, of one sperm right into the oocyte cytoplasm (Fig. 11.12). It

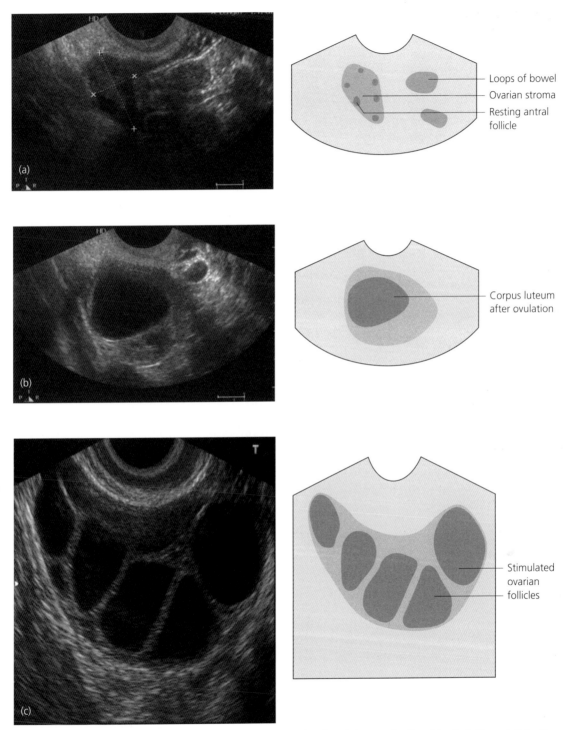

Fig. 11.10 Transvaginal ultrasound photographs of: (a) a resting ovary at baseline, during menstruation; (b) a single 20 mm follicle, after ovulation in an unstimulated cycle; (c) multiple 15–20 mm follicles during a gonadotrophin-stimulated cycle.

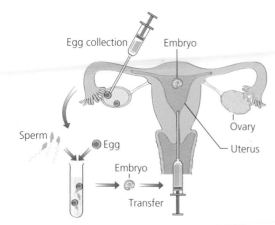

Fig. 11.11 Process of an *in vitro* fertilization (IVF) cycle.

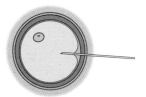

Fig. 11.12 Intracytoplasmic sperm injection (ICSI).

is a laboratory adjunct to IVF. It is useful for male factor infertility when there are not enough motile sperm available to incubate a sufficiently high concentration with each oocyte for standard IVF. Prior to the development of ICSI in the 1990s, such couples could only be treated with donor insemination. Now they can achieve the same pregnancy rates as couples with no male factor infertility undergoing IVF. Sperm can be retrieved from the testes, frozen and then thawed during a fresh IVF cycle and used for ICSI.

Oocyte donation

Some women cannot conceive with their own eggs either naturally or with IVF because of ovarian failure, older age or genetic disease. With oocyte donation, a donor goes through a full stimulated IVF cycle. Her retrieved oocytes are fertilized with the sperm of the recipient woman's partner. The recipient woman receives oestrogen and progesterone to prepare her endometrium for transfer of the fresh embryos. As there is a shortage of anonymous oocyte donors, 'egg sharing' is commonly performed in which women who themselves need IVF agree to share or donate half of their oocytes anonymously to a recipient couple.

Preimplantation genetic diagnosis (PGD)

Blastocysts (day 5–6 preimplantation embryos) generally contain >100 cells. With PGD 3–5 cells are removed from the trophectoderm (area which becomes the placenta) of the blastocyst, which is then frozen, and the DNA examined using the techniques of karyomapping or polymerase chain reaction (PCR) to look for genetic abnormalities. Unaffected embryos are then thawed and replaced in the uterus in a subsequent menstrual cycle either with or without exogenous hormone therapy. Biopsy is less commonly performed at the oocyte (polar body biopsy) or cleavage (day 3) stage. PGD is used for couples who are carriers of single-gene defects such as cystic fibrosis or who have chromosome translocations placing them at a high risk of conceiving a child with aneuploidy. Embryos can also be sexed to avoid the replacement of male embryos that may be affected by, for example, haemophilia. Embryo sexing for 'social reasons' is not permitted in the UK.

All couples produce a proportion of embryos containing abnormal numbers of chromosomes. The rate increases with advancing maternal and (to a lesser degree) paternal age and explains most failed implantations and miscarriages. Women can have their IVF blastocysts biopsied, frozen and 'screened' using PGS to identify chromosomally 'normal' embryos for later transfer in an attempt to overcome the age-related decline in IVF live birth rates. Molecular techniques used include next generation sequencing (NGS) and array- comparative genomic hybridization (CGH). The extent to which PGS improves IVF outcome in healthy couples with no genetic disease is debated (*Hum Reprod* 2015; **30**: 473–483).

Surrogacy

Some women are unable to carry a pregnancy because of problems with their uterus (absent due to congenital anomaly or hysterectomy) or health (e.g. renal failure or immunological disease requiring teratogenic drugs). Surrogacy can be used in which another woman, the surrogate, carries the pregnancy and delivers the child who is then adopted by the commissioning couple. Either the surrogate's own eggs can be fertilized by insemination of the patient's partner's sperm (straight surrogacy) or, if the patient's ovaries are functioning, she can go through IVF, have her oocytes collected and fertilized, and the embryos are then transferred to the womb of the surrogate (host surrogacy). There are a number of difficult ethical issues surrounding surrogacy.

Complications of assisted conception

Superovulation: Multiple pregnancy and ovarian hyperstimulation are discussed above. The former are producing a significant impact on obstetric and neonatal services.

Egg collection: Intraperitoneal haemorrhage and pelvic infection may complicate the ultrasound-guided aspiration of mature follicles necessary for IVF although the risk is low (<1%).

Pregnancy complications: In addition to increased multiple pregnancies, the rates of ectopic pregnancy are also higher. Recent data suggest a slight but significant increase in perinatal mortality and morbidity following IVF, even allowing for multiple pregnancies, although the cause is unclear. It may be that couples who require IVF have an inherently higher risk of adverse outcome than those who conceive naturally (*Reprod Biomed Online* 2014; **28**: 162–182). A small increase in chromosomal and gene abnormalities is reported with ICSI although this appears to be related to a higher rate of genetic abnormality in men with severe male factor infertility.

Fertility preservation

Men or adolescent boys whose fertility is at risk because of disease or the treatment for the disease (e.g. testicular cancer or leukaemia) can urgently freeze sperm samples. The sperm is thawed at a later date and used during an IVF cycle to inseminate the partner's eggs.

The situation is more complex for a woman facing a sterilizing disease or treatment. Currently, to preserve fertility, she needs to complete a standard IVF cycle and have her eggs (if single) or embryos (if in a relationship) frozen for later use. If embryos are stored then, when the time comes for them to be thawed for replacement, both partners must give their consent. If the couple have separated, the male partner could withdraw his consent and the embryos will need to be destroyed even though the woman may now be infertile. The success rate of fertility preservation in women is very dependent on age. The chance of having a baby in the future following a single IVF cycle and egg or embryo freezing is around 30–50% for women <37 years of age, reducing with age.

A more recent development is the *cryopreservation of ovarian tissue* removed at laparoscopy before sterilizing treatment for cancer in females regardless of whether they are pre- or postpubertal. Following successful oncology treatment, the ovarian biopsy is first confirmed to be free of metastases and then grafted back into the woman's pelvis (*Hum Reprod* 2015; **30**: 2838–2845). *Cryopreservation of testicular tissue* from prepubertal boys (not yet able to produce sperm) may similarly allow preservation of fertility.

Social egg freezing: With improvements in the success rate of egg freezing and with women progressively delaying childbearing, there are increasing requests for 'social' fertility preservation. During a standard IVF cycle, the woman's eggs are frozen (*vitrified*) and potentially years later, thawed and fertilized to produce embryos for transfer.

Further reading

Jayasena CN, Franks S. The management of patients with polycystic ovary syndrome. *Nature Reviews Endocrinology* 2014; **10**: 624–636.

National Institute for Health and Care Excellence. *Fertility Assessment and Treatment for People with Fertility Problems*. Clinical Guideline No. 156. Available at: www.NICE.org.uk/guidance/cg156 (accessed 11 July 2016).

Subfertility at a glance

Definition	Failure to conceive after a year Primary: female never conceived. Secondary: previously conceived	
Epidemiology	15% of couples	
Aetiology	Anovulation (30%)	Polycystic ovary syndrome (PCOS), hypothalamic hypogonadism, hyperprolactinaemia, thyroid dysfunction, ovarian failure
	Male factor (25%)	Idiopathic, varicocoele, antibodies, genetic, drug/chemical exposure, many others
	No fertilization	Tubal factor (25%): infection, endometriosis, surgery Cervical factor (<5%) Sexual factor (5%)
	Unexplained (30%)	
Investigations	Detect ovulation	Mid-luteal phase progesterone, ultrasound scan, urine luteinizing hormone (LH) testing
	Cause of anovulation	Follicle-stimulating hormone (FSH), LH, testosterone, prolactin, thyroid-stimulating hormone (TSH)
	Detect male factor	Semen analysis
	Detect tubal factor	Laparoscopy and dye or hysterosalpingogram/HyCoSy
Treatment	General	Ensure correct weight. Give folic acid
	If anovulation	Treat specific disorder PCOS: clomifene, metformin, letrozole, gonadotrophins, ovarian diathermy
	If male factor	Treat specific disorder (generally not possible). Intrauterine insemination (IUI), *in vitro* fertilization (IVF) with or without intracytoplasmic sperm injection (ICSI), donor insemination (DI)
	If tubal factor	Laparoscopic surgery if mild/endometriosis IVF if fails or with severe disease
	If unexplained	IUI/IVF

Polycystic ovary syndrome (PCOS) at a glance

Definition	Polycystic ovary (PCO) is multiple (>12) small follicles within enlarged ovaries PCOS is 2 out of 3 of: PCO on scan; irregular periods; hirsutism (raised serum androgens and/or acne/excess body hair)
Epidemiology	20% of women have PCO; 5% have PCOS; 80% of anovulatory infertility due to PCOS
Aetiology	PCO is genetic; development of syndrome poorly understood. Peripheral insulin resistance, so raised fasting insulin (worsened by obesity). Increased luteinizing hormone (LH) secretion and increased androgen production
Features	Asymptomatic, anovulatory infertility, oligo-/amenorrhoea, obesity, hirsutism, acne

Investigations Ultrasound scan of ovaries

Blood	Often raised testosterone
	Normal follicle-stimulating hormone (FSH) (high with ovarian failure and low with anorexia)
	Low luteal phase progesterone if anovulatory

Treatment

None if chance finding	Weight loss if appropriate
If infertility	Clomifene; metformin, letrozole, ovarian diathermy, gonadotrophins. If failed, *in vitro* fertilization (IVF)
If menstrual problems	Combined oral contraceptive or the Mirena IUS
If acne/hirsutism	Cosmetic treatments, contraceptive pill ± cyproterone acetate, spironolactone, eflornithine facial cream

Complications	Infertility, obesity, miscarriage Long-term risks: diabetes, endometrial carcinoma if persistent anovulation

CHAPTER 12

Contraception

Contraception is the prevention of pregnancy. On an individual basis, it is important to ensure that all pregnancies are wanted or intended (www.fpa.org.uk). It is also important on a global scale because the world population is rapidly increasing. Millions of women worldwide would prefer to delay or avoid pregnancy but lack access to safe and effective contraception. Contraceptive methods also help reduce the spread of disease due to, for example, human immunodeficiency virus (HIV) and chlamydia.

The ideal contraceptive

The ideal contraceptive does not exist but would have the following characteristics. It would be 100% effective, safe and reversible, free from side effects, independent of intercourse, cheap/ free, free from medical intervention, acceptable to all cultures and religions and would prevent sexually transmitted infections. Long-acting reversible contraceptives (LARC) come closest.

Efficacy of contraception

This is measured as the risk of pregnancy per 100 woman-years of using the given contraceptive method, and is called the Pearl Index (PI). If the PI of a contraceptive is 2 then, of 100 women using it for a year, two will be pregnant by the end. The effectiveness of a contraceptive is also determined by the user's compliance. With user-dependent contraceptives such as the pill, and particularly condoms, efficacy with 'perfect use' will be greater than with 'typical use'.

Safety of contraception

Most methods of contraception have been the subject of adverse publicity. Some are less safe than others, or are contraindicated in particular women. By taking a full medical history, the doctor can consider and discuss with the woman whether the benefits of a particular method outweigh the risks. It is important that measurements of safety are compared with the safety of pregnancy; for instance, the diabetic woman is at increased risk of complications with the 'pill', but pregnancy (e.g. through not using the 'pill') risks more complications. Similarly, smoking is considerably more hazardous than using the 'pill'.

Compliance with contraception

This is a major problem. Contraception must be appropriate to the woman's lifestyle; if it is disliked or misunderstood, it will not be used. The woman must be fully counselled about any proposed contraceptive: its major problems and minor side effects. This will enable the woman to know what to expect, and may prevent discontinuation of the chosen method. In the past, media 'scares' over the 'pill' have led to inappropriate discontinuation and unwanted pregnancies.

Special patient groups

Contraception for the adolescent

In the UK, one-third of 16 year olds have had sexual intercourse; indeed, 1% of 13–15 year olds become pregnant every year. Nevertheless, there has been a

Obstetrics & Gynaecology, Fifth Edition. Lawrence Impey, Tim Child.
© 2017 John Wiley & Sons, Ltd. Published 2017 by John Wiley & Sons, Ltd.

reduction in teenage pregnancies. About half of teenage conceptions end in legal termination; continuing pregnancies have increased perinatal mortality. If non-barrier methods such as the 'pill' are chosen then the use of condoms should be encouraged so as to prevent sexually transmitted disease. Depo-Provera largely overcomes compliance issues but, given the associated loss in bone density, other forms of contraceptive should be considered first. Young people should be made aware of emergency contraceptive options, how they are used and where they are accessed. The UK legal situation and ethics of contraception for <16 years olds are discussed in Chapter 35.

Contraception in women with inflammatory bowel disease (IBD)

Small bowel disease and associated malabsorption can lead to decreased efficacy of oral contraception. Alternative forms of contraception should be used such as combined patches, progesterone-only injectables and implants, intrauterine and vaginal methods (see Combined vaginal ring, below). As women with IBD are at increased risk of osteoporosis, Depo-Provera should not be the first-line option in patients under 18 years of age.

Contraception in breastfeeding women

Breastfeeding delays the return of ovulation. In women who are fully breastfeeding, amenorrhoeic and less than 6 months postpartum, breastfeeding is >98% effective in preventing pregnancy. If the woman has unprotected intercourse before day 21 postpartum, she will not require emergency contraception. The combined pill affects breast milk volume and is avoided before 6 weeks postpartum and is relatively contraindicated between 6 weeks and 6 months postpartum. Progestogen-only methods have no effect on milk production and can be used in the first 6 weeks postpartum and thereafter. The intrauterine device (IUD) can be inserted from 4 weeks postpartum.

Contraception in later life

Although fertility is reduced after 40 years of age (mainly due to increased oocyte and embryo aneuploidy), most women with regular cycles still ovulate.

During the perimenopause, ovulation, and therefore periods, become irregular and often very infrequent. Women under the age of 50 years are advised to continue contraception for at least 2 years after the last period, and if over 50 continue contraception for 1 year after the last period; nevertheless, pregnancy without egg donation after 47 years is extremely rare. All methods of contraception can be used, including a low-dose combined oral contraceptive in non-smoking women with no other risk factors. Intrauterine devices are particularly appropriate and, if fitted after the age of 40 years, may not need to be replaced. The hormone-releasing intrauterine system (IUS) will, in addition, greatly reduce menstrual loss. Despite this, many women seek sterilization.

Contraception in the developing world

Where education and access to healthcare are poor, the practical requirements of a contraceptive are different. Minimal medical supervision, prevention of sexually transmitted disease, cost and duration of treatment are important. This means that reversible depot methods, such as Nexplanon and vaccines, have more potential. Breastfeeding (see above) has important contraceptive benefits where contraception is scarce.

Hormonal contraception

Oestrogens and progestogens can be used for contraception in the following ways.

1 Progestogen as a tablet: the progestogen-only pill ('mini-pill').

2 Progestogen as a depot: Nexplanon, Depo-Provera or in the levonorgestrel-containing IUS.

3 Combined hormonal contraception (CHC): contains both oestrogen and progestogen:
- combined oral contraceptive (COC; the 'pill'): mono/bi/triphasic
- transdermal patch
- vaginal ring.

Combined oral contraceptives

Combined oral contraceptives (COCs) act mainly by exerting a negative feedback effect on gonadotrophin release and thereby inhibiting ovulation. They also thin the endometrium and thicken cervical mucus. A single

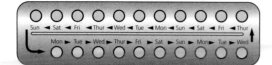

Fig. 12.1 The combined oral contraceptive.

tablet, containing both an oestrogen and a progestogen, is taken every day for 3 weeks and then stopped for 1 week (Fig. 12.1). Most COC preparations contain the synthetic oestrogen ethinyloestradiol. Newer types of COC, such as Qlaira and Zoely, contain the natural oestrogen oestradiol valerate, which is metabolized in the body to the naturally occurring hormone oestradiol. Vaginal bleeding occurs at the end of the pill packet as a result of withdrawal of the hormonal stimulus on the endometrium. The cycle is then restarted. Pill packets can be taken consecutively without a break ('back to back') to reduce the frequency of the withdrawal bleed although increased irregular spotting may occur.

Types of COC

Containing ethinyloestradiol: Most are monophasic pills, delivering the same dose of oestrogen and progestogen every day. The content of the synthetic oestrogen ethinyloestradiol ranges from 20 to 40 μg, with 'standard-dose' pills containing 30–35 μg and 'low-dose' pills 20 μg. The usual preparations of choice are the 30 or 35 μg pills (e.g. Microgynon 30). Oral contraceptives are also grouped in four 'generations', depending on the dose of ethinyloestradiol used and type of progestogen. Bleeding patterns are determined more by the type of progestogen used than the oestrogen dose or the type of phasic regimen.
Containing oestradiol valerate: This natural oestrogen is now combined with a synthetic progestogen in monophasic (Zoely) or phasic (Qlaira) preparations. Long-term data are limited: risks are assumed to be similar to the other COCs.

Contraceptive efficacy

Taken properly, combined hormonal contraception is highly effective, with a failure rate of 0.2 per 100 woman-years. If less care is taken, failure rates are much higher. The low-dose COC preparations containing 20 μg ethi-

nyloestradiol have similar contraceptive efficacy to 'standard' 30–35 μg pills (*Cochrane* 2013; CD003989).

Common side effects of sex hormones	
Progestogenic	*Oestrogenic*
Depression	Nausea
Premenstrual tension-like symptoms	Headaches
	Increased mucus
Bleeding; amenorrhoea	Fluid retention and weight gain
Acne	Occasionally hypertension
Breast discomfort	Breast tenderness and fullness
Weight gain	Bleeding
Reduced libido	

Indications

All women without major contraindications may use combined oral contraception ('from menarche to menopause'). It is suitable for the teenager (in conjunction with condoms) and the older woman with no cardiovascular risk factors until the age of 50. It is also useful for menstrual cycle control, menorrhagia, premenstrual symptoms, dysmenorrhoea, acne/hirsutism and prevention of recurrent simple ovarian cysts.

The COC pill in practice

Reduced absorption of the pill can occur if suffering from diarrhoea, vomiting or if taking some oral antibiotics. If the woman has diarrhoea, she should continue taking the pills but follow the missed pill instructions (see below) for each day of the illness. If she vomits within 2 hours of taking the pill, she should take another or follow the rules for missed pills. If she is taking broad-spectrum antibiotics, she should continue the pills but use condoms during and for 7 days after the antibiotic course. With liver enzyme-inducing drugs (e.g. anticonvulsants), the oestrogen dose may need to be increased.
The missed pill: For standard-strength preparations (30–35 μg ethinyloestradiol), one or two missed pills anywhere in the pack are not a problem. For low-dose preparations (20 μg), only one pill can be missed. The forgotten pill should be taken as soon as possible and then the packet continued as normal. If more pills have been missed, the packet should be continued as normal but condoms should be used for 7 days. If there are

fewer than seven pills remaining in the packet, the next packet should be started straight after the last, avoiding a pill-free break. Advice for missed pills is different and more complex for Qlaira and Zoely (see product information).

The pill and surgery: The pill is normally stopped 4 weeks before major surgery because of its prothrombotic risks, but the risks of pregnancy should also be considered. The pill is not discontinued prior to minor surgery.

Counselling the woman starting on the combined oral contraceptives

Advise of major complications and benefits
Advise to stop smoking
Advise to see doctor if symptoms suggestive of major complications
Advise about poor absorption with antibiotics and sickness and what to do about missed pill(s) (give leaflet)
Stress the importance of follow-up and blood pressure measurement

---

Disadvantages

Major: complications

These are very rare. In general, the risks of pregnancy (including termination of an unwanted pregnancy) outweigh the risks of CHC. The estimated excess annual risk of death for women taking the pill is 2–5 per million users for women <35 years of age. This can be minimized by careful selection and follow-up of women. *Venous thrombosis* and *myocardial infarction* are the most important complications (www.fsrh.org). The risk is further multiplied by smoking, increased age and obesity (absolute contraindication if body mass index [BMI] >40, or age >35 years and smokes >15 cigarettes per day; relative contraindication if BMI 35–39). *Venous thromboembolism* is more common with 'third-generation' pills containing the progestogens gestodene or desogestrel than with the more widely prescribed second-generation preparations containing norithisterone or levonorgestrel, although the absolute risk remains low. Other problems include a slightly increased risk of *cerebrovascular accidents, focal migraine, hypertension, jaundice,* and *liver, cervical and breast carcinoma* (Fig. 12.2).

Minor: side effects

Both oestrogenic and progestogenic side effects may occur. The most common are nausea, headaches and

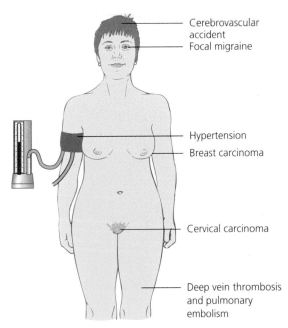

Fig. 12.2 Major complications of the combined oral contraceptive.

Cerebrovascular accident
Focal migraine
Hypertension
Breast carcinoma
Cervical carcinoma
Deep vein thrombosis and pulmonary embolism

breast tenderness. Breakthrough bleeding is common in the first few months, but has usually settled after 3 months. If not, then consider changing the pill to one containing a more potent progestogen or if using a 20 μg ethinyloestradiol pill, increase it to a 30 μg preparation. Lactation is partly suppressed so the pill is contraindicated during the first 6 weeks of breastfeeding.

Advantages

Contraceptive: Despite the rare complications, COC is a very effective and acceptable method of contraception. It has been the subject of considerable research and in appropriate women it is very safe.

Non-contraceptive benefits: Useful effects include more regular, less painful and lighter menstruation. There is protection against simple ovarian cysts, benign breast cysts, fibroids and endometriosis. Hirsutism and acne may improve: the COC need not be prescribed merely for contraception. The risk of pelvic inflammatory disease (PID), but not HIV, is reduced possibly because of thicker cervical mucus. Longer term, there is reduction in the incidence of ovarian, endometrial and bowel cancer.

Contraindications to combined hormonal (including oral) contraception	
Absolute	History of venous thrombosis
	History of cerebrovascular accident, ischaemic heart disease, severe hypertension
	Migraine with aura
	Active breast/endometrial cancer
	Inherited thrombophilia
	Pregnancy
	Smokers >35 years and smoking >15 cigarettes/day
	Body mass index (BMI) >40
	Diabetes with vascular complications
	Active/chronic liver disease
Relative	Smokers
	Chronic inflammatory disease
	Renal impairment, diabetes
	Age >40 years
	BMI 35–40
	Breastfeeding up to 6 months postpartum

Risk of non-fatal venous thromboembolism for users of combined oral contraceptives	
User category	*Incidence per 100 000 women per year*
All women not using 'pill'	5
Pregnant women	60
Women using older 30 µg 'pill'	15
Women using new 30 µg 'pill'	25
Women smoking and using 'pill'	60

Other combined hormonal contraception

These are non-oral combined preparations of oestrogen and progestogens. Safety, side effects and efficacy are similar to combined oral preparations.

Combined transdermal patch (Evra)

Evra is a transdermal adhesive patch that releases ethinyloestradiol (34 µg) plus the progestogen norelgestromin. A new patch is applied weekly for 3 consecutive weeks, this is followed by a patch-free week. Efficacy, side effects and contraindications to use are similar to the COC.

Combined vaginal ring (Nuvaring)

The latex-free Nuvaring releases a daily dose of 15 µg of ethinyloestradiol and 120 µg of the progestogen etonogestrel to inhibit ovulation. The ring is easily inserted into the vagina by the patient and worn for 3 weeks. It is then removed to allow for a 7-day ring-free break and a withdrawal bleed. A new ring is then inserted. This may be better tolerated than the COC due to lower systemic oestrogenic side effects. It is recommended that the ring not be removed during intercourse but, if necessary, may be removed for a maximum of 3 hours. When used properly, the efficacy of the ring is equivalent to the COC. It has the same metabolic and coagulation effects as other combined hormonal methods (*Contraception* 2011; **83**: 107–15).

Progestogen-only pill (POP)

The standard progestogen-only pill ('mini-pill') contains a low dose (e.g. 350 µg norethisterone: Micronor) and must be taken every day without a break and at the same time (±3 hours). It makes cervical mucus hostile to sperm and in 50% of women inhibits ovulation too. Failure rates are 1 per 100 woman-years, higher than the combined pill. Side effects are progestogenic: vaginal spotting (breakthrough bleeding), weight gain, mastalgia and premenstrual-like symptoms are most common. Functional ovarian cysts can occur. It is less effective than the combined pill, and the need for meticulous timing can spell failure, especially in younger women. It is particularly suitable for older women and those in whom the combined pill is contraindicated, such as lactating mothers. There is no increased risk of thrombosis and it can be used in almost all the situations where the combined pill is contraindicated. If a pill is missed by more than 3 hours then another should be taken as soon as possible and condoms used for 2 days. The POPs are not affected by broad-spectrum antibiotics.

Cerazette and Cerelle are different preparations to standard mini-pills, contain a higher dose of the third-generation progestogen *desogestrel*, and inhibit ovulation in over 95% of cycles. They are more effective and can be taken within a 12-hour window.

Counselling before using the 'mini-pill'
Advise woman about bleeding patterns
Emphasize the importance of meticulous timekeeping

Long-acting reversible contraceptives (LARCs)

With depot administration methods, progestogens are slowly released, bypassing the portal circulation. The mode of action is similar to that of the 'mini-pill' but ovulation is normally also prevented; consequently they protect against functional ovarian cysts and ectopic pregnancy. The LARCs demonstrate many of the features of an ideal contraceptive. In particular, they are not user dependent and have high efficacy rates. The LARC methods are more cost-effective than the COC after 12 months of use. However, current usage rates are low.

Depo-Provera, Noristerat and Sayana Press

Depo-Provera, containing medroxyprogesterone acetate (150 mg), is administered by intramuscular injection every 3 months. The failure rate is <1.0 per 100 woman-years. It often causes irregular bleeding in the first weeks, but this is usually followed by amenorrhoea. Other progestogenic side effects may occur. Prolonged amenorrhoea may follow its cessation and women should be warned of this, particularly if they are considering pregnancy in the near future. Bone density decreases over the first 2–3 years of use, then stabilizes, and is regained after stopping. Consequently, other contraceptives are preferable in teenagers (before peak bone mass is achieved) and in women at risk of osteoporosis, e.g. older women. It is useful during lactation and when compliance is a problem.

Noristerat is an IM depot preparation containing norethisterone enantate, with similar efficacy to Depo-Provera, which is given every 8 weeks. Noristerat is recommended as a short-term interim contraception, for example whilst waiting for a vasectomy to become effective.

Sayana Press is a subcutaneous preparation of medroxyprogesterone acetate, licensed for self-administration, which provides cover for 13 weeks.

All three depot preparations may be used in breastfeeding women, although it is recommended that medroxyprogesterone acetate be given no sooner than 6 weeks after birth.

Nexplanon

This consists of a single 40 mm flexible rod containing progestogen (etonogestrel), which is inserted in

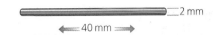

Fig. 12.3 Nexplanon.

the upper arm subdermally with local anaesthetic (Fig. 12.3). The failure rate is <1.0 per 100 woman-years. It will last 3 years and female satisfaction is high. Side effects include progestogenic symptoms, particularly irregular bleeding in the first year. There is no drop in bone density. Removal is usually easy and there is a rapid resumption of fertility. Because it is simple and long-acting, it may have a particular role in the developing world.

Progestogen-impregnated intrauterine system

This is discussed below.

Emergency contraception

In emergency contraception, a drug or IUD is used shortly after unprotected intercourse in an attempt to prevent pregnancy. A number of different regimes are available, over the pharmacy counter, in the UK.

The 'morning-after pill'

It is vital to arrange future contraception and to consider screening for sexually transmitted infections (STIs), depending on circumstances. If the next period is late, the woman should be advised to perform a pregnancy test.

The chance of conception after unprotected intercourse can be reduced by taking the 'morning-after pill'. Two types are available, either with or without prescription.

Levonelle contains a single 1.5 mg dose of the progestogen levonorgestrel. It is best taken within 24 hours, and no later than 72 hours, after unprotected intercourse. It affects sperm function and endometrial receptivity and if given just prior to ovulation, may prevent follicular rupture. The method has a 95% success rate if used within 24 hours, reduced to 58% if delayed until 72 hours. Vomiting can occur plus menstrual disturbances in the following cycle.

Ulipristal (ellaOne) is a selective progesterone receptor modulator (SPRM), like mifepristone. It prevents or delays ovulation, and may also reduce embryo implantation. It is at least as effective as Levonelle and, further, can be used up to 120 hours after unprotected intercourse. As it blocks the action of progesterone, ellaOne will reduce the effectiveness of progesterone-containing contraceptives and so women should use condoms or avoid unprotected intercourse until the next period.

Intrauterine device

Insertion of an IUD usually prevents implantation and is the most efficacious method of emergency contraception. The IUD can be inserted up to 5 days after either the episode of unprotected intercourse or the expected day of ovulation (so if intercourse occurred, for example, 2 days before expected ovulation, the IUD could be inserted 7 days later). Antibiotic prophylaxis is usually given at the time of insertion.

Barrier contraception

Barrier methods physically prevent the sperm from getting through the cervix. A principal advantage, especially with condoms, is the protection against STIs.

Male condom

This consists of a sheath (latex or not) that fits onto the erect penis (Fig. 12.4). The failure rate is 2–15 per 100 woman-years; this is dependent on using it properly. It affords the best protection against disease, including HIV, and should always be used for casual intercourse, even if in conjunction with other methods.

Female condom

This fits inside the vagina. Failure rates are similar to the male condom but it is less well accepted. It too protects against STIs.

Diaphragms and caps

These are fitted before intercourse and must remain *in situ* for at least 6 hours afterwards. Cervical caps fit over the cervix (Fig. 12.5a), whilst the spring of the latex

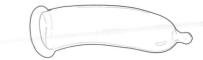

Fig. 12.4 The male condom.

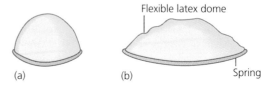

Fig. 12.5 (a) The cervical cap. (b) The diaphragm.

dome of the diaphragm holds it between the pubic bone and the sacral curve, covering the cervix (Fig. 12.5b). Types and sizes vary, and selection should be determined by trained personnel. Failure rates are about 5 per 100 woman-years and dependent on the type used. Although some protection against PID is gained, there is less protection against HIV. Some women find them inconvenient, and they are best suited to a woman with good motivation.

Spermicides

Barrier methods are used in conjunction with a spermicide containing *nonoxynol-9*, in the form of a jelly, cream or pessary. Spermicides are not recommended for use on their own.

Intrauterine contraceptive devices ('the coil')

These devices are put into the uterine cavity and are of two types: copper or progestogen bearing. Thin plastic strings protrude through the cervix and are pulled to remove the device. They are changed every 5–10 years.

Types of IUDs

Copper-containing devices operate primarily by preventing fertilization, the copper ion being toxic to sperm. They also act to block implantation. The copper is either wound around an inert frame which sits within the uterine cavity (Fig. 12.6a) or threads which are attached to the fundus (Fig. 12.6c).

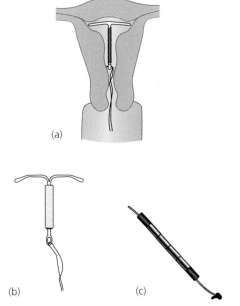

(a)

(b)   (c)

Fig. 12.6 Intrauterine devices (IUDs). (a) Copper T in uterus, (b) intrauterine system (IUS), (c) Gynefix.

Hormone-containing devices contain the progestogen levonorgestrel, which is slowly released locally over several years. This is called the intrauterine system (IUS). *Jaydess* and *Levosert* need to be replaced every 3 years while *Mirena* needs to be replaced every 5 years (Fig. 12.6b). Its main contraceptive effects are local, through changes to the cervical mucus and uterotubal fluid which impair sperm migration, backed by endometrial changes impeding implantation. In addition, it reduces menstrual loss and pain. The blood levels of levonorgestrel are much less than that of the progestogen mini-pill so systemic side effects are low. Irregular light bleeding is the main problem but satisfaction and contraceptive efficacy rates are high. Return of fertility after removal is rapid and complete.

Contraceptive efficacy

With high copper content and progestogen-releasing devices, the failure rate is <0.5 per 100 woman-years. A major advantage is the lack of user dependence.

Indications

The IUD is used by 20% of sexually active French women but only 5% in the UK. It is safe, effective and reversible and can be used in a number of situations when hormonal contraception is contraindicated, particularly in older women. Coils are normally inserted during the first half of the cycle, but can be used straight after termination of pregnancy or in the puerperium. The progestogen-releasing IUS is also used for non-contraceptive indications such as menorrhagia or dysmenorrhoea.

Complications

Pain or cervical shock (due to increased vagal tone) can complicate insertion. The device can be *expelled*, usually within the first month. *Perforation* of the uterine wall (<0.5%) can occur at insertion, or the device may migrate through the wall afterwards. Expulsion or perforation will cause the threads to disappear, but they may also have been cut too short. If the threads are not visible at the cervix, an ultrasound scan is performed to look for the IUD within the uterus. If it is not present then an abdominal X-ray will reveal the IUD if it is within the abdomen; if so then a laparoscopy is indicated to remove it. *Heavier or more painful menstruation* can occur (except with progestogen devices). Women with asymptomatic STIs in the cervix are at increased risk of PID during the first 20 days after insertion. The risk of *infection* (10%) is mainly limited to younger women with multiple partners and is reduced by screening for infection first.

If pregnancy occurs despite the presence of an IUD, it is more likely to be *ectopic*, but the overall ectopic rate is still lower than in a woman using no contraception. If ectopic pregnancy has been excluded, the IUD should be removed early so as to reduce the risk of miscarriage, particularly mid-trimester loss.

Contraindications to the intrauterine device	
Absolute	Endometrial or cervical cancer Undiagnosed vaginal bleeding Active/recent pelvic infection Current breast cancer (for progestogen intrauterine system (IUS)) Pregnancy

Relative	Previous ectopic pregnancy
	Excessive menstrual loss (unless
	    progestogen IUS)
	Multiple sexual partners
	Young/nulliparous
	Immunocompromised, including human
	    immunodeficiency virus (HIV) positive

Advantages

The IUD is extremely safe. The woman does not need to remember to use other contraception. Menstrual loss is reduced if progestogen-containing devices are used (IUS). The IUD can be used as emergency contraception if inserted within 5 days of ovulation.

Counselling before inserting an intrauterine device	
Advise of the major risks	
Advise to inform her doctor if:	She bleeds intermenstrually
	She experiences pelvic pain or a vaginal discharge, or if she feels she might be pregnant
Advise about checking for strings after each period	

Female sterilization

In the UK, 10% of couples rely on female and 20% on male sterilization for contraception. Between 2000 and 2010, the number of sterilization procedures decreased by 75% and 50% for women and men respectively. The minimum that needs to be done for female sterilization is interruption of the fallopian tubes so that sperm and egg cannot meet. The most common technique uses clips (e.g. Filshie clip; Fig. 12.7). These are applied to the tubes laparoscopically, completely occluding the lumen. This normally involves a general anaesthetic. Sometimes sterilization is performed at the time of caesarean section when a portion of each tube is excised, though the rates of regret are higher than when performed later.

An alternative is transcervical sterilization involving the hysteroscopic placement of microinserts into the proximal part of each tubal lumen (e.g. Essure; Fig. 12.8). The inserts expand and cause fibrosis and occlusion of the lumen, confirmed 3 months later with a hysterosalpingogram.

Contraceptive efficacy

The Filshie clip and Essure both have failure rates of around 0.5%, i.e. about 1 in 200 women will become pregnant at some time, though data for Essure are less established.

Indications

Both doctor and woman must be satisfied that there will be no regret. Therefore it is usually used in an older woman whose family is complete, or when disease contraindicates pregnancy.

Counselling a woman before sterilization
The woman, and preferably her partner, must be certain
Alternative contraception is discussed
Warn of 1 in 200 lifetime risk of failure
Risk of ectopic if pregnancy
Reversal not possible with hysteroscopic sterilization and not guaranteed with Filshie clips. Reversal unavailable on the NHS
Risks of surgery and of possible laparotomy

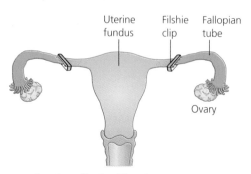

Fig. 12.7 Female sterilization. View of uterine fundus with Filshie clips on tubes.

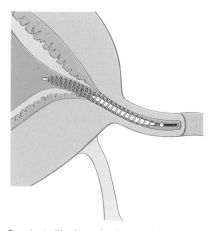

Fig. 12.8 Female sterilization: microinserts placed hysteroscopically into fallopian tubes.

Complications

Laparoscopic sterilization is a safe procedure (*Cochrane* 2015; CD003034), but perioperative complications include the risks of laparoscopy (primarily visceral damage) and inadequate access to the tubes. Postoperative pain is reduced by using local anaesthetic on the tubes and in the skin incisions. If pregnancy does occur, it is more likely to be ectopic. Requests for reversal should be rare with adequate woman selection and counselling. Reversal is performed using microsurgical techniques via a laparotomy or, occasionally, laparoscopy. Successful reversal is less likely if a portion of the tube has been removed, for example if performed at caesarean section. *In vitro* fertilization (IVF) is an alternative to reversal.

The efficacy of transcervical hysteroscopic sterilization (Essure) is less well established and reoperation rates are higher than with laparoscopic sterilization (*NEJM* 2015; **373**: e17).

Male sterilization

Vasectomy is more effective than female sterilization (1 in 2000 lifetime risk after two negative semen analyses) and involves ligation and removal of a small segment of the vas deferens, thereby preventing release of sperm. It can be performed under local anaesthetic. Sterility is not assured until azoospermia is confirmed by two semen analyses and may take up to 6 months to achieve. Complications (5%) include failure, postoperative haematomas and infection, and chronic pain. Natural conception following successful reversal is often prevented by antisperm antibody formation which restricts motility. Such sperm can be washed and used during an insemination or IVF cycle. Surgical sperm retrieval followed by IVF is an alternative to vasectomy reversal.

Male hormonal contraception

Spermatogenesis can be halted by depot administration of progestogens through central effects at the hypothalamus and pituitary. The gonadotrophin drive to the testes is reduced (in a similar way to the effects of depot progestogen in women causing anovulation). However, this also switches off androgen production so additional exogenous testosterone replacement therapy is required.

Despite 2015 marking the 55th year of COC use in women, there is still no equivalent pharmacological male method available. Surveys suggest both men and women would welcome the development of male hormonal contraception. Trial results are promising and the development of a reliable male hormonal contraception is likely (*Cochrane* 2012; CD004316).

Natural contraception

This is less reliable than most methods and offers no protection against STIs. It is only suitable for monogamous women who would not be concerned by pregnancy. *Lactation* has a major contraceptive role in the developing world. The *'rhythm' method* avoids the fertile period around ovulation and over-the-counter kits can help this. Some kits (e.g. Persona) measure urine levels of luteinizing hormone and oestrogen and from this calculate 'safe' days for intercourse. *'Withdrawal'* involves removal of the penis just before ejaculation, but is not recommended because sperm can be released before orgasm.

Further reading

Faculty of Sexual and Reproductive Healthcare, Royal College of Obstetricians and Gynaecologists (source of excellent contraception guidelines and reviews): www.fsrh.org

Family Planning Association (sexual health charity): www.fpa.org.uk

Contraception at a glance

Combined hormonal contraceptive	Women:	Any, except smoker >35 years, BMI >40, history of venous thromboembolism, cerebrovascular disease and cerebrovascular accident, hypertension or inherited thrombophilia, current breast cancer
	Failure:	Pearl Index (PI) 0.1 (perfect use); 5.0 (typical use)
	Mode of action:	Inhibits ovulation
	How to use:	Start on day 1 of cycle, 3 weeks, then 1 week break
	Rare major problems:	Deep vein thromboses, ischaemic heart disease, cerebrovascular accident, hypertension, breast and cervical carcinoma
	Common side effects:	Breast tenderness, bleeding, headaches, nausea
	Benefits:	Good contraception, cycle control, well accepted. Reduces risk of developing fibroids, and ovarian, endometrial, bowel cancer
	Drawbacks:	Major side effects and contraindications. User dependent so failure rate increased
Progestogen-only pill	Women:	Any. Need to be well motivated
	Failure:	PI 0.5 (perfect use); 5.0 (typical use) (Cerazette/Cerelle similar to combined pill)
	Mode of action:	Cervical mucus and sometimes inhibition of ovulation
	How to use:	Continuous, every day at same time (Cerazette/Cerelle 12 h window)
	Side effects:	Vaginal spotting, other progestogenic effects
	Benefits:	Few contraindications, lactation
	Drawbacks:	Compliance and failure rate. User dependent
Depot progestogens	Women:	Any. When compliance a problem
	Failure:	PI <0.5
	Mode of action:	As above, and ovulation usually inhibited
	How to use:	Depo-Provera intramuscularly every 3 months, Noristerat every 8 weeks, Nexplanon every 3 years
	Side effects:	Progestogenic; prolonged amenorrhoea and reversible bone loss with Depo-Provera
	Benefits:	Woman can 'forget about it' (i.e. no user-dependent failures)
	Drawbacks:	Progestogenic side effects
Intrauterine devices (IUDs)	Women:	Older, multiparous, monogamous
	Failure:	PI <1.0 depending on type (PI 0.1 for progestagen intrauterine system (IUS))
	Mode of action:	Prevents implantation/fertilization
	How to use:	Insert into uterus, change every 3–10 years
	Side effects:	Pelvic infection, menstrual disturbance, perforation

(Continued)

Contraception at a Glance (Continued)

	Benefits:	Woman can 'forget about it'; IUS reduces blood loss
	Drawbacks:	Pelvic infection, increased menstrual bleeding and pain with copper IUD
Condoms	Person:	Any, essential for casual intercourse
	Failure:	PI 2.0 (perfect use); 15 (typical use)
	Benefits:	Non-hormonal, safe, protection against sexually transmitted infection (STIs)
	Drawbacks:	Inconvenience, poor technique
Caps/diaphragms	Woman:	Any, well motivated, usually monogamous
	Failure:	PI 5.0 (perfect use); 15 (typical use)
	How to use:	Insert before intercourse, with spermicide, remove 6 h later
	Benefits:	Non-hormonal, woman has control
	Drawbacks:	Failure rates, inconvenience, limited protection against STIs
Sterilization	Person:	Older, multiparous, family finished
	Failure:	1 in 200 (female); 1 in 2000 (male) lifetime risk
	How to do:	Female: laparoscopic clip best, hysteroscopic
		Male: ligation and removal of segment of vas deferens (vasectomy)
	Side effects:	Perioperative complications
	Benefits:	'Permanent'
	Drawbacks:	Reversal expensive and limited success. Common source of litigation

CHAPTER 13

The menopause and postreproductive health

Definitions

Menopause is the permanent cessation of menstruation resulting from loss of ovarian follicular activity. It occurs at a median age of 51 years. Natural menopause is recognized to have occurred after 12 consecutive months of amenorrhoea (Fig. 13.1).

Perimenopause includes the time beginning with the first features of the approaching menopause, such as vasomotor symptoms and menstrual irregularity, and ends 12 months after the last menstrual period.

Postmenopause should be defined as dating from the final menstrual period. However, it cannot be determined until after 12 months of spontaneous amenorrhoea.

Premature menopause is arbitrarily defined as menopause occurring before the age of 40 and affects 1% of women. In most women no cause is found. Some will have a *surgical menopause* following bilateral oophorectomy perhaps performed during hysterectomy. Other causes include infections, autoimmune disorders, chemotherapy, ovarian dysgenesis and metabolic diseases. Hormone replacement therapy (HRT), which is increasingly known as menopausal hormone therapy (MHT), is indicated at least until the age of 50. Oocyte donation is required for fertility treatment.

Postmenopausal bleeding

Definition

Vaginal bleeding occurring at least 12 months after the last menstrual period.

Causes

Postmenopausal bleeding is an important clinical problem. The main point is to exclude carcinoma of the endometrium or cervix and premalignant endometrial hyperplasia with cytological atypia, which account for about 20% of cases. Withdrawal bleeds occur with sequential menopausal hormonal therapy and, so long as they are regular, do not warrant investigation. Bleeding may also occur from a poorly oestrogenized vaginal wall ('atrophic vaginitis') but this should be a diagnosis of exclusion. A purulent blood-stained vaginal discharge in a postmenopausal woman should be investigated to rule out endometrial cancer or, uncommonly, a diverticular abscess draining via the uterus or vagina.

Causes of postmenopausal bleeding (PMB)
Endometrial carcinoma
Endometrial hyperplasia ± atypia and polyps
Cervical carcinoma
Atrophic vaginitis
Cervicitis
Ovarian carcinoma
Cervical polyps

Management

All women should undergo a bimanual and speculum examination and a cervical smear if one has not been taken according to the national screening programme. *Transvaginal sonography* (TVS) has become a routine procedure for initial assessment. It measures

Obstetrics & Gynaecology, Fifth Edition. Lawrence Impey, Tim Child.
© 2017 John Wiley & Sons, Ltd. Published 2017 by John Wiley & Sons, Ltd.

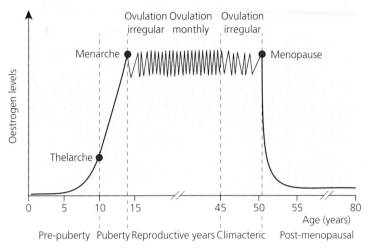

Fig. 13.1 Oestrogen levels in a lifetime.

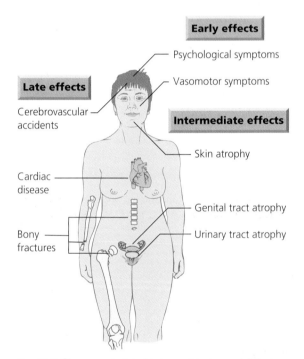

Fig. 13.2 Changes and clinical features of oestrogen deficiency.

endometrial thickness and also gives information on other pelvic pathology, such as fibroids and ovarian cysts. TVS is less invasive than endometrial biopsy or hysteroscopy but does not give a histological diagnosis. A thickened endometrium or a cavity filled with fluid indicates an increased risk of malignancy or other pathology (hyperplasia or polyps).

If the endometrial thickness is 4 mm or less on TVS and there was only a single episode of PMB then endometrial biopsy ± hysteroscopy is not required. If the endometrium is thicker or there have been multiple bleeds an *endometrial biopsy ± hysteroscopy* should be performed. If undertaken as an outpatient procedure, endometrium can be obtained using a Pipelle suction device. Outpatient hysteroscopy can also be performed and may employ paracervical local anaesthesia. If an endometrial polyp is found on scan, if the woman is anxious about having an outpatient procedure, or if vaginal access is expected to be difficult (for instance, due to an atrophic vagina) then hysteroscopy and endometrial biopsy is performed under general anaesthetic as a day case procedure. Once malignancy is excluded, atrophic vaginitis can be treated with topical oestrogen or oral ospemifene (a selective estrogen receptor modulator (SERM)).

Symptoms and consequences of the menopause (Fig. 13.2)

Cardiovascular disease

Cardiovascular disease (CVD) (coronary heart disease and stroke) is the number one cause of death globally and now the number two cause in the UK (second only to cancer). In the UK, CVD accounts for about one-quarter of all deaths in women (Fig. 13.3), the same proportion as for men.

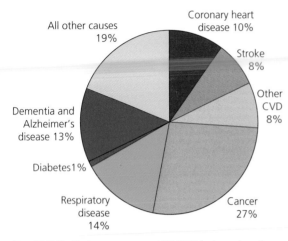

Fig. 13.3 Deaths by cause, women, UK 2014 (redrawn from the British Heart Foundation). CVD, cardiovascular disease.

Vasomotor symptoms

Hot flushes and night sweats are the most common symptoms of the menopause and affect about 70% of Western women. Night sweats can cause sleep disturbance leading to tiredness and irritability. They may begin before periods stop and usually are present for less than 5 years. However, some women will continue to flush in their 60s and 70s.

Urogenital problems

Oestrogen deficiency can cause vaginal atrophy and urinary problems. The condition is termed genitourinary syndrome of menopause. Vaginal atrophy can also affect women taking systemic HRT. It can be extremely uncomfortable and can result in dyspareunia, cessation of sexual activity, itching, burning and dryness. Urinary symptoms include frequency, urgency, nocturia, incontinence and recurrent infection. Women may suffer in silence and not seek medical help.

Sexual problems

Sexual problems affect about half of all women and become more common with age. Interest in sex declines in both sexes with increasing age and this change is more pronounced in women. The term female sexual dysfunction (FSD) is now used and an international classification system employed. Sexual problems are classified into various types: loss of sexual desire, loss of

sexual arousal, problems with orgasm and sexual pain, e.g. dyspareunia.

Osteoporosis

Osteoporosis is 'a skeletal disorder characterized by compromised bone strength predisposing to an increased risk of fracture'. It is a major problem, with 1 in 3 women over 50 years having one or more osteoporotic fractures. Bone strength reflects the integration of two main features: bone density and bone quality. *Bone density* is expressed as grams of mineral per area or volume and, in any given individual, is determined by peak bone mass and amount of bone loss. *Bone quality* refers to architecture, turnover, damage accumulation (e.g. microfractures) and mineralization.

The World Health Organization (WHO) definitions of osteoporosis, classified according to bone mineral density (BMD), are shown below. The T score is that number of standard deviations (SD) by which a particular bone differs from the young normal mean.

Definitions of osteoporosis according to the WHO	
Description	*Definition*
Normal	BMD value between –1 SD and +1 SD of the young adult mean (T score –1 to +1)
Osteopenia	BMD between –1 and –2.5 SD from the young adult mean (T score –1 to –2.5)
Osteoporosis	BMD ≥ –2.5 SD from the young adult mean (T score –2.5 or lower)

Osteoporotic fractures

Fractures are the clinical consequences of osteoporosis. The most common sites are the wrist or Colles' fracture, the hip and the spine. Fractures have a major impact on quality of life, result in a significant economic burden and, in the case of hip fractures, are associated with considerable mortality (30% in the year after a hip fracture).

Risk factors for the development of osteoporosis

Most important in clinical practice are prior fracture, parental history of fracture (particularly hip fracture), early menopause, chronic use of corticosteroids (oral and possibly inhaled), smoking and prolonged immobilization. The FRAX tool has been developed by the WHO to give the 10-year probability of fracture based on individual patient clinical factors and their BMD (www.shef.ac.uk/FRAX/).

Risk factors for osteoporosis	
Genetic	Family history of fracture (particularly a first-degree relative with hip fracture)
Constitutional	Low body mass index Early menopause (<45 years of age)
Environmental	Cigarette smoking Alcohol abuse Low calcium intake Sedentary lifestyle
Drugs	Corticosteroids, >5 mg/day prednisolone or equivalent
Diseases	Rheumatoid arthritis Neuromuscular disease Chronic liver disease Malabsorption syndromes Hyperparathyroidism Hyperthyroidism Hypogonadism

Investigations of the menopause

Follicle-stimulating hormone (FSH)

Follicle-stimulating hormone levels give an estimate of the degree of ovarian reserve remaining (Fig. 13.4). Increased levels suggest fewer oocytes remaining in the ovaries. Levels are helpful with suspected *premature ovarian failure*, but in women over the age of 45 who are having hot flushes the diagnosis is usually clear. FSH levels vary daily during the perimenopause and are not a guide to fertility status or when the last period is likely to occur and therefore are of limited value. FSH levels can be measured in women whether or not they have had a hysterectomy. If not, they are best measured between days 2 and 5 of the cycle (day 1 is the first day of menstruation) in order to avoid the mid-cycle preovulatory increase and the luteal phase suppression of FSH. In women with oligomenorrhoea or amenorrhoea or who have undergone hysterectomy, two samples, 2 weeks apart, are obtained. FSH levels are of little value in monitoring HRT.

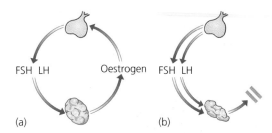

Fig. 13.4 Ovarian responsiveness to pituitary hormones. (a) Reproductive years: feedback control between ovary and hypothalamic–pituitary axis. (b) Postmenopausal years: unresponsive ovaries produce no oestrogen or inhibin. Lack of feedback on hypothalamus–pituitary axis causes high levels of follicle-stimulating hormone (FSH) and luteinizing hormone (LH).

Anti-mullerian hormone

Anti-mullerian hormone (AMH) is produced by small ovarian follicles and gives a direct measurement of ovarian reserve, low levels being consistent with ovarian failure. AMH levels are stable throughout the menstrual cycle and so can be measured on any day. The measurement of AMH is rapidly becoming established in assisted conception. Its interpretation in predicting age of menopause needs to be made in the clinical context, and validated age-specific normal ranges, quality assurance and standardization of measurement are required (*Menopause* 2016; **23**: 224–232).

Other blood tests

Thyroid function tests (free T4 and thyroid-stimulating hormone [TSH]) are checked if there is an inadequate symptomatic response to MHT, as thyroid disease can cause hot flushes.

Catecholamines and 5-hydroxyindoleacetic acid, raised in phaeochromocytoma and carcinoid syndrome, can also be measured in these circumstances.

Luteinizing hormone, oestradiol and progesterone: Oestradiol is naturally low early in the menstrual cycle in women with normal ovarian function. A low progesterone level indicates anovulation which can be secondary to many causes, most commonly polycystic ovary syndrome (PCOS).

Bone density estimation

Population screening is of little value: it is best to target women at risk of osteoporosis (see box above). The main sites for measurement are the lumbar spine and the hip. Since the spine may have falsely increased values due to osteophytes from osteoarthritis, kyphosis, scoliosis and aortic calcification, the best site to measure is the hip. Bone density changes slowly and the frequency of follow-up scans is controversial. Initially, follow-up scans may be undertaken every 2–3 years to assess response to treatment.

Dual-energy X-ray absorptiometry (DEXA) is an X-ray based system that uses two different energies to differentiate between soft tissue and bone. Values for BMD may be quoted as g/cm^2 (see Fig. 13.6) or converted into values that relate to either the average young female (or male) peak bone mass (T score) or that of the patient's age group (Z score).

Biochemical markers of bone metabolism

Biochemical markers of bone turnover are classified as markers of resorption or formation. Biochemical markers of bone turnover can be used to monitor response to therapy such as bisphosphonates (see below) because significant suppression of bone turnover occurs far more rapidly than detectable changes in bone mineral density. Significant changes can occur within 3–6 months of initiation of therapy. Bone markers are not used to diagnose osteoporosis.

Treatment: hormone replacement therapy

Hormone replacement therapy consists of oestrogen alone in women who have had a hysterectomy, but is combined with a progestogen in those who have not. Progestogens are given cyclically or continuously with the oestrogen. Systemic oestrogens can be delivered orally, transdermally (patch or gel) or subcutaneously (implant) (Fig. 13.5). Topical oestrogens are given vaginally. Progestogens can be delivered orally, transdermally (patch) or directly into the uterus (intrauterine system (IUS)). Many preparations are available with different combinations, strengths and routes of administration. Regimens may vary between countries. A new development is the combination of the SERM bazedoxifene with an oestrogen for women with a uterus.

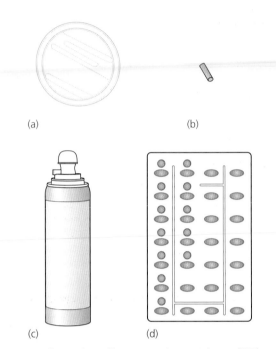

Fig. 13.5 Preparations of hormone replacement therapy (HRT): (a) patch, (b) implant, (c) gel and (d) pills.

Oestrogens

Two types of oestrogen are available: synthetic and natural. Natural oestrogens include oestradiol, oestrone and oestriol. These are synthesized from soya beans or yams and are chemically identical to the natural human hormones. Conjugated equine oestrogens are derived from pregnant mares' urine. Synthetic oestrogens, such as ethinyloestradiol used in the combined oral contraceptive pill, are not used for HRT because of their greater metabolic impact.

Progestogens

The progestogens used in HRT, such as levonorgestrel and norethisterone, are also derived from plant sources such as soya beans or yams. The levonorgestrel intrauterine system (Mirena IUS) is licensed for endometrial protection when oestrogen HRT is being given. This method of delivery also provides a solution to the problem of contraception in the perimenopause and is also the only way in which a 'no bleed' HRT regimen can be achieved in perimenopausal women.

Tibolone

Tibolone is a synthetic steroid compound that is inert but is converted *in vivo* to metabolites with oestrogenic, progestogenic and androgenic actions. It is used in post-menopausal women who desire amenorrhoea and treats vasomotor, psychological and libido problems. It conserves bone mass and reduces the risk of vertebral fracture.

Androgens

Testosterone can be used to improve libido but is not successful in all women, as other factors may be involved. Availability of testosterone preparations in female doses is limited and varies worldwide.

Regimens of HRT

Oestrogen alone: women after hysterectomy

These women should be given oestrogen alone. There may be concerns about a remnant of endometrium in the cervical stump in women who have had a sub-total hysterectomy. If this is suspected, the presence or absence of bleeding induced by monthly sequential HRT is a useful diagnostic test.

Combined oestrogen and progestogen: women with a uterus

Progestogens are added to oestrogens to reduce the increased risk of endometrial hyperplasia and carcinoma, which occurs with unopposed oestrogen. Progestogen can be given 'sequentially' for 10–14 days every 4 weeks or for 14 days every 13 weeks, or it can be used 'continuously', i.e. every day. The first leads to monthly bleeds, the second to 3-monthly bleeds and the last aims to achieve amenorrhoea: 'no-bleed' or 'continuous combined' HRT. Progestogen must still be given to women who have undergone endometrial ablative techniques for menorrhagia such as transcervical resection of endometrium (TCRE), as not all the endometrium may have been removed.

Menopausal status: perimenopausal women

Women receiving MHT who are still menstruating or are within 12 months of their last spontaneous menstrual period can be given sequential or cyclic therapy.

Alternatively, intrauterine levonorgestrel with oral or patch oestrogen is useful in women with heavy menstrual bleeding or needing contraception.

Menopausal status: postmenopausal women

Women are considered to be postmenopausal 12 months after their last menstrual period, although this definition is difficult to apply in clinical practice. Continuous combined regimens should be used because of the lack of induced bleeding and because they probably reduce the risk of endometrial cancer compared with sequential regimens. Continuous combined therapy induces endometrial atrophy. Intrauterine delivery of levonorgestrel can be continued but it may be technically more difficult to insert the intrauterine device in older women. The combination of bazedoxifene and oestrogen is approved for postmenopausal women where treatment with progestogen-containing therapy is not appropriate

Topical oestrogens/ospemifene

These are used to treat urogenital symptoms. The topical oestrogen options available are vaginally administered low-dose natural oestrogens, such as oestriol by cream or pessary, or oestradiol by tablet or ring. Long-term treatment is required since symptoms return on cessation of therapy. These low-dose preparations do not elevate systemic oestrogen levels, so additional progestogen to protect the endometrium is not required. Oral ospemifene (a SERM) is used for moderate-to-severe symptomatic vulvovaginal atrophy in postmenopausal women who are not candidates for local vaginal oestrogen therapy.

Benefits, risks and uncertainties of oestrogen-based HRT

Benefits

Menopausal symptoms: Oestrogen is effective in treating hot flushes, usually within 4 weeks. Relief of hot flushes is the most common indication for HRT, which is often used for less than 5 years. Vaginal dryness, soreness, superficial dyspareunia, urinary frequency and urgency respond well to oestrogens, which may be given either topically or systemically or both together. Sexuality may be improved with oestrogen alone but

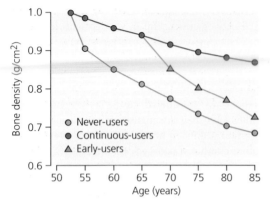

Fig. 13.6 Bone density in oestrogen users and non-users.

may need testosterone in addition, especially in young oophorectomized women. Availability of testosterone preparations in female-appropriate doses is variable.

Osteoporosis: HRT reduces the risk of both spine and hip as well as other osteoporotic fractures (Fig. 13.6). MHT is effective and appropriate for the prevention of osteoporosis-related fractures in at-risk women before the age of 60 or within 10 years after menopause.

Colorectal cancer: HRT reduces the risk of colorectal cancer by about one-third. However, little is known about the risk when treatment is stopped, and use of HRT as preventive therapy is not currently recommended.

Risks

Breast cancer: Combined, but not oestrogen alone, HRT slightly increases the risk, as an extra 4 per 1000 cases after 5 years combined HRT use. This effect is not seen in women who start HRT early for a premature menopause, indicating that it is the duration of lifetime sex hormone exposure that is relevant. Breast cancer risk falls on stopping combined therapy: after 5 years it is no greater than that in women who have never taken MHT.

Endometrial cancer: Unopposed (non-vaginal) oestrogen replacement therapy increases endometrial cancer risk. This is why a progestogen is added to regimens for non-hysterectomized women.

Venous thromboembolism: Oral HRT increases risk of venous thromboembolism (VTE) twofold from a background (not taking HRT) risk of 1.7 per 1000 in women over 50, with the highest risk occurring in the first year of use. Transdermal patches and gel HRT may be associated with a lower risk. Advancing age, obesity and an underlying thrombophilia significantly increase the risk.

Gallbladder disease: Oral HRT increases the risk of gallbladder disease.

HRT and cancer	
↑ risk:	Breast (not if oestrogen only)
	Endometrial (if oestrogen only)
↓ risk	Colon (role uncertain)

Uncertainties

Cardiovascular disease (coronary heart disease and stroke): HRT should not be used primarily for primary or secondary cardiovascular disease prevention. The timing, dose and possibly type of HRT (tablets or patches) appear to influence cardiovascular effects.

Dementia and cognition: While oestrogen may delay or reduce the risk of Alzheimer's disease (AD), the evidence is contradictory, and it should not be used for this indication. It does not improve established disease.

Ovarian cancer: The evidence is conflicting, with some studies showing an increased risk and others not. If there is an increased risk, it is small.

Quality of life: The evidence is conflicting.

Duration of therapy

Menopausal symptoms: Treatment is usually continued for up to 5 years and then stopped to evaluate whether symptoms recur with sufficient severity to warrant continuation.

Osteoporosis: HRT is effective and appropriate for the prevention of osteoporosis-related fractures in at-risk women before the age of 60 or within 10 years after menopause. Treatment may need to be lifelong.

Bone mineral density falls when treatments are stopped (see Fig. 13.6). Women may later change to other agents, such as bisphosphonates, because of the increased risk of breast cancer with longer-term combined HRT.

Premature menopause: Women are usually advised to continue with HRT until the median age of the natural menopause (i.e. 51 years).

Other treatments for the menopause

Non-oestrogen-based therapies

These should be considered for women who do not wish to take HRT or have a contraindication to therapy.

For hot flushes and night sweats

Progestogens such as 5 mg/day norethisterone or 40 mg/day megestrol acetate can be effective.

Clonidine, a centrally acting alpha-adrenoceptor agonist, is of limited value.

Selective serotonin reuptake inhibitors (SSRIs) and serotonin and noradrenaline reuptake inhibitors, such as paroxetine, fluoxetine, citalopram and venlafaxine, are effective in treating hot flushes in short-term studies.

Gabapentin is used to treat epilepsy, neuropathic pain and migraine. Limited evidence shows that it may be effective.

For vaginal atrophy

A variety of lubricants and moisturizers are available without prescription but are less effective than oestrogen.

Prevention and treatment of osteoporosis

All pharmacological interventions except for parathyroid hormone and strontium ranelate act mainly by inhibiting bone resorption. Information on prevention in perimenopausal women or those with premature ovarian failure is scant.

Bisphosphonates, e.g. alendronate, risedronate, zoledronic acid and ibandronate, are used in the prevention and treatment of osteoporosis. The principal side effect is irritation of the upper gastrointestinal tract with oral therapies. Bisphosphonates remain in bone for many years, may affect the fetal skeleton and are not advised in women desiring pregnancy.

Strontium ranelate decreases the risk of vertebral and hip fractures (use is restricted because of increased risk heart disease).

Raloxifene and *bazedoxifene*, SERMs, reduce the incidence of osteoporosis-related vertebral fracture in women with established osteoporosis.

Parathyroid hormone peptides reduce the risk of vertebral but not hip fractures. Expensive, they are reserved for severe osteoporosis in those unable to tolerate or unresponsive to other treatments. Use is limited to 2 years as there is an increased risk of osteosarcoma in rats.

Denosumab is a fully human monoclonal antibody to RANKL and reduces osteoclast activity. Given by subcutaneous injection every 6 months, it reduces the risk of fractures in postmenopausal women with osteoporosis. It is most useful where oral bisphosphonates are contraindicated or with malabsorption.

Calcium and vitamin D supplements are useful if insufficiency exists, especially in the elderly. However, the effects on fractures are contradictory and controversial, and in women whose diet is replete there may be an increased risk of renal stones and coronary heart disease.

Alternative and complementary therapies

There is little evidence that these improve menopausal symptoms or have the same benefits as HRT or non-oestrogen-based treatments, but they are nevertheless widely used. Concerns include production quality, drug interactions and the presence, in some, of oestrogenic compounds.

Phyto-oestrogens are plant substances with effects similar to oestrogens. The most important groups are called isoflavones and lignans. Isoflavones are found in soya beans and chickpeas, lignans particularly in oilseeds.

Herbal remedies include black cohosh, kava kava, evening primrose, dong quai, gingko, ginseng and wild yam cream.

Progesterone transdermal creams have not been proven to be effective for menopausal symptoms or skeletal protection, and are not protective of the endometrium.

Further reading

British Menopause Society: information and education for healthcare professionals: www.thebms.org.uk

Compston J, Bowring C, Cooper A, *et al.* Diagnosis and management of osteoporosis in postmenopausal women and older men in the UK: National Osteoporosis Guideline Group (NOGG) update 2013. *Maturitas* 2013; **75**: 392–396.

Dreisler E, Poulsen L, Antonsen S, *et al.* EMAS clinical guide: assessment of the endometrium in peri and postmenopausal women. *Maturitas* 2013; **75**: 181–190.

National Institute for Health and Care Excellence. *Menopause: Diagnosis and Management.* Clinical Guideline No. 23. Available at: https://www.nice.org.uk/guidance/ng23?unlid=42553257020164112121 (accessed 12 July 2016).

Neves-e-Castro M, Birkhauser M, Samsioe G, *et al.* EMAS position statement: the ten point guide to the integral management of menopausal health. *Maturitas* 2015; **81**: 88–92.

The menopause at a glance

Definition	The last menstrual period
Median age	51 years. Premature if <40 years
Perimenopause	Time preceding menopause, menstruation often erratic
Features	Early changes: hot flushes, insomnia, psychological Later changes: skin and breast atrophy, hair loss, atrophic vaginitis, prolapse, urinary symptoms, osteoporosis, cardiovascular disease
Investigations	Usually none as diagnosis based on clinical grounds. Low anti-mullerian hormone (AMH). Follicle-stimulating hormone (FSH) raised, but may be normal initially
Treatment	Not mandatory or universal. Consider menopausal hormone therapy (MHT) to alleviate symptoms and prevent osteoporosis (or bisphosphonates), but beware of risks

Hormone replacement therapy (HRT) at a glance

Definition	Use of exogenous oestrogens when endogenous secretion is absent
Preparations	Oestrogen alone for hysterectomized women, combined with a progestogen in women whose uterus is intact Oral, patch, gel, implant, topical (vaginal cream, tablet or ring) depending on availability
Advantages	Relief from menopausal symptoms Protects against osteoporosis Reduces urinary symptoms Treatment of choice in women with a premature menopause
Disadvantages	Menstruation unless 'period-free' preparation Oestrogenic and progestogenic side effects Increased risk of breast cancer (with progestogen MHT) and venous thromboembolism (oral)

CHAPTER 14

Disorders of early pregnancy

Physiology of early pregnancy

The oocyte is fertilized in the ampulla of the fallopian tube to form a zygote. Mitotic division occurs as the zygote is swept toward the uterus by ciliary action and peristalsis (Fig. 14.1a). Tubal damage will impair movement and render tubal implantation and ectopic pregnancy more likely. The zygote normally enters the uterus on day 4, at the multicellular morula stage. The morula becomes a blastocyst by developing a fluid-filled cavity within. Its outer layer becomes the trophoblast, which will form the placenta, and from the sixth to 12th days, this invades the endometrium to achieve implantation (Fig. 14.1b). Fifteen per cent of embryos are lost at this stage though this is too early to be considered a miscarriage.

The trophoblast produces hormones almost immediately, notably human chorionic gonadotrophin (hCG) (detected in pregnancy tests), which will peak at 12 weeks. This ability to invade and produce hCG is reflected in gestational trophoblastic disease. Nutrients are gained from the secretory endometrium, which turns deciduous (rich in glycogen and lipids) under the influence of oestrogen and progesterone from the corpus luteum which is maintained by hCG from the trophoblast. Trophoblastic proliferation leads to formation of chorionic villi. On the endometrial surface of the embryo, this villous system proliferates (chorion frondosum) and will ultimately form the surface area for nutrient transfer, in the cotyledons of the placenta. Placental morphology is complete at 12 weeks. A heartbeat is established at 4–5 weeks and is visible on transvaginal ultrasound a week later.

Spontaneous miscarriage

Definition and epidemiology

The fetus dies or delivers dead before 24 completed weeks of pregnancy. The majority occur before 12 weeks. Fifteen per cent of clinically recognized pregnancies spontaneously miscarry; more will be so early as to go unrecognized. The rate of miscarriage increases with maternal age (Fig. 14.2).

Types of miscarriage

Threatened miscarriage: There is bleeding but the fetus is still alive, the uterus is the size expected from the dates and the cervical os is closed (Fig. 14.3a). Only 25% will go on to miscarry.

Inevitable miscarriage: Bleeding is usually heavier. Although the fetus may still be alive, the cervical os is open. Miscarriage is about to occur.

Incomplete miscarriage: Some fetal parts have been passed, but the os is usually open (Fig. 14.3b).

Complete miscarriage: All fetal tissue has been passed. Bleeding has diminished, the uterus is no longer enlarged and the cervical os is closed.

Septic miscarriage: The contents of the uterus are infected, causing endometritis. Vaginal loss is usually offensive, the uterus is tender, but a fever can be absent. If pelvic infection occurs there is abdominal pain and peritonism.

Missed miscarriage: The fetus has not developed or died *in utero*, but this is not recognized until bleeding occurs

Obstetrics & Gynaecology, Fifth Edition. Lawrence Impey, Tim Child.
© 2017 John Wiley & Sons, Ltd. Published 2017 by John Wiley & Sons, Ltd.

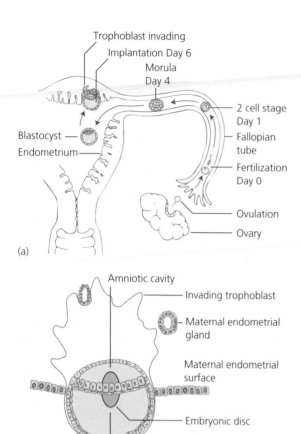

Fig. 14.1 (a) Fertilization and development of the blastocyst. (b) Implantation: day 6.

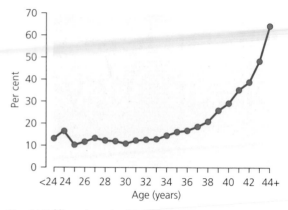

Fig. 14.2 Miscarriage rates by maternal age.

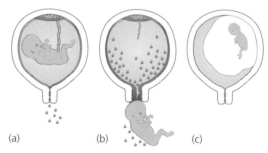

Fig. 14.3 (a) Threatened miscarriage. (b) Incomplete miscarriage. (c) Missed miscarriage.

or ultrasound is performed. The uterus is smaller than expected from the dates and the os is closed (Fig. 14.3c).

Aetiology of sporadic miscarriage

Isolated non-recurring chromosomal abnormalities account for >60% of 'one-off' or sporadic miscarriages. However, if three or more miscarriages occur, then the rarer recurrent causes are more likely. Exercise, intercourse, 'stress' and emotional trauma do not cause miscarriage.

Clinical features

History: Bleeding is usual unless a missed miscarriage is found incidentally at ultrasound examination.

Pain from uterine contractions can cause confusion with an ectopic pregnancy.

Examination: Uterine size and the state of the cervical os are dependent on the type of miscarriage. Severe tenderness is unusual.

Investigations

Early pregnancy assessment units (EPAU) should be available at least 5, ideally 7, days per week and easily accessible by GPs. EPAUs streamline management, and reduce costs and the number and duration of admissions.

Ultrasound will show if a fetus is in the uterus and if it is viable (Fig. 14.4), and it may detect retained fetal tissue (products). If there is doubt, the scan should be repeated a week later, as long as the woman is clinically stable, as non-viable pregnancies can be confused with a very early pregnancy, especially where the date of the last menstrual period is uncertain or periods irregular. Ultrasound does not always allow visualization of an

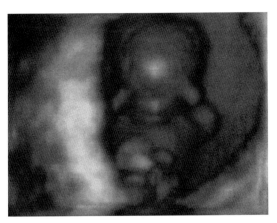

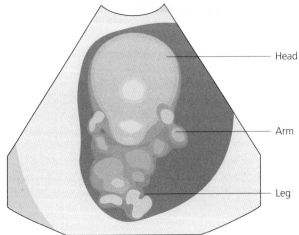

Head

Arm

Leg

Fig. 14.4 Three-dimensional image of live fetus at 11 weeks' gestation.

ectopic pregnancy, but if a fetus is seen in the uterus, coexistent ectopic pregnancy (heterotopic pregnancy) is extremely unlikely unless conception followed *in vitro* fertilization (IVF) treatment with the replacement of multiple embryos. Sometimes it is not possible to initially differentiate between an early viable or failing intrauterine pregnancy, a complete miscarriage or an ectopic pregnancy, all of which can show an empty uterine cavity and no abnormal adnexal masses or fluid (blood) – this is termed *pregnancy of unknown location (PUL)*. Women with PUL could have an ectopic pregnancy until the location is determined.

Blood tests: hCG levels in the blood normally increase by >63% in 48 hours with a viable intrauterine pregnancy. This helps differentiate between ectopic and viable pregnancies when no intrauterine gestation sac is visible on scan. A decline in hCG of greater than 50% suggests a non-viable pregnancy. A change in hCG over 48 hours between a 50% decline and a 63% rise is suggestive of ectopic pregnancy. The *full blood count* (FBC) and *Rhesus group* should also be checked.

Management

Admission is necessary if ectopic pregnancy is suspected and the woman symptomatic, if the miscarriage is septic or there is heavy bleeding.

Resuscitation is occasionally required. Products of conception in the cervical os cause pain, bleeding and vasovagal shock and are removed via a speculum using polyp forceps. Intramuscular *ergometrine* will reduce bleeding by contracting the uterus, but is only used if the fetus is non-viable. If there is a fever, swabs for bacterial culture are taken and intravenous antibiotics are given. *Anti-D* is given to women who are rhesus negative if the miscarriage is treated surgically or medically, or if there is bleeding after 12 weeks' gestation. This reduces the risk of isoimmunization and Rhesus disease in future pregnancies.

Viable intrauterine pregnancy (threatened miscarriage)

Ninety per cent of women in whom fetal heart activity is detected at 8 weeks will not miscarry. Bed rest or hormone treatment with progesterone or hCG do not prevent miscarriage.

Non-viable intrauterine pregnancy

Options include *expectant, medical* or *surgical management*.

Expectant management can be continued as long as the woman is willing and there are no signs of infection. It is successful within 2–6 weeks in >80% of women with incomplete miscarriage and in 30–70% of women with missed miscarriage. A large intact sac is associated with lower success rates.

Medical management is with vaginal, or oral, prostaglandin (misoprostol). Medical management is successful in

>80% of women with incomplete miscarriage (similar to expectant management) and 40–90% of women with missed miscarriage. A urine pregnancy test should be repeated 3 weeks after medical management to exclude an ectopic or molar pregnancy.

Surgical management: Surgical management of miscarriage (SMM) (previously known as evacuation of retained products of conception (ERPC)) is carried out under anaesthetic using vacuum aspiration. Evacuation is suitable if the woman prefers it, if there is heavy bleeding or signs of infection (performed under antibiotic cover). Success rates are >95% for both incomplete and missed miscarriage. Tissue is examined histologically to exclude molar pregnancy.

Complications

Vaginal bleeding with *expectant* or *medical* management can be heavy and painful so women must have 24-hour direct access to an emergency gynaecological service for advice/treatment. Risks of *expectant* and *medical* management include the need for surgical evacuation (10–40%). Infection rates are similar (3%) between *expectant, medical or surgical* management. If infection becomes systemic, septic shock occasionally ensues. Surgical evacuation can partially remove the endometrium, causing Asherman's syndrome, or perforate the uterus (<1%). Long-term conception rates do not differ between the management options (*BMJ* 2009; **339**: b3827), although surgical management is more expensive.

Counselling after miscarriage

Patients should be told that the miscarriage was not the result of anything they did or did not do and could not have been prevented. Reassurance as to the high chance of successful further pregnancies is important. Referral to a support group may be useful (www.miscarriageassociation.org.uk). Because miscarriage is so common, further investigation is usually reserved for women who have had three miscarriages or miscarriage after 12 weeks.

Recurrent miscarriage

Definition and epidemiology

Recurrent miscarriage is when three or more miscarriages occur in succession; 1% of couples are affected. The chance of miscarriage in a fourth pregnancy is still only 40%, but a recurring cause is more likely and investigations and support should be arranged (*NEJM* 2010; **363**: 1740–1747).

Causes and their management

Whilst investigation may reveal a possible cause, few treatments are of proven value. These patients are often extremely distressed and support is vital. This involves emotional support for both partners in the form of counselling as well as a clearly defined management plan during pregnancy in terms of ultrasound monitoring (*Hum Reprod* 2011; **26**: 873–877). In later pregnancy, 'high-risk' monitoring is important because late pregnancy complications are more common.

Antiphospholipid antibodies can cause recurrent miscarriage. Thrombosis in the uteroplacental circulation is likely to be the mechanism. Treatment is with aspirin and low-dose low molecular weight heparin (*Curr Opin Rheum* 2011; **23**: 299–304).

Parental chromosomal defects: Fetal miscarriage tissue is karyotyped and if this shows an unbalanced abnormality then parental karyotyping is performed. Referral to a clinical geneticist allows for full explanation of abnormal parental findings and a discussion regarding karyotyping of other family members who may have inherited the same rearrangement. Prenatal diagnosis using chorionic villus sampling (CVS) or amniocentesis is offered. The use of donor oocytes or sperm (all donors are routinely karyotyped) or preimplantation genetic diagnosis (PGD) of IVF embryos are alternative options.

Anatomical factors: Uterine abnormalities are diagnosed with ultrasound (and subsequent magnetic resonance imaging (MRI) or hysterosalpingogram if abnormal). They are more common with late miscarriage. Many, however, are incidental findings and surgical treatment could lead to uterine weakness or adhesion formation. Cervical problems contribute to late (>16 weeks) miscarriage as well as preterm labour.

Infection: This is not a cause of recurrent early miscarriage but is implicated in preterm labour and late (>16 weeks) miscarriage, where early treatment of bacterial vaginosis reduces the incidence of fetal loss.

Hormonal factors: Thyroid dysfunction, particularly in the presence of thyroid autoantibodies, is associated with recurrent miscarriage and so should be tested and treated. Polycystic ovary syndrome (PCOS) may be associated with an increased rate of pregnancy loss though this is probably through raised body mass index (BMI).

Others: Obesity, smoking and excess caffeine intake have been implicated and should all be addressed. Older maternal age is one of the main factors affecting the chance of a single pregnancy miscarrying and therefore the chance of having consecutive losses.

A recent large randomized controlled trial (RCT) has demonstrated that, for women with a history of unexplained recurrent miscarriage, vaginal progesterone from pregnancy test until 12 weeks' gestation does not increase the live birth rate compared to placebo (*NEJM* 2015; **373**: 2141–2148).

Investigation of recurrent miscarriage

Antiphospholipid antibody screen (repeat at 6 weeks if positive)
Karyotyping of fetal miscarriage tissue
Thyroid function
Pelvic ultrasound (and MRI or hysterosalpingogram (HSG) if abnormal)

Unwanted pregnancy and therapeutic abortion

Definition

Induced abortion or termination of pregnancy (TOP) is a very common gynaecological procedure. The World Health Organization (WHO) estimates that about 30% of all pregnancies end in an induced abortion: approximately 50 million world-wide. Legislation about abortion varies throughout the world, can vary within different states of an individual country and is illegal in some countries. The upper time limit for legal induced abortion also varies. In countries where abortion is legal, the large majority of abortions (typically >90%) occur before the end of 12 weeks' gestation. Over 200 000 procedures are performed each year in Britain and at least one-third of British women will have had a termination by the age of 45 years. The statutory grounds for termination of pregnancy in England, Scotland and Wales are detailed in the box below. The legal time limit for abortion is 24 weeks for clauses C and D. However, abortions after 24 weeks are allowed if there is grave risk to the life of the woman, evidence of severe fetal abnormality or risk of grave physical and mental injury to the woman.

Statutory grounds for termination of pregnancy in England, Scotland and Wales

A	The continuance of the pregnancy would involve risk to the life of the pregnant woman greater than if the pregnancy were terminated
B	The termination is necessary to prevent grave permanent injury to the physical or mental health of the pregnant woman
C	The pregnancy has *not* exceeded its 24th week and continuance of the pregnancy would involve risk, greater than if the pregnancy were terminated, of injury to the physical or mental health of the pregnant woman
D	The pregnancy has *not* exceeded its 24th week and continuance of the pregnancy would involve risk, greater than if the pregnancy were terminated, of injury to the physical or mental health of any existing child(ren) of the family of the pregnant woman
E	There is a substantial risk that if the child were born it would suffer from such physical or mental abnormalities as to be seriously handicapped

---

Methods of abortion

The method of TOP available depends on the gestation of the pregnancy and the woman's choice. The procedures offered also vary from one centre to another. Blood tests should be taken for haemoglobin, blood group and Rhesus status and testing for haemoglobinopathies as indicated. Rhesus-negative women should receive anti-D within 72 hours of TOP. Women are screened for chlamydia and undergo a risk assessment for other sexually transmitted infections (STIs) and are screened for them if appropriate. Contraception should be discussed at the initial consultation. It can be administered at the time of surgical TOP and most methods can be safely used following medical TOP, either initiated on the day of misoprostol administration (oral pills, condoms, injectables, implants) or following the next menstrual cycle (intrauterine device or sterilization).

Surgical methods

Suction curettage is generally used between 7 and 12–14 weeks. Before 7 weeks, failure rates are higher than with medical abortion. Above 14 weeks, medical methods are usually employed, although surgical abortion by *dilatation and evacuation* (D&E) is safe and effective when undertaken by appropriately skilled, experienced practitioners. The cervix is 'prepared' with preoperative vaginal misoprostol and antibiotic prophylaxis given.

Medical methods

The antiprogesterone *mifepristone*, plus *prostaglandin* (misoprostol or gemeprost, prostaglandin E1 analogues) 36–48 hours later, is the most effective method of abortion at gestations of less than 7 weeks and can also be used at any gestation as an alternative to surgical termination. It is also the usual and most effective method for mid-trimester abortion (13–24 weeks' gestation). From 22 weeks, feticide is performed first to prevent live birth, using KCl into the umbilical vein or fetal heart. Such later terminations are usually only performed where a fetal abnormality is present.

Selective abortion

This is occasionally performed with high-order multiple pregnancies to reduce the risk, particularly, of preterm birth, or where a fetus of a multiple pregnancy is abnormal.

Complications of therapeutic abortion

Complications of TOP include *haemorrhage* (1 in 1000 overall, greater risk with later gestations), *infection* (up to 10% of cases and reduced by screening and prophylactic antibiotics), *uterine perforation* (1–4 in 1000 surgical abortions), *cervical trauma* at the time of surgical abortion, and failure (<5% of surgical and medical abortions require a further intervention, for example to remove retained tissue, and <1% of abortions fail to end the pregnancy). Multiple surgical abortions are associated with an increased risk of subsequent preterm delivery. Psychological sequelae are common but may also reflect underlying problems before the termination.

'Unsafe abortion' is defined as a procedure for terminating an unwanted pregnancy performed either by persons lacking the necessary skills or in an environment lacking the minimal medical standards, or both. Worldwide, nearly 50% of all abortions are considered unsafe and 98% of these occur in developing countries. Unsafe abortion causes approximately 35 000 deaths worldwide each year (www.who.int/reproductivehealth/ topics/unsafe_abortion/magnitude/en/). Promoting the knowledge of, and access to, effective contraception reduces the need for pregnancy termination.

Ectopic pregnancy

Definition and epidemiology

An ectopic pregnancy is when the embryo implants outside the uterine cavity and occurs in 1 in 60–100 pregnancies. The mortality rate for ectopic pregnancy in the UK is reducing and is currently 16.9/100 000 estimated ectopic pregnancies. It is more common with advanced maternal age and lower socioeconomic class.

Pathology and sites of ectopic pregnancy

The most common site is in the fallopian tube (95%), although implantation can occur in the cornu, the cervix, the ovary and the abdominal cavity (Fig. 14.5). The thin-walled tube is unable to sustain trophoblastic invasion: it bleeds into its lumen or may rupture, when intraperitoneal blood loss can be catastrophic. The ectopic can also be naturally aborted either within the tube or extruded through the fimbrial end.

Aetiology

Often no cause is evident, but any factor which damages the tube can cause the fertilized oocyte to be caught. Commonly, this is pelvic inflammatory disease, usually from sexually transmitted infection. Assisted conception and pelvic, particularly tubal, surgery are

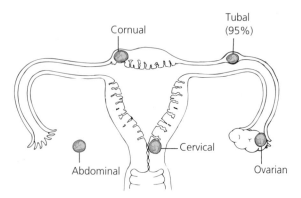

Fig. 14.5 Sites of ectopic pregnancy.

additional risks, as is having had a previous ectopic and being a smoker. An ectopic pregnancy must be urgently excluded in a woman who conceives despite having a copper intrauterine device (IUD) in place; this prevents most intrauterine pregnancies but not those destined to implant in the tube.

Clinical features

The diagnosis is easily missed. Abnormal vaginal bleeding, abdominal pain or collapse in any woman of reproductive age should all arouse suspicion and a urine pregnancy test should be performed. Increasing numbers of women are now diagnosed early and when asymptomatic, because of routine ultrasound.

History: Usually, lower abdominal pain is followed by scanty, dark vaginal bleeding. One may, however, be present without the other. The pain is variable in quality, often initially colicky as the tube tries to extrude the sac, and then constant. Syncopal episodes and shoulder tip pain suggest intraperitoneal blood loss. The 'classic' presentation of collapse with abdominal pain accounts for <25%. Amenorrhoea of 4–10 weeks is usual, but the patient may be unaware that she is pregnant and may interpret a vaginal bleed as a period.

Examination: Tachycardia suggests blood loss, and hypotension and collapse occur only *in extremis*. There is usually abdominal and often rebound tenderness. On pelvic examination, movement of the uterus may cause pain (cervical excitation) and either adnexum may be tender. The uterus is smaller than expected from the gestation and the cervical os is closed.

Investigations

A pregnancy test (urine hCG) *must* be performed on *all* women of reproductive age who present with pain, bleeding or collapse, whatever the medical specialty to which the woman presents. It is almost invariably positive with an ectopic pregnancy. Modern urine pregnancy tests are very sensitive and are positive even before the day of the missed period.

Ultrasound (preferably transvaginal) does not always visualize an ectopic pregnancy (Fig. 14.6), but it should detect an intrauterine pregnancy. If the latter is not present, the gestation is either too early (<5 weeks) or there has been a complete miscarriage, or the pregnancy is elsewhere, i.e. ectopic. In the adnexae a blood clot may be seen, 'free fluid' (i.e. blood), or a gestation sac with or without a fetus within. The probe may elicit tenderness.

Quantitative serum hCG is useful if the uterus is empty. If the maternal level is >1000 IU/mL then, if an intrauterine pregnancy is present, it will normally be visible on transvaginal ultrasound. If the level is lower than this, but rises by more than 63% in 48 hours, an earlier but intrauterine pregnancy is likely. Declining or slower

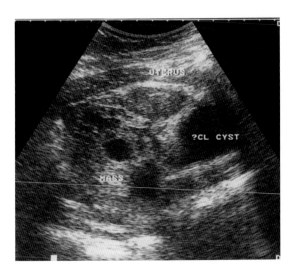

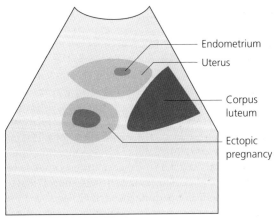

Fig. 14.6 Ultrasound of ectopic pregnancy. It is unusual to visualize the ectopic pregnancy with ultrasound.

rising levels ('plateauing') suggest an ectopic or non-viable intrauterine pregnancy. Caution is still required as, particularly with assisted conception, an intrauterine and an ectopic pregnancy can occasionally coexist (heterotopic pregnancy).

Laparoscopy is the most sensitive investigation, but it is invasive. The combination of hCG and ultrasound allows for fewer 'negative' laparoscopies.

Management of the symptomatic suspected ectopic pregnancy
Nil by mouth Full blood count (FBC) and cross-match blood Pregnancy test Ultrasound Laparoscopy or consider medical management if criteria met Intravenous access

Management

Where symptoms are present, the patient should be admitted. Intravenous access is inserted and blood is cross-matched. Anti-D is given if the patient is Rhesus negative.

Acute presentations

If the patient is haemodynamically unstable, expedient resuscitation and surgery are required. Laparoscopy may be suitable for experienced operators but laparotomy is often performed. The affected tube is removed (salpingectomy) (Fig. 14.7).

Subacute presentations

Surgical management: This is appropriate if a woman is unable to return for follow-up or has an ectopic pregnancy plus any of the following: significant pain, adnexal mass >35 mm, visible fetal heart activity or a serum hCG level >5000 IU/mL. Laparoscopy is standard and is preferable to laparotomy because recovery is faster and subsequent fertility rates are equivalent or better (Fig. 14.8). At laparoscopy, the ectopic is either removed from the tube (salpingostomy) or the whole tube including the ectopic is removed (salpingectomy). If salpingostomy is performed, there is both a 10% chance that repeat surgery for persisting ectopic will be required (detected by failure of serum hCG to fall on

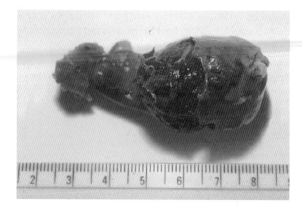

Fig. 14.7 The ectopic pregnancy (in Fig. 14.6) removed by salpingectomy.

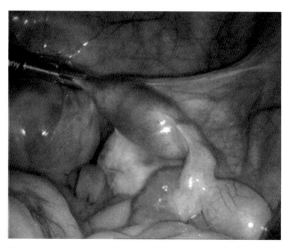

Fig. 14.8 Laparoscopic photograph of an unruptured tubal ectopic pregnancy.

follow-up) and an increased risk of repeat ectopic since the damaged tube remains. If the contralateral tube is damaged then salpingostomy may allow for future spontaneous conception (and possibly ectopic) whereas salpingectomy will require IVF. If the contralateral tube appears normal then the subsequent intrauterine pregnancy rates are similar between salpingostomy or salpingectomy. It is important to discuss these two surgical approaches with the patient preoperatively.

Medical management: This is appropriate if the patient is able to return for follow-up, has no significant pain with an unruptured ectopic pregnancy, has an adnexal mass <35 mm with no fetal heart activity seen, plus no coexisting intrauterine pregnancy. The lower the hCG (must be <5000 IU/mL but ideally <1500 IU/mL) then the higher the success rate. Systemic single-dose methotrexate can be used without recourse to laparoscopy. Serial hCG levels are subsequently monitored to confirm that all trophoblastic tissue has gone; a second dose (15% of women) or surgery (10%) may be required. Outcomes with systemic methotrexate are equivalent to laparoscopic salpingostomy.

Complications

Women treated with salpingostomy or medical management must have serial hCG measurements until <20 IU/mL to confirm ectopic resolution. They must have clear information on warning signs and be within easy reach of the hospital treating them. Particular support must be given to women with ectopic pregnancy, who have not only 'lost their baby' through a life-threatening condition but have also undergone surgery and had their fertility reduced. Seventy per cent will subsequently have a successful pregnancy and up to 10% will have another ectopic pregnancy. Patient support groups are useful (www.ectopic.org.uk).

Hyperemesis gravidarum

Definition and epidemiology

Hyperemesis gravidarum is when nausea and vomiting in early pregnancy are so severe as to cause severe dehydration, weight loss or electrolyte disturbance. This occurs in only 1 in 750 women. However, vomiting in pregnancy is a common cause of hospital admission, but most patients are only mildly dehydrated and therefore have 'moderate' nausea and vomiting of pregnancy (NVP). It seldom persists beyond 14 weeks and is more common in multiparous women.

Nausea and vomiting of pregnancy (NVP)	
Mild NVP	Nausea and occasional morning vomiting 50% of pregnant women No treatment required
Moderate NVP	More persistent vomiting 5% of pregnant women Often admitted to hospital
Severe NVP	Hyperemesis gravidarum

Management

Predisposing conditions, particularly urinary infection and multiple or molar pregnancy, are excluded. Intravenous rehydration is given, with antiemetics such as metoclopramide, cyclizine and even ondansetron, and thiamine (to prevent neurological complications of vitamin depletion such as Wernicke's encephalopathy). There is little evidence for acupuncture, ginger or vitamin B6 (*Cochrane* 2015; CD007575). Steroids have been used in severe cases. Psychological support is essential, particularly as many of these women have social or emotional problems.

Gestational trophoblastic disease

Definitions, pathology and epidemiology

In this condition, trophoblastic tissue, which is the part of the blastocyst that normally invades the endometrium, proliferates in a more aggressive way than is normal. hCG is usually secreted in excess. Proliferation can be localized and non-invasive: this is called a *hydatidiform mole* and is considered a premalignant condition. Hydatidiform mole can be subdivided into *complete* and *partial* mole based on genetic and histopathological features. *A complete mole* is entirely paternal in origin, usually when one sperm fertilizes an empty oocyte and undergoes mitosis. The result is diploid tissue, usually 46 XX. There is no fetal tissue, merely a proliferation of swollen chorionic villi. A *partial mole* is usually triploid, derived from two sperms entering one oocyte. There is variable evidence of a fetus.

Alternatively, the proliferation may have characteristics of malignant tissue. If invasion is only present locally within the uterus, this is an *invasive mole*; if metastasis occurs, it is a *choriocarcinoma*. The least common form of gestational trophoblastic disease (GTD) is *placental site trophoblastic tumour* (PSTT) which, in contrast to other types of trophoblastic disease (which normally present soon after the index pregnancy), presents an average of 3.4 years later.

Gestational trophoblastic disease (which includes premalignant hydatidiform mole (complete and partial), and the malignant invasive mole, choriocarcinoma, and PSTT) occurs in 1 in 500–1000 pregnancies, is more common at the extremes of reproductive age and is twice as common in Asian women.

Clinical features

Examination: The uterus is often large. Early pre-eclampsia and hyperthyroidism may occur.
History: Vaginal bleeding is usual and may be heavy. Severe vomiting (hyperemesis) may occur. The condition may be detected on routine ultrasound.

Investigations

Ultrasound characteristically shows a 'snowstorm' appearance of the swollen villi with *complete moles* (Fig. 14.9), but the diagnosis can only be confirmed histologically. Serum hCG levels may be very high.

Management and follow-up

The trophoblastic tissue is removed by suction curettage (ERPC) and the diagnosis confirmed histologically. Bleeding is often heavy. Thereafter, serial blood or urine hCG levels are taken; persistent or rising levels are suggestive of malignancy. In the UK, women with a molar pregnancy should be registered with a supraregional centre (London, Sheffield and Dundee: www.hmole-chorio.org.uk/) who will guide management and follow-up. Oral contraception can be used after ERPC for a molar pregnancy whilst hCG levels are being monitored. Pregnancy is avoided until after completion of the surveillance period.

Complications

Recurrence of molar pregnancy occurs in about 1 in 60 subsequent pregnancies. After every future pregnancy, further hCG samples are required to exclude disease recurrence.

Gestational trophoblastic neoplasia, as an *invasive mole* or *choriocarcinoma*, follows 15% of complete moles and 0.5% of partial moles. However, molar pregnancy precedes only 50% of malignancies, because malignancy can also follow miscarriages and normal pregnancies, usually presenting as persistent vaginal bleeding. The diagnosis of malignancy is made from persistently elevated or rising hCG levels, persistent vaginal bleeding or evidence of blood-borne metastasis, commonly to the lungs. The tumour is highly malignant, but is normally very sensitive to chemotherapy. Patients are scored into 'low-risk' and 'high-risk' categories according to prognostic variables. Low-risk patients receive methotrexate with folic acid, whereas higher risk patients receive combination chemotherapy. Five-year survival rates approach 100%.

Further reading

National Institute for Health and Care Excellence. *Ectopic Pregnancy and Miscarriage: Diagnosis and Initial Management in Early Pregnancy of Ectopic Pregnancy and Miscarriage*. Clinical Guideline No. 154. Available at: www.nice.org.uk/guidance/cg154 (accessed 12 July 2016).

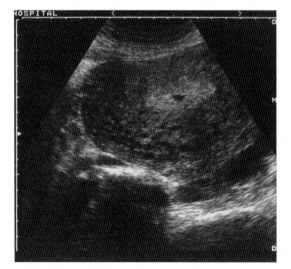

Fig. 14.9 Ultrasound of a molar pregnancy.

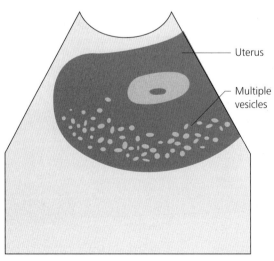

Uterus

Multiple vesicles

National Institute for Health and Care Excellence. Clinical Knowledge Summaries. *Nausea/Vomiting in Pregnancy*. Available at: http://cks.nice.org.uk/nauseavomiting-in-pregnancy (accessed 12 July 2016).

Royal College of Obstetricians and Gynaecologists. *The Management of Gestational Trophoblastic Disease*. Green-top Guideline No. 38. Available at: www.rcog.org.uk/globalassets/documents/guidelines/gtg_38.pdf (accessed 12 July 2016).

Royal College of Obstetricians and Gynaecologists. *The Care of Women Requesting Induced Abortion*. Evidence-Based Clinical Guideline No. 7. Available at: www.rcog.org.uk/globalassets/documents/ guidelines/abortion-guideline_web_1.pdf (accessed 12 July 2016).

Royal College of Obstetricians and Gynaecologists. *The Investigation and Treatment of Couples with Recurrent First-Trimester and Second-Trimester Miscarriage*. Green-top Guideline No. 17. Available at: www.rcog.org.uk/globalassets/documents/guidelines/gtg_17.pdf (accessed 12 July 2016).

Royal College of Obstetricians and Gynaecologists. *The Investigation and Management of the Small-for-Gestational-Age Fetus*. Green-top Guideline No. 31. Available at: www.rcog.org.uk/globalassets/documents/guidelines/gtg_31.pdf (accessed 12 July 2016).

Spontaneous miscarriage at a glance

Definition	Expulsion or death of the fetus before 24 weeks
Epidemiology	15% of recognized pregnancies
Aetiology	Increasing maternal age; >50% chromosomal abnormalities, usually sporadic. Recurrent miscarriage also associated with antiphospholipid antibodies, uterine abnormalities and parental chromosome abnormalities
Pathology	Products can be retained and cause haemorrhage and/or infection
Features	Heavy vaginal bleeding, often with pain. Cervix may be open. Little tenderness
Investigations	Ultrasound to confirm intrauterine site and fetal viability
Management	Anti-D if Rhesus negative and spontaneous miscarriage from 12 weeks' gestation or if treated medically or surgically at any gestation Surgical management of miscarriage (SMM) (formerly evacuation of retained products of conception (ERPC)) if heavy bleeding or infection Expectant or medical management an alternative for incomplete or missed miscarriage
Complications	Haemorrhage and infection, and of surgery

Ectopic pregnancy at a glance

Definition	Embryo implants outside the uterus
Epidemiology	1%+ of pregnancies in UK
Aetiology	Idiopathic, tubal damage from pelvic inflammatory disease or surgery
Pathology	95% in fallopian tube. Occasionally cornu, cervix, ovary, abdomen Tubal implantation can lead to tubal rupture and intraperitoneal bleeding

(Continued)

Ectopic pregnancy at a glance (Continued)

Features	At 4–10 weeks of amenorrhoea Acute: collapse with abdominal pain and bleeding, patient shocked Subacute: abdominal pain, scanty dark per vaginam (PV) loss. Lower abdominal tenderness, cervical excitation, adnexal tenderness usual Incidental: detected at ultrasound
Investigations	Pregnancy test and transvaginal ultrasound, human chorionic gonadotrophin (hCG) Laparoscopy to confirm and treat unless diagnosis certain and medical management proposed
Management	Surgical: to stop/prevent bleeding: salpingectomy/salpingostomy Medical: methotrexate if criteria met Anti-D if Rhesus negative
Complications	Haemorrhage can be fatal; repeat ectopic, subfertility

CHAPTER 15
Gynaecological operations

There are three main routes to gain access to the pelvic organs, which can be combined.

1 The abdominal route involves opening the abdominal wall through a lower transverse (Pfannenstiel) or, occasionally, a vertical mid-line incision.

2 The vaginal route is used both to inspect and operate on the inside of the uterus and for vaginal and pelvic surgery.

3 Laparoscopic surgery, using a video-monitor via a laparoscope with a camera attached; this and the instruments are inserted through small incisions (ports) in the abdominal wall.

Endoscopy and endoscopic surgery

Diagnostic hysteroscopy

The uterine cavity is inspected with a rigid or flexible hysteroscope passed through the cervical canal. The cavity is distended using carbon dioxide or saline (Fig. 15.1). This can be performed without anaesthetic, or with a cervical local anaesthetic block or under general anaesthetic. It is used as an adjunct to endometrial biopsy or if menstrual problems do not respond to medical treatment.

Hysteroscopic surgery

An operating hysteroscope is used in which small instruments are passed down a parallel channel. Using cutting diathermy and glycine irrigation fluid, the endometrium (transcervical resection of endometrium (TCRE) (Fig. 15.2) or intracavity fibroids (transcervical resection of fibroid (TCRF)) and polyps are removed. If a uterine septum is present, this can be resected up to the fundus of the cavity. The complications of uterine perforation and fluid overload are unusual with experienced surgeons. With TCRE and/or TCRF, most patients have a significant reduction in blood loss. TCRE is best used with bleeding that is heavy but regular and not painful, in women approaching the menopause. Sterility is not ensured so sometimes a laparoscopic tubal sterilization is performed at the same time. Endometrial roller-ball diathermy, laser ablation or heating with an intrauterine hot balloon or microwave probe produce similar effects and may be safer but, because no specimen is produced, prior biopsies are essential.

Diagnostic laparoscopy

The peritoneal cavity is insufflated with carbon dioxide after carefully passing a small hollow Veress needle through the abdominal wall. This enables a sharp trocar to be inserted through the umbilicus with less risk of damaging organs or major blood vessels. A laparoscope is then passed down the trocar to enable visualization of the pelvis (Figs 15.1, 15.3). Laparoscopy is used to assess macroscopic pelvic disease in the management of pelvic pain and dysmenorrhoea, infertility (when dye is passed through the cervix to assess tubal patency: 'lap and dye'), suspected ectopic pregnancy and pelvic masses.

Laparoscopic surgery

Instruments to grasp or cut tissue are inserted through separate ports in the abdominal wall. Laparoscopic surgery is commonly performed to sterilize, to remove adhesions or areas of endometriosis, or remove an ectopic pregnancy, but virtually every gynaecological operation has now been performed laparoscopically. The advantages are better visualization of tissues, less tissue handling, less infection, reduced hospital stay

Obstetrics & Gynaecology, Fifth Edition. Lawrence Impey, Tim Child.
© 2017 John Wiley & Sons, Ltd. Published 2017 by John Wiley & Sons, Ltd.

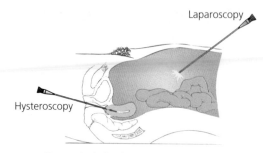

Fig. 15.1 Gynaecological endoscopy.

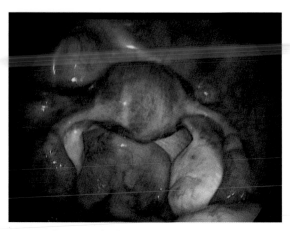

Fig. 15.3 Laparoscopic photograph of a normal pelvis. The right ovary contains a 2 cm preovulatory follicle.

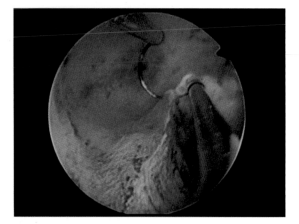

Fig. 15.2 Transcervical resection of endometrium (TCRE). The monopolar cutting loop creates 'trenches' within the endometrium until it is completely removed.

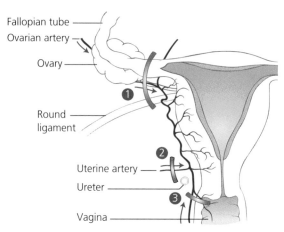

Fig. 15.4 Hysterectomy. (1) Blood: the anastomosis between uterine and ovarian arteries. If the ovaries are removed, the ovarian artery and vein are ligated instead. Ligament: the round ligament. (2) Blood: the main uterine artery. Ligament: the cardinal ligament. The bladder is first dissected off the cervix and upper vagina, to prevent injury to it or to the ureters, which are close. (3) Blood: the cervicovaginal branches of the uterine artery supplying the cervix and upper vagina. Ligament: the uterosacral ligament.

and faster postoperative recovery with less pain. However, serious visceral damage can occur, particularly in less experienced hands and/or with more complicated and extensive surgery. Three-dimensional 'robotic' surgery can be undertaken in which the surgeon sits at a console (potentially some distance from the patient), wears 3D glasses whilst looking at a special monitor, and controls the intra-abdominal instruments, which are able to rotate through greater degrees of freedom, potentially giving greater precision than standard laparoscopic instruments, by moving joysticks with each hand. Whilst many hospitals have a 'robot', the benefits of their use in gynaecological surgery over the standard laparoscopic approach have yet to be demonstrated.

Hysterectomy

This is the most common major gynaecological operation (Fig. 15.4). The fallopian tubes are usually also removed (bilateral salpingectomy) to reduce the risk of

ovarian cancer (see Chapter 5) and the ovaries also, in older women or those with a history of cysts (bilateral oophorectomy). Hysterectomy is most commonly performed for menstrual disorders, fibroids, endometriosis, chronic pelvic inflammatory disease and prolapse; the treatment of pelvic malignancies also includes hysterectomy. Advances in medical management, for example of abnormal uterine bleeding (such as the intrauterine system (IUS)) should make the operation rarer and should be tried before this last resort.

Types of hysterectomy

Total abdominal hysterectomy (TAH) is removal of the uterus and cervix through an abdominal incision. The steps are performed from above, and therefore in the order 1, 2, 3 shown in Fig. 15.4. Specific indications include malignancy (ovarian and endometrial, in conjunction with a full laparotomy), a very large or immobile uterus and when abdominal inspection is required. In a subtotal hysterectomy, the cervix is retained and step 3 (see Fig. 15.4) is omitted. This reduces the risk of damaging the ureters or bladder since less extensive dissection is required. However, the patient will need to continue with regular cervical smears, so the procedure is inappropriate if there is a history of abnormal smears. Some will continue to have menstrual spotting from small amounts of endometrium remaining in the cervical canal.

Vaginal hysterectomy (VH) is removal of the cervix and uterus after incising the vagina from below, and therefore in the order 3, 2, 1 (see Fig. 15.4). The vaginal vault is closed after hysterectomy is complete. The specific indication is uterine prolapse, but absence of prolapse and moderate enlargement are not contraindications in experienced hands. VH has a lower morbidity and quicker recovery than abdominal hysterectomy.

Laparoscopic hysterectomy can involve steps 1 and 2 (see Fig. 15.4) from above with laparoscopic instruments, with step 3 completed vaginally (*laparoscopic-assisted vaginal hysterectomy* (LAVH)), or be performed completely from above with the vault closed with laparoscopic sutures (*total laparoscopic hysterectomy* (TLH)). This is an alternative to TAH but not VH, since if there is sufficient prolapse, the latter operation is cheaper with similar recovery times. A subtotal hysterectomy can be performed laparoscopically and the uterine body removed from the peritoneal cavity with a morcellator instrument. This should be undertaken with care in women after the age of 40 with abnormal bleeding since an underlying unsuspected endometrial malignancy could be present and potentially spread through morcellation. It is good practice to confirm normal endometrial pathology preoperatively in such women by performing a Pipelle endometrial biopsy.

Wertheim's (radical) hysterectomy involves removal of the parametrium, the upper third of the vagina and the pelvic lymph nodes. The usual indication is stage 1a(ii)–2a *cervical carcinoma*. Occasionally, radical hysterectomy is performed vaginally (Schauta's radical hysterectomy).

Complications of hysterectomy	
Mortality	1 in 10 000
Immediate	Haemorrhage, bladder or ureteric injury
Postoperative	Venous thromboembolism (use prophylactic low molecularweight heparin), pain, retention and infection of urine, wound and chest infection (use prophylactic antibiotics), pelvic haematoma
Long term	Prolapse, genuine stress incontinence, premature menopause, pain and psychosexual problems

Other common gynaecological problems

Dilatation and curettage (D&C)

The cervix is dilated with steel rods (Hegar dilators) of increasing size; the endometrium is then curetted to biopsy it (Fig. 15.5). This is a diagnostic procedure and inferior to hysteroscopy because the cavity is not inspected. It is now not commonly performed.

Evacuation of retained products of conception (ERPC)

The cervix is dilated and a retained non-viable fetus or placental tissue is removed using a suction curette. Surgical therapeutic abortion before 12 weeks' gestation uses a similar method.

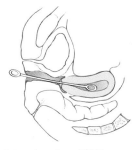

Fig. 15.5 Dilatation and curettage (D&C).

Operations for cervical intraepithelial neoplasia

Large loop excision of the transformation zone (LLETZ): This involves using cutting diathermy, under local anaesthetic, to remove the transformation zone of the cervix where cervical intraepithelial neoplasia (CIN) is present. The risk of subsequent preterm delivery is slightly increased.

Cone biopsy: This removes the transformation zone and much of the endocervix by making a circular cut with a scalpel or loop diathermy in the cervix. It is used to stage apparently early cervical carcinoma and is sufficient treatment for stage 1a(i) disease. A general or epidural/spinal anaesthetic is required. The increased cervical damage means the risk of subsequent preterm delivery is considerably increased.

Operations for prolapse

'Repair' operations: An anterior repair (cystocoele) involves excision of prolapsed vaginal wall and plication of the bladder base and fascia. The vagina is then closed. A posterior repair (rectocoele) is similar, the levator ani muscle on either side being plicated between rectum and vagina. These operations are often performed together, or with a vaginal hysterectomy for uterine prolapse. Specific complications include retention of urine and overtightening of the vagina, so it is important to ascertain if the patient is sexually active.

Hysteropexy is resuspension of the prolapsed uterus using a strip of non-absorbable bifurcated mesh to lift the uterus and hold it in place (Fig. 15.6). One end of the mesh is attached to the cervix and the other to the

anterior longitudinal ligament over the sacrum. This can be done as an open or laparoscopic procedure. The theoretical advantages of this operation over hysterectomy, as well as preservation of fertility, are a stronger repair, with less risk of recurrent prolapse. Cuts to the vagina itself are also avoided so there is probably less risk of subsequent sexual problems.

Sacrocolpopexy is used for prolapse of the vaginal vault after hysterectomy; the mesh is attached from the vaginal vault to the sacrum. This can be performed by the open or laparoscopic approach.

Sacrospinous fixation, using a blind vaginal approach, is also used for vault prolapse. It is less effective than sacrocolpopexy.

Operations for urinary stress incontinence

The principle is to elevate the bladder neck to allow it to be compressed when abdominal pressure rises.

Tension-free vaginal tape (TVT): The tape, made of polypropylene mesh, is approximately 1 cm wide and fixed to a trocar at each end. A small 2 cm vertical incision is made on the anterior vaginal wall over the mid-urethral section. After lateral dissection around the urethra, the tape is introduced vaginally with the trocars entering the retropubic space. The trocars are brought out through small transverse suprapubic incisions with the tape in position without tension and the vaginal skin is closed over (Fig. 15.7a). A cystoscopy is performed to ensure that the bladder has not been perforated. If the tape has been overtightened, postoperative urinary retention can occur. The tension on the tape can be adjusted within the first 2 weeks after insertion.

Transobturator tape (TOT): This is a variation of the TVT, in which the tape is passed through the obturator canal (Fig. 15.7b).

Burch colposuspension involves dissection through an abdominal incision in the extraperitoneal space over the bladder and anterior vaginal wall. The vaginal wall on either side of the bladder neck is hitched up to the iliopectineal ligament on either side of the symphysis pubis with non-absorbable sutures. The operation is usually performed now for failed tape procedures.

Operations for fibroids (see Chapter 3)

Myomectomy can be performed through the cervix (TCRF) or abdominally (laparoscopic or open approach).

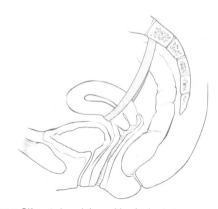

Fig. 15.6 Bifurcated mesh in position for hysteropexy.

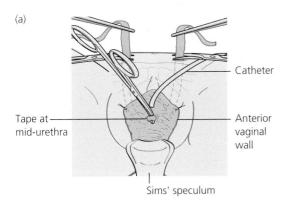

(a)

Catheter

Tape at mid-urethra

Anterior vaginal wall

Sims' speculum

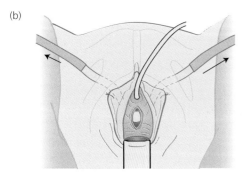

(b)

Fig. 15.7 (a) Tension-free vaginal tape (TVT). The mid-urethra and bladder neck are supported by the tape. (b) Transobturator tape (TOT).

Risks include adhesion formation, uterine rupture during labour (greater with laparoscopc approach) and peroperative haemorrhage occasionally requiring hysterectomy. There is a remote risk of spread of an unsuspected leiomyosarcoma during laparoscopic morcellation.

Uterine artery embolization is an alternative to hysterectomy for women with fibroids. The effect on fertility is variable and pregnancy complications appear more common.

Precautions in major gynaecological surgery

Thromboembolism

The combined oral contraceptive is usually stopped 4 weeks prior to major abdominal surgery. If MHT is not stopped, low molecular weight heparin (LMWH) must be used. All women should be mobilized early, given thromboembolic disease stockings (TEDS) and kept hydrated; LMWH is given according to risk assessment (see box), which should be routine.

Thromboprophylaxis in gynaecological surgery	
Low risk	Minor surgery or major surgery <30 min, no risk factors
Moderate risk	*Consider* antiembolus stockings and/or subcutaneous heparin for: surgery >30 min, obesity, gross varicose veins, current infection, prior immobility, major current illness
High risk	*Use* LMWH prophylaxis for 5 days or until mobile for: cancer surgery, prolonged surgery, history of deep vein thrombosis/ thrombophilia, ≥3 of moderate risk factors above

Infection

Prophylactic antibiotics are used for major abdominal or vaginal surgery.

Urinary tract

Routine catheterization is performed before most operations. An indwelling transurethral catheter (e.g. Foley catheter) is left overnight after major vaginal and abdominal procedures. Following surgery for genuine stress incontinence, a suprapubic catheter is often used so that the ability to pass urine urethrally can be assessed before catheter removal.

Further reading

www.websurg.com/index.php (free online surgical site with video tutorials and demonstrations).

Baggish MS, Karam MM. *Atlas of Pelvic Anatomy and Gynecologic Surgery*, 4th edn. Philadelphia: Saunders, 2015.

Royal College of Obstetricians and Gynaecologists. *Preventing Entry-related Gynaecological Laparoscopic Injuries.* Green-top Guideline No. 49. Available at: http://bsge.org.uk/wp-content/uploads/2016/03/ GtG-no-49-Laparoscopic-Injury-2008.pdf (accessed 2 August 2016).

Obstetrics

CHAPTER 16

The history and examination in obstetrics

The obstetric 'patient' is usually a healthy woman undergoing a normal life event. The history and examination are to enable the doctor or midwife to safeguard both mother and fetus during this event, and are different from other specialities. Nevertheless, you need to develop a consistent system of history taking and examination to obtain the necessary information.

The obstetric history

Personal details

Ask the woman's name, age, occupation, gestation and parity.

Presenting complaint/present circumstances

If she is an inpatient, why is she in hospital? Common reasons for admission are hypertension, pain, antepartum haemorrhage, unstable lie and possible ruptured membranes. If the pregnancy has hitherto been uncomplicated, say so.

History of present pregnancy

Dates: Was conception spontaneous or from *in vitro* fertilization (IVF)? What was the first day of her last menstrual period (LMP)? What was the length of her menstrual cycle and was it regular? How many weeks' gestation is she? (If a woman is at 38 weeks' gestation, it is actually 36 weeks since conception.) To estimate the expected day of delivery (EDD), subtract 3 months from the date of the LMP, add 7 days and 1 year (Nägle's rule). In practice, this can be quickly calculated using an obstetric 'wheel' (Fig. 16.1). If a cycle is >28 days, the EDD will be later and needs to be adjusted: the number of days by which the cycle is longer than 28 is added to the date calculated using Nägle's rule. The reverse applies if the cycle is shorter than 28 days. If a woman has recently stopped the combined oral contraceptive, her cycles can be anovulatory and LMP is less useful.

In the UK, ultrasound between 11 and 13 + 6 weeks is routine and considered more accurate even than 'certain' dates, unless the pregnancy follows IVF. The EDD is therefore calculated from the crown–rump length (CRL) at this scan.

Estimation of gestational age

From LMP, allowing for cycle length.
Ultrasound scan:
1 Measurement of crown–rump length between 9 and 13 + 6 weeks (preferred method in UK) (Fig. 16.2).
2 Head circumference between 14 and 20 weeks if no early scan and LMP unknown.
Measurements to calculate gestational age are of little use beyond 20 weeks.

Complications of pregnancy: Has there been any bleeding or hypertension, diabetes, anaemia, urine infections, concerns about fetal growth or other problems? Has she been admitted to hospital in the pregnancy?
Tests: What tests have been performed (e.g. ultrasound scans, blood tests, prenatal diagnostic tests)?

Obstetrics & Gynaecology, Fifth Edition. Lawrence Impey, Tim Child.
© 2017 John Wiley & Sons, Ltd. Published 2017 by John Wiley & Sons, Ltd.

Past obstetric history

Take details of past pregnancies in chronological order. Ask what was the mode and gestation of delivery and, if operative, why. Ask the birth weight and sex of the baby, and if the mother or the baby had any complications.

Parity: This is the number of times a woman has delivered potentially viable babies (in UK law this is defined as beyond 24 completed weeks). A woman who has had three term pregnancies is 'para 3', even if she is now in her fourth pregnancy. A suffix denotes the number of pregnancies that have miscarried (or been terminated) before 24 weeks; for example, if the same woman had had two prior miscarriages at 12 weeks, she would be described as 'para 3 + 2'. A nulliparous woman has never delivered a potentially live baby, although she may have had miscarriages or abortions; a multiparous woman has delivered at least one baby at 24 completed weeks or more.

Gravidity: This describes the number of times a woman has been pregnant. The woman above would be gravida 6, encompassing her three term deliveries, two miscarriages and the present pregnancy. The use of the term 'gravid' is less descriptive and is best avoided.

Nulliparity and multiparity	
Nulliparous	Has delivered no live/potentially live babies
Multiparous	Has delivered live/potentially live (>24 week) babies

Other history

Past gynaecological history: This should be brief. Ask the date of the last cervical smear and if she has been treated for an abnormal smear. Ask about prior contraception and any difficulty in conceiving.

Past medical history: Ask about operations, however distant. Ask about heart disease, hypertension, diabetes, psychiatric disease, epilepsy and other chronic illnesses. Ask 'have you ever been in hospital?'.

If the woman is from a country/culture where female genital mutilation (FGM) is practised, this must be sensitively considered. The words 'circumcision' or 'cutting' are best understood; disclosure, especially to a male or in front of family, may be a problem.

Systems review: Ask the usual cardiovascular, respiratory, abdominal and neurological questions.

Drugs: What drugs was she taking at conception? What was she taking before (she might have stopped a drug)

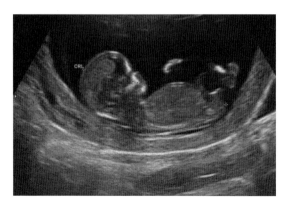

Fig. 16.1 The obstetric 'wheel'.

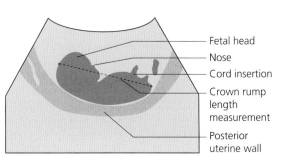

Fig. 16.2 Crown–rump length of fetus at 12+ weeks.

and what now? Ask specifically about low-dose aspirin (LDA) and vitamin D.

Family history: Is there a first-degree history of diabetes, pre-eclampsia, autoimmune disease, venous thromboembolic disease or thrombophilia, mental illness or any inherited disorder?

Personal history: Does she smoke or drink alcohol and how much? Ask, sensitively, about other drugs.

Social history: Is there social support? You may need to sensitively ask about domestic abuse and child safeguarding issues.

Allergies: Ask specifically about penicillin and latex.

Venous thromboembolic (VTE) risk: Consider her risk factors for this major cause of maternal mortality. A risk assessment form is routinely used in pregnancy and must be completed at booking, at any admission, and postnatally.

Other questions

Now ask: 'Is there anything else you think I ought to know?'. The patient may be knowledgeable about her condition and she may help you if you have not discovered all the important facts.

Presenting the history

Start by summing up the important points, including important facts about any presenting complaint:

This is . . . aged . . . , who is . . . weeks into her . . . pregnancy and has been admitted to hospital because of . . .

Example: This is X, aged 30 years, who is 38 weeks into her previously uncomplicated second pregnancy and has been admitted to hospital because of a painless antepartum haemorrhage.

N.B. You have demonstrated your understanding by mentioning the absence of pain, an important factor in the differential diagnosis of antepartum haemorrhage.

Now go through the history in some detail.

Then sum up again, in one sentence, including any important findings in the history.

Why routinely palpate the abdomen?

<24 weeks	To check dates, twins
>24 weeks	To assess well-being by assessing size and liquor
>36 weeks	To also check lie, presentation and engagement

The obstetric examination

General examination

General: *appearance*, temperature, pulse rate, oedema and possible anaemia are assessed. At the booking visit, the weight, height (calculate and record the body mass index (BMI)), chest, breasts, cardiovascular system and legs are also examined. The *blood pressure* and *urinalysis* tests should be performed together so that they are not forgotten (Fig. 16.3). The patient lies comfortably with her back semi-prone at 45°. Diastolic blood pressure is recorded as Korotkoff V (when the sound disappears). If the blood pressure is raised or if there is proteinuria, examine elsewhere also (e.g. for epigastric tenderness).

Mood should be routinely assessed at booking, and postnatally. The 'Whooley questions' are useful: 'During the past month, have you often been bothered by feeling down, depressed or hopeless?' 'During the past month, have you often been bothered by having little interest or pleasure in doing things?' If the answers are positive, ask whether she would like help.

Patients and actors in exams

Make eye contact
Introduce yourself and ensure you know her name
Smile and talk to her
Make sure she is comfortable, e.g. neck supported
Be gentle and watch her face when you examine
Her assessment is as important as the examiner's

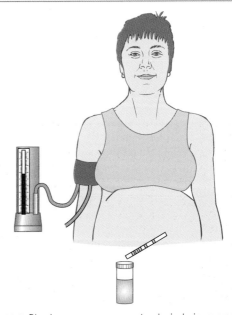

Fig. 16.3 Blood pressure measurement and urinalysis are essential.

Abdominal examination

The patient should lie semi-prone, avoiding aortocaval compression, discreetly exposed from just below the breasts to the symphysis pubis. Talk to her, make eye contact and be gentle. The uterus is normally palpable abdominally at 12 weeks. By 20 weeks, the fundus is usually at the level of the umbilicus. Before 20 weeks, a uterus that is larger than expected could be due to incorrect dates, a full bladder, multiple pregnancy, uterine fibroids or a pelvic mass.

Inspection

Look at the size of the pregnant uterus and look for striae, the linea nigra and scars, particularly in the suprapubic area (Fig. 16.4). Fetal movements are often visible in later pregnancy.

Palpation

This is purposeful and firm, but must be gentle. As you palpate, ask yourself the reasons why you are doing it:
1 Is the fetus adequately grown?
2 Is the liquor volume normal?
3 Is the lie longitudinal?
4 Is the presentation cephalic and, if so, is it engaged?
Palpation can be considered as consisting of three steps (Figs 16.5–16.7).
Step 1: Find the fundus using the fingers and ulnar border of the left hand. *Measure the distance to the symphysis pubis* with a tape measure (see Fig. 16.5), facing the abdomen to avoid 'cheating'. After 24 weeks, the symphysis–fundal height in centimetres approximately corresponds to the gestation ±2 cm. This is the best clinical test for detecting the 'small-for-dates' fetus, but the sensitivity is <70%. Plot the symphysis fundus height on a chart to assess consistency of enlargement. Also look for tenderness or uterine irritability.
Step 2: Next, facing the mother, use both hands to palpate down the fetus towards the pelvis (see Fig. 16.6). Use 'dipping' movements to *palpate fetal parts* and *estimate the liquor volume*. Imagine a large potato in a small plastic bag containing water. Pressing on the outside of the bag will allow palpation of the potato, and the feel of the water is exactly how liquor feels. If none is present, the contents are easy to feel; if fluid volume is excessive (polyhydramnios), the bag will be tense and the fingers will need to dip in far to feel anything. Try to ascertain

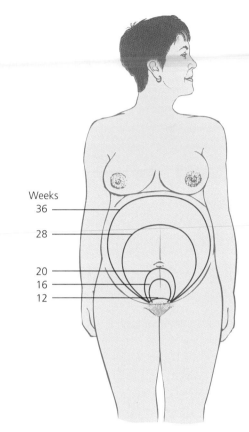

Weeks
36
28
20
16
12

Fig. 16.4 Abdominal palpation of uterine size.

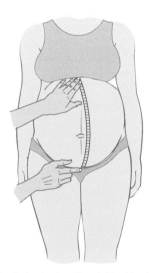

Fig. 16.5 Abdominal palpation. Step 1: Fundal palpation and measurement of symphysis–fundal height.

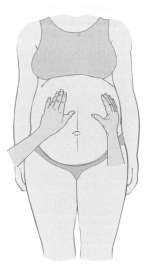

Fig. 16.6 Abdominal palpation. Step 2: Examination of fetal parts.

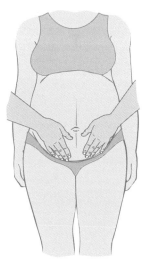

Fig. 16.7 Abdominal palpation. Step 3: Examination of presentation.

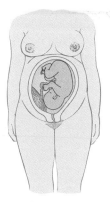

Fig. 16.8 Longitudinal lie (cephalic presentation in this instance).

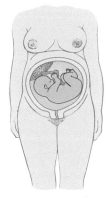

Fig. 16.9 Transverse lie.

what you are feeling: the head is hard and, if free, can be gently 'bounced' or balloted between two hands, whereas the breech is softer and less easy to define.

The lie refers to the relationship between the fetus and the long axis of the uterus. If longitudinal, the head and buttocks are palpable at each end (Fig. 16.8). If transverse or oblique, the fetus is lying across the uterus and the pelvis will be empty (Fig. 16.9).

Step 3: Turn to face the pelvis and press the fingers of both hands firmly down just above the symphysis pubis to assess the presentation: the fetal part that occupies the lower segment or pelvis (see Fig. 16.7). With a longitudinal lie (see Fig. 16.8), it is the head, or occasionally the buttocks.

Engagement of the head (Fig. 16.10) occurs when the widest diameter descends into the pelvis: descent is described as 'fifths palpable'. If only two-fifths of the head is palpable abdominally, then more than half has entered the pelvis and so the head must be engaged. If more than two-fifths of the head is palpable, it is not engaged. If you are still unsure of the presentation, grasp the presenting fetal part between the thumb and index finger of the examining hand (Pawlik's grip). This can be uncomfortable for the patient and is seldom necessary.

Common causes of polyhydramnios
Diabetes/gestational diabetes Fetal abnormality Idiopathic

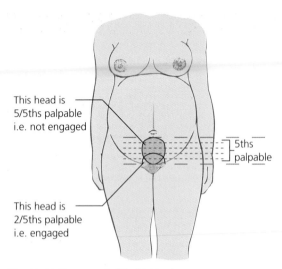

This head is
5/5ths palpable
i.e. not engaged

5ths
palpable

This head is
2/5ths palpable
i.e. engaged

Fig. 16.10 Engagement of the fetal head.

Attempting to determine the *position* or *attitude* of the fetus is not a useful part of antenatal palpation of the abdomen. If a woman has complained of pain or antepartum haemorrhage, it is important to look for areas of tenderness and uterine irritability (it contracts when palpated).

Auscultation

Listening over the anterior shoulder (usually palpable between the head and the umbilicus), the fetal heart should be heard; after 28 weeks this should be possible with a Pinard's stethoscope. Place this flat over the shoulder, press it on the abdomen with your ear, keeping both hands free and time the heart rate with your watch. It should be 110–160 beats/minute.

Other features of relevance

Consider examination of fundi, reflexes, temperature, epigastrium, legs, chest, etc. if clinically indicated from the history or other examination findings. Vaginal examination is not a useful part of routine antenatal examination, unless labour is suspected or is to be induced, and is described in the chapters on labour.

Abdominal findings in pregnancy	
Uterine size	Fundus palpable at 12–14 weeks
	At umbilicus at 20 weeks
	At xiphoid sternum at 36 weeks
	Fundal height increases approx. 1 cm/ week after 24 weeks
Presentation	Breech in 30% at 28 weeks
	Breech in 3% after 37 weeks
Engagement	Common in nulliparous after 37 weeks
	Multiparous usually not engaged

Presenting the examination

Present the examination findings, including relevant positive or negative findings:

X looks . . . (describe general appearance sensitively), *her blood pressure is . . . and urinalysis shows. . . . Her abdomen is distended compatible with pregnancy, the symphysis–fundal height is . . . , the lie is . . . and the presentation is . . . and is . . .* (engagement). *The fetal heart is audible and is . . .* (rate). *There is . . .* (any important other positive or negative findings).

Example: X looks well, but has severe ankle and sacral oedema; her blood pressure is 150/110 mmHg and urinalysis shows 2+ of protein. Her abdomen is distended compatible with pregnancy and the symphysis–fundal height is 32 cm. The presentation is cephalic and the head is engaged. The fetal heart is 130 beats/minute. She has no epigastric tenderness.

N.B. You have shown understanding that this woman has pre-eclampsia by mentioning important negative findings (epigastric tenderness) pertinent to this diagnosis.

Management plan: You will now need to decide on a course of action. Plan what investigations (if any) are needed and what course of action (if any) is most appropriate.

The postnatal history and examination

History

Ascertain the name and age of the mother and the number of days since delivery.

Delivery: Ask about the gestation and mode of delivery, and if instrumental or caesarean, ask why. Ask about the mode of onset (e.g. spontaneous or induced), length of labour and analgesia. What was the blood loss?

Infant: Ask about the infant's name, sex, birth weight and Apgar scores, cord pH if taken, and mode of feeding. Was vitamin K given?

History of puerperium so far: Ask about lochia (volume, any odour), have her bowels opened yet, is she passing urine normally, or is there difficulty, leaking or dysuria? Does she have pain, particularly in the perineum?

Drugs: what is she taking, including analgesics?

Plans for the puerperium: What contraception does she intend to use? (Progesterone-only contraception is suitable for breastfeeding mothers; the combined pill can be started at 4–6 weeks if bottle feeding.) What help is available at home?

History of pregnancy and obstetric history: This should be brief, but ask about her parity and major antenatal complications, e.g. pre-eclampsia, diabetes.

Social/ personal history: Consider home conditions for the neonate.

Venous thromboembolic (VTE) risk: update her risk assessment for VTE.

Presenting the postnatal history

Summarize her labour, delivery, and her and the neonate's current health:

X, aged . . . had a . . . delivery . . . (if not normal, state indication, i.e. *for . . .*) day*s ago and delivered a . . .* (sex) *infant, weighing . . . kilograms, with Apgar of . . . and . . . labour was . . .* (mode of onset) *at . . . weeks' gestation and lasted . . . hours. This was her . . . pregnancy, which . . .* (state any major complications). *She is currently . . .* (brief assessment of her health: blood pressure, anaemia, uterine involution), *is . . .* (bottle or breast) *feeding and plans to use . . . as contraception. Her risk assessment for VTE is . . . and so fragmin prophylaxis is . . . required.*

Example: X, aged 32 years, had a caesarean delivery for prolonged labour 2 days ago and delivered a girl weighing 3.7 kg. Labour was spontaneous at 40 weeks' gestation and lasted 9 h. This was her first pregnancy and was uncomplicated. She is comfortable, afebrile, her blood pressure is 120/80 mmHg, her uterus is well contracted, she is breastfeeding and plans to use the progesterone-only pill. She is at moderate risk for thromboembolism and a week's fragmin is recommended.

Management/discharge plans: Mention anti-D and rubella vaccination if relevant.

Apgar scoring

Sign	0	1	2
Heart rate	Absent	<100	>100
Respiratory effort	Absent	Weak	Strong cry
	irregular		
Muscle tone	Absent	Limb flexion	Active motion
Colour	All blue/pale	Extremities blue	All pink
Reflex irritability (stimulate foot)	No response	Grimace	Cry

Total score out of 10, at 1 and 5 min
1-min Apgar gives indication of need for resuscitation, but has little prognostic value
5-min Apgar correlates very vaguely with subsequent neurological outcome

Examination

General examination: Assess mood and appearance, temperature, pulse, blood pressure, possible anaemia. Also examine chest, breasts, any wound or intravenous site and legs if fever or tachycardia (Fig. 16.11). The 'Whooley questions' should again be used.

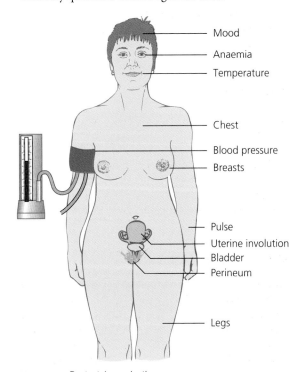

Fig. 16.11 Postnatal examination.

Abdominal examination: Look for uterine involution and a palpable bladder. Inspect the perineum if there is discomfort.

Neonatal examination	
General	Colour (pallor/jaundice/cyanosis), features (dysmorphism/evidence of trauma/birthmarks/any abnormalities), posture, behaviour and feeding movement (abnormal or restricted), respiration
Measure	Heart rate, temperature, head measurements, weight
Examine	Look for primitive reflexes (grasp, Moro, rooting)
	Inspect back and spine with baby prone
	Heart, check all pulses equal (e.g. radiofemoral delay)
	Abdomen, genitalia (undescended testes/hernias/ambiguous genitalia), anus
	Look and examine for congenital dislocation of the hip and talipes
Investigations	Serum bilirubin (SBR) if jaundiced. Day 7: Guthrie (phenylketonuria, thyroid)

Basic neonatal assessment

History: Review the family history, antenatal course, labour course and delivery method and if resuscitation was required. Review birth weight, birth weight centile and weight gain/loss.

Examination: Examine the neonate in the presence of his/her mother. Undress the baby fully. Handle gently and wrap the neonate up after examination.

Further reading

FGM guidance: www.nhs.uk/NHSEngland/About-NHSservices/sexual-health-services/Pages/fgm-for-professionals.aspx (accessed 13 July 2016).

National Institute for Health and Care Excellence. *Antenatal and Postnatal Mental Health: Clinical Management and Service Guidance*. Clinical Guideline No. 192. Available at: www.nice.org.uk/guidance/cg192/chapter/1-recommendations (accessed 13 July 2016).

Obstetric history at a glance

Personal details	Name, age, occupation, gestation, parity
Presenting complaint or present circumstances	
History of present pregnancy	Dates: last menstrual period (LMP), cycle length. Calculate expected day of delivery (EDD), from ultrasound if performed. Check current gestation
	Complications: specific complications, hospital admissions
	Tests done, e.g. ultrasound scan, prenatal diagnosis, booking bloods
Obstetric history	Past pregnancies: year, gestation, mode of delivery, complications, birth weight, ante/intra/postpartum complications
Gynaecological history	Intermenstrual bleeding (IMB), postcoital bleeding (PCB), last cervical smear, contraception, subfertility
Medical history	Operations, major illnesses, particularly diabetes, hypertension, cardiac disease, mental illness. Female genital mutilation if appropriate

Obstetric history at a glance

Personal details	Name, age, occupation, gestation, parity
Systems review	
Drugs	At conception and since conception
Personal	Smoking and alcohol, drugs of abuse
Social	Home conditions, accommodation. Consider child safeguarding issues
Allergies	
Venous thromboembolism risk assessment	
Is there anything else you think I should know?	

Obstetric examination at a glance

General	Appearance, pulse, temperature, weight, oedema (full examination at booking), blood pressure, urinalysis. Mood using 'Whooley questions'	
Abdomen	Inspect	Size, scars, fetal movements
	Palpate	Measure symphysis–fundal height and plot on serial measurement chart. Assess (after 24 weeks) lie and presentation, liquor volume, engagement of presenting part
	Listen	Fetal heart over anterior shoulder
Vaginal examination	Not usually indicated antenatally	
Other features	If relevant	

CHAPTER 17

Antenatal care

Pregnancy and childbirth are physiological events; most women are healthy and few need medical intervention. The main purpose of antenatal care is to identify mothers who do need medical attention, to prevent maternal and fetal morbidity and mortality. Recent reports (MBRRACE-UK 2014: www.rcog.org.uk) emphasize the importance of hitherto poorly appreciated risks such as language barriers, obesity and mental illness. Whilst some women at risk are identifiable at the booking visit, most show no indication of the problems that can develop in pregnancy, labour or the puerperium. Therefore risk needs to be constantly re-evaluated throughout pregnancy and after. Failure of professionals to identify risk or follow recommendations is a major contributor to adverse outcomes; on this, the teachings of Dr Atul Gawande are recommended (see Further reading).

The aims of antenatal care

1 Detect and manage pre-existing maternal disorders that may affect pregnancy outcome.
2 Prevent or detect and manage maternal complications of pregnancy.
3 Prevent or detect and manage fetal complications of pregnancy.
4 Detect congenital fetal problems, if requested by the parents.
5 Plan, with the mother, the circumstances of pregnancy care and delivery to ensure maximum safety for the mother and baby, and maximum maternal satisfaction.
6 Provide education and advice regarding lifestyle and 'minor' conditions of pregnancy.

Preconceptual care and counselling

Many of the aims of antenatal care could be better fulfilled before conception. *Previous pregnancies* may have been traumatic and the implications of another can be discussed. The *health check* is better performed before conception and hitherto undetected problems such as cervical smear abnormalities or cardiac disease can be treated. *Rubella status* can be checked so that immunization can occur before pregnancy. Health in women with chronic disease can be optimized; for instance, strict preconceptual *glucose control in diabetics* reduces the incidence of congenital abnormalities. *Medication* can be optimized for pregnancy; for instance, certain antiepileptics, e.g. lamotrigine, are safer than others, e.g. sodium valproate. Routine preconceptual administration of 0.4 mg/day *folic acid* reduces the chance of neural tube defects.

The booking visit

The first appointment should be before 10 weeks' gestation. The most important purpose is to screen for possible complications that may arise in pregnancy, labour and the puerperium. 'Risk' is therefore assessed, using the history and examination and the investigations that are a standard feature of the booking visit. Decisions about pregnancy care must be constantly re-evaluated as the pregnancy proceeds. At the same time, the gestation of the pregnancy is checked, appropriate prenatal screening is discussed and a general health check is accompanied by health advice.

History

Age: Women below the age of 17 years and above the age of 35 years have an increased risk of obstetric and

---

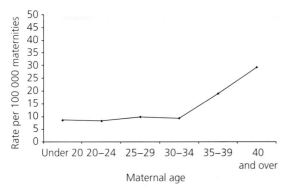

UK maternal mortality according to age

Fig. 17.1 UK maternal mortality according to age. Source: Centre for Child and Maternal Enquiries (CMACE). *BJOG* 2011; **118** (Suppl. 1): 1–203. Reproduced with permission of John Wiley & Sons Ltd.

medical complications in pregnancy (Fig. 17.1). Chromosomal trisomies are more common with advancing maternal age.

History of present pregnancy: In the UK, early ultrasound (usually 11–13 + 6 weeks) is used to date all except *in vitro* fertilization (IVF) pregnancies.

Past obstetric history: Many *obstetric disorders* have a significant recurrence rate. These include preterm labour, the small-for-gestational age and the 'growth-restricted' fetus, stillbirth, antepartum and postpartum haemorrhage, some congenital anomalies, Rhesus disease, pre-eclampsia and gestational diabetes.

Past gynaecological history: Past gynaecological surgery (e.g. myomectomy) may influence delivery recommendations (e.g. loop diathermy) or increase preterm labour risk.

Past medical history: Women with a history of hypertension, diabetes, autoimmune disease, haemoglobinopathy, thromboembolic disease, cardiac or renal disease, or other serious illnesses are at an increased risk of pregnancy problems and need input from the appropriate specialist. Past mental illness increases suicide risk.

Drugs: Contraindicated drugs should be changed to those considered to be safe. Ideally, this should have occurred at a preconceptual counselling visit.

Family history: Gestational diabetes is more common if a first-degree relative is diabetic. Hypertension, thromboembolic and autoimmune disease and pre-eclampsia are also familial.

Immigration and language issues: Access to appropriate information and advice is essential.

Personal/social history: The possibility of domestic violence should always be considered.

Examination

General health and nutritional status are assessed. The body mass index (BMI) is calculated; if >30 (20% of women), maternal and fetal complications are more common. A baseline blood pressure enables comparison if hypertension occurs in later pregnancy. If pre-existing hypertension is found, the risk of subsequent pre-eclampsia is increased. Incidental disease such as breast carcinoma may occasionally be detected.

Abdominal examination before the third trimester is limited. From 12 weeks, the fetal heart can be auscultated with an electronic monitor. Routine vaginal examination is inappropriate. If a smear has not been performed for 3 years it is usually done 3 months postnatally.

Booking visit investigations

Ultrasound scan

Ultrasound between 11 and 13 + 6 weeks is offered. In the UK, all women are 'dated' using crown–rump length (CRL) if <14 weeks, unless the pregnancy is from IVF. This scan also detects multiple pregnancy and enables screening for chromosomal abnormalities with nuchal translucency measurement, in conjunction with blood levels of human chorionic gonadotrophin beta-subunit (β-hCG) and pregnancy-associated plasma protein A (PAPPA), as the 'combined test'.

Blood tests

A *full blood count* (FBC) identifies pre-existing anaemia.

Serum antibodies (e.g. anti-D) identify those at risk of intrauterine isoimmunization.

Glucose tolerance test: In women at risk, this is planned for later in the pregnancy.

Blood tests for syphilis are still routine because of the serious implications for the fetus.

Rubella immunity is checked: vaccination, if required, will be offered postnatally.

Human immunodeficiency virus (HIV) and *hepatitis B* counselling and screening are offered.

Haemoglobin electrophoresis is performed in at-risk women. *Sickle cell anaemia* is common in Afro-Caribbean women, the *thalassaemias* in Mediterranean and Asian women. The partner should be tested if the woman is a carrier, to identify women who should be offered prenatal diagnosis.

Other tests

Screening for infections implicated in preterm labour (e.g. chlamydia, bacterial vaginosis) could be performed at this stage, in women at increased risk. These are not routinely recommended in the UK. Toxoplasmosis and cytomegalovirus (CMV) screening are not recommended in the UK because of their rarity and absence of treatment respectively.

Urine microscopy and culture are performed because asymptomatic bacteriuria in pregnancy commonly (20%) leads to pyelonephritis.

Urinalysis for glucose, protein and nitrites screen for underlying diabetes, renal disease and infection, respectively.

Routine booking investigations
Urine culture
Full blood count (FBC)
Antibody screen
Serological tests for syphilis
Rubella immunoglobulin G
Offer human immunodeficiency virus (HIV) and hepatitis B
Ultrasound scan
Screening for chromosomal abnormalities
±Haemoglobin electrophoresis

Health promotion and advice

Drugs

Medications are generally avoided in the first trimester, but teratogenicity is rare. Regular medication should ideally be adjusted preconceptually.

Folic acid supplementation, with 0.4 mg/day folic acid, should continue until at least 12 weeks. Increased dosage of 5 mg is recommended for women with a BMI >30, with diabetes, sickle disease or malabsorption, and those on antiepileptics.

Vitamin D supplementation is recommended for all women (10 μg/day), and at 25 μg/day in those with a BMI >30, of South Asian or Afro-Caribbean origin or with low sunlight exposure, and in women at increased risk of pre eclampsia.

Aspirin 75 mg is also recommended for women at increased risk of pre-eclampsia.

Immunization against seasonal influenza and, after 28 weeks, against pertussis must be strongly advised.

Lifestyle

Diet in pregnancy should be balanced, with a daily energy intake of about 2500 calories. *Alcohol* is best avoided, particularly in the first 12 weeks. *Smoking advice* is given. Nicotine replacement therapy (NRT) may be used. *A dental check-up* is advised. *Coitus* is not contraindicated except when the placenta is praevia or the membranes have ruptured. Avoidance of infection with *Listeriosis* is avoided by drinking only pasteurized or UHT milk, by avoiding soft and blue cheeses, paté and uncooked or partially cooked ready-prepared food.

Other: Exercise in pregnancy is advised: swimming is ideal; contact sports or very heavy exercise should be avoided. When driving, a seatbelt should be worn, above and below the 'bump'. Sleeping should be in the left lateral position from 28 weeks.

Preparation for birth

Antenatal classes educate women and their partners about pregnancy and labour. Knowledge and understanding help alleviate fear and pain, and allow women more control and informed choice. In addition, intrapartum techniques of posture, breathing and pushing can be taught (Fig. 17.2).

Risk assessment and planning pregnancy care

In the UK, most pregnancies are supervised by community midwives, acting according to guidelines. Input from medical staff is required where there is pre-existing

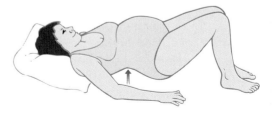

Fig. 17.2 Pelvic tilt at antenatal classes.

illness or an increased risk of pregnancy complications and adverse maternal or fetal outcomes. The degree of medical involvement will depend on the pregnancy risk and the occurrence of complications.

Optimum risk assessment for maternal and fetal complications would allow any preventive treatment and appropriate usage of additional tests and intervention. It would have a high sensitivity (i.e. identify most women at risk of problems) and a high specificity (i.e. not misclassify women as high risk when they are at low risk). Because additional surveillance and intervention in pregnancy are expensive, may 'medicalize' a normal pregnancy and even cause harm (e.g. unnecessary caesarean section or preterm delivery), they need to be used selectively. History and examination are used but are limited in their usefulness: most bad things happen to apparently normal pregnancies.

An example of this is risk assessment for stillbirth. This is rare (approximately 1 in 200), but in some cases preventable, including by iatrogenic delivery before term. Less than a quarter of affected women can be identified as being at increased risk by history at booking; early delivery is not appropriate for all women, or even a quarter. The use of additional tests, particularly where integrated with each other and other risk factors, should ultimately allow better risk assessment, as has been developed for Down's syndrome. This could radically alter the planning of pregnancy care. In the meantime, most risk assessment is based on history and the presence or absence of established risk factors.

Early pregnancy risk assessments

Target disorder	Action if high risk
Venous thromboembolism	Low molecular weight heparin
Pre-eclampsia	Aspirin 75 mg
Increased blood pressure monitoring	
Chromosomal abnormalities	Non-invasive prenatal diagnosis or invasive testing
Fetal growth restriction	Serial ultrasound of fetal growth
Gestational diabetes	Glucose tolerance test

Routine later pregnancy tests

Ultrasound for structural abnormalities

An ultrasound examination should be offered at around 20 weeks. This 'anomaly scan' enables detection of most structural fetal abnormalities, although reported success rates vary widely.

Ultrasound screening for risk assessment

Ultrasound cervical length measurement at around 20 weeks can be used for risk assessment of preterm delivery in otherwise low-risk women. This is currently not recommended for all women in the UK. However, progesterone administration to women who have a short cervix but are otherwise 'low risk' probably halves their risk of preterm delivery (*AJOG* 2012; **206**(2): 124. e1–19).

Ultrasound measurement of uterine artery resistance can be used as a screening test for intrauterine growth restriction and pre-eclampsia. This is currently not recommended for all women in the UK. However, it identifies women at risk better than history.

Other routine later pregnancy tests

Full blood count and an *antibody assessment* are performed at 28 weeks; the FBC is repeated later if treatment for anaemia is given.

Non-invasive prenatal testing (NIPT) is now recommended in the UK to determine which Rhesus-negative mothers are carrying a Rhesus-positive baby. Unless the fetal status is unknown (e.g. missed test), only those with a positive baby are given anti-D.

Glucose tolerance testing is used for all women at increased risk, the most common indications being increased BMI, ethnicity and a first-degree family history of diabetes.

Continuing antenatal care

Frequency of antenatal visits

The woman is seen at decreasing intervals through the pregnancy because complications are more common later in the pregnancy. The frequency with which she is seen is dependent on the likelihood of complications

Investigations

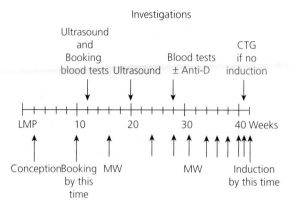

Fig. 17.3 Basic antenatal care in nulliparous women. CTG, cardiotocography; LMP, last menstrual period; MW, midwife.

and on the apparent fetal and maternal health as assessed in subsequent visits. In the UK, NICE recommends an antenatal appointment schedule (Fig. 17.3) for uncomplicated pregnancies of 10 appointments for nulliparous and seven for multiparous women. More frequent visits are appropriate for many 'high-risk' pregnancies. Less intensive care is less well accepted by women and health carers alike.

Conduct of antenatal visits (Fig. 17.4)

At each visit, the history is briefly reviewed. The woman is asked about her physical and mental state and given the opportunity to ask questions. Routine weighing is of little use. The blood pressure is taken and the urine is

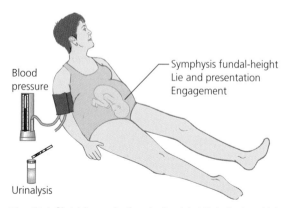

Fig. 17.4 Obstetric examination at antenatal visits in the late third trimester.

checked for protein, glucose and nitrites. Urine culture is performed if the latter are detected. The abdomen is examined in the normal manner, but presentation is variable and unimportant until 36 weeks. Listening to the fetal heart is reassuring. A reassessment of pregnancy risk is undertaken.

The following is the basic antenatal schedule recommended by NICE, and more intensive surveillance is appropriate for pregnancies at risk of, or who develop, complications.

- *16 weeks*: the results of screening tests for chromosomal abnormalities and booking blood tests should specifically be reviewed. If screening for chromosomal abnormalities was missed, an alternative 'triple test' is offered.
- *18–21 weeks*: the anomaly scan is performed. A further scan is at 32 weeks if the placenta is low.
- *25 weeks (recommended for nulliparous women only)*: this is to exclude early-onset pre-eclampsia. A glucose tolerance is performed if indicated.
- *28 weeks*: fundal height is measured. The FBC and antibodies are checked. Anti-D is given to Rhesus-negative women with a baby of unknown or Rhesus-positive status.
- *31 weeks* (nulliparous women only): fundal height is measured.
- *34 weeks*: fundal height is measured. The full blood count is rechecked if the haemoglobin was low.
- *36, 38 and 40 weeks*: fundal height is measured and the fetal lie and presentation are checked. Referral for external cephalic version (ECV) is offered if the presentation is breech. Pelvic examination is inappropriate unless induction is contemplated or there is suspicion of obstruction.
- *41 weeks*: fundal height is measured and the fetal lie and presentation are checked. Membrane sweeping is offered, as is induction of labour by 42 weeks.

'Minor' conditions of pregnancy

Itching is common in pregnancy. The sclerae are checked for jaundice, and liver function tests and bile acids are assessed. Although rare, liver complications in pregnancy often present with itching.
Pelvic girdle pain (formerly symphysis pubis dysfunction) is common and causes varying degrees of discomfort in the pubic and sacroiliac joints. Physiotherapy, corsets, analgesics and even crutches may be used. Care

with leg abduction is required. It is usually, but not invariably, cured after delivery.

Abdominal pain is universal to some degree in pregnancy; it is usually benign and unexplained. However, medical and surgical problems are no less common in pregnancy, and may have a worse prognosis, particularly appendicitis and pancreatitis. Urinary tract infections and fibroids can cause pain in pregnancy.

Heartburn affects 70% and is most marked in the supine position. Extra pillows are helpful; antacids are not contraindicated, ranitidine can be used in severe cases. Pre-eclampsia can present with epigastric pain.

Backache is almost universal and may cause sciatica. Most cases resolve after delivery. Physiotherapy, advice on posture and lifting, a firm mattress and a corset may all help.

Constipation is common and exacerbated by oral iron. A high fibre intake is needed. Stool softeners are used if this fails.

Ankle oedema is common, worsens towards the end of pregnancy and is an unreliable sign of pre-eclampsia. However, a sudden increase in oedema warrants careful assessment and follow-up of blood pressure and urinalysis. Benign oedema is helped by raising the foot of the bed at night; diuretics should not be given.

Leg cramps affect 30% of women. Treatments are unproven but sodium chloride tablets, calcium salts or quinine may be safely tried.

Carpal tunnel syndrome is due to fluid retention compressing the median nerve. It is seldom severe and is usually temporary. Splints on the wrists may help.

Vaginitis due to candidiasis is common in pregnancy and more difficult to treat. Imidazole vaginal pessaries (e.g. clotrimazole) are used for symptomatic infection.

Tiredness is almost universal and is often incorrectly attributed to anaemia.

Further reading

National Institute for Health and Care Excellence. *Antenatal Care for Uncomplicated Pregnancies.* Clinical Guideline No. 62. Available at: www.nice.org.uk/guidance/cg62/ (accessed 13 July 2016).

Dr Atul Gawande: www.bbc.co.uk/programmes/b00729d9/episodes/downloads (accessed 13 July 2016).

Physiological changes in pregnancy at a glance

Weight gain	10–15 kg
Genital tract	Uterus weight increase from 50 to 1000 g Muscle hypertrophy, increased blood flow and contractility Cervix softens, may start to efface in late third trimester
Blood	Blood volume: 50% increase Red cell mass: increase Haemoglobin: decrease (normal lower limit 11.0 g/dL) White blood cell count (WBC) increase
Cardiovascular system	Cardiac output: 40% increase Peripheral resistance: 50% reduction Blood pressure: small mid-pregnancy fall
Lungs	Tidal volume: 40% increase Respiratory rate: no change
Others	Renal blood flow: glomerular filtration rate 40% increase, so creatinine/urea decrease Reduced gut motility: delayed gastric emptying/constipation Thyroid enlargement

CHAPTER 18

Congenital abnormalities and their identification

Congenital abnormalities affect 2% of pregnancies (1% major). They can be *structural deformities* (e.g. diaphragmatic hernia) or *chromosomal abnormalities* (most commonly trisomies, e.g. Down's syndrome) or *inherited diseases* (e.g. cystic fibrosis), or are the result of *intrauterine infection* (e.g. rubella) or *drug exposure* (e.g. antiepileptics).

Abnormalities account for <25% of perinatal deaths and are a major cause of disability in later life. Prenatal identification of such abnormalities is important to prepare the parents, to allow delivery to be at an appropriate time and place, to prepare neonatal services and to enable the parents to terminate the pregnancy if they wish. Further, some conditions can be treated *in utero*. Parental attitudes vary with age, religion and social background; counselling must be non-directive. The parents must be given the facts to allow their choice to be informed. This applies to when an abnormality is found, or whether the abnormality should be sought in the first place. Screening for Down's syndrome, for instance, should only be performed if the parents would wish to know. The facts about and implications of the available tests should be discussed at the booking visit.

The difference between screening and diagnostic tests

A *screening test* is available for all women and gives a measure of the risk of the fetus being affected by a particular disorder. The 'higher-risk' patient can then be offered a diagnostic test. A result might be: 'the risk of Down's syndrome in this pregnancy is 1 in 50'.

A *diagnostic test* is performed on women with a 'high risk' to confirm or refute the possibility, e.g. 'this fetus does not have Down's syndrome'.

Screening and diagnostic tests

These aim to identify subjects at increased risk for a given condition. In pregnancy, they are usually offered to all women. A good screening test is *cheap*, has a *high sensitivity* (i.e. does not miss affected individuals) and *specificity* (i.e. not many false positives) and is *safe*. There must also be an *acceptable diagnostic test* for the disorder for which it is screening and the implications of being affected by the condition *should be serious enough* to warrant the test. This diagnostic test must diagnose or refute the condition. Diagnostic tests are not always offered as a first line because they may be expensive or have complications. By performing diagnostic tests only in women identified as high risk, the impact of these is minimized.

Terms describing screening tests

The *sensitivity* is the proportion of subjects with the condition classified by the test as screen positive for the condition. The *negative predictive value* (NPV) is the probability that a subject who is screen negative will not have the condition. The *specificity* is the proportion of subjects without the condition who are classified as screen negative.

The *screen-positive rate* is the proportion of subjects who are classified as high risk by the test. The *positive predictive value* (PPV) is the probability that a subject who is screen positive will have the condition. In practice, the PPV is often low; most screen positives do not have the condition, and the screen-positive rate is similar to the *false-positive rate* (FPR), the number classified as high risk who do not nevertheless have the condition.

Obstetrics & Gynaecology, Fifth Edition. Lawrence Impey, Tim Child.
© 2017 John Wiley & Sons, Ltd. Published 2017 by John Wiley & Sons, Ltd.

Performance of screening tests

The sensitivity and specificity are related. For instance, Down's syndrome [→ p.159] is more common in older mothers, so maternal age can be used alone as a screening test. The performance of the test will depend on what maternal age is considered 'screen positive'.

Although age is a risk factor, most babies with Down's syndrome will be born to younger mothers because, although their individual risks are lower, they are more likely to be pregnant. If we were to call all women over 30 years screen positive, the test would detect most Down's babies, or have a high sensitivity and high NPV. However, at this age cut-off about half of the population would be classified as screen positive, so the test would have a low specificity and PPV, and a high false-positive rate. Sensitivity is therefore quoted at a given screen-positive rate, often 3% or 5%.

Integration of risk factors

Age alone is a poor screening test for Down's syndrome, with it and some other conditions there are several potential screening tests. If these tests are independent of each other, they can be 'integrated' or used together to create a more accurate overall single screening test. This is now the principle behind all Down's syndrome screening.

Methods of prenatal testing for congenital abnormalities

Maternal blood testing

As a screening test

Chromosomal abnormalities: The levels of several maternal blood markers are also altered where the fetus has a chromosomal abnormality such as Down's syndrome. These include human chorionic gonadotrophin beta-subunit (β-hCG), pregnancy-associated plasma protein A (PAPP-A), alpha fetoprotein (AFP), oestriol and inhibin A. The results of these can be integrated with other risk factors such as maternal age and ultrasound measurements (e.g. nuchal translucency) to screen for the trisomies 21 (Down's syndrome), 18 and 13. Maternal serum alpha fetoprotein (MSAFP) assessment is no longer recommended.

As a diagnostic test

Non-invasive prenatal diagnosis (NIPT) from free fetal DNA in the maternal circulation is now allowing non-invasive antenatal diagnosis of chromosomal abnormalities. The accuracy is not quite 100%, but the tests take >1 week and currently remain expensive. The use of NIPT is increasing rapidly and is likely to be routinely recommended in the UK in most women at increased risk of aneuploidy.

Ultrasound

To confirm dates

Ultrasound is used to determine the gestation and pregnancy site and exclude multiple pregnancy.

As a screening test for abnormalities

Ultrasound remains the cornerstone of screening for trisomies. The nuchal 'translucency' (the space between skin and soft tissue overlying the cervical spine) between 11 and 13 + 6 weeks is measured (Fig. 18.1) and the larger it is, the higher the risk (Figs 18.2, 18.3). A larger nuchal translucency also indicates a higher risk of structural, particularly cardiac, abnormalities. In addition, 50% of fetuses with trisomies have structural abnormalities, e.g. exomphalos.

To aid other diagnostic tests

Amniocentesis and chorionic villus sampling (CVS) are performed under ultrasound vision.

As a diagnostic test

Structural abnormalities are usually diagnosed around 20 weeks, at the 'anomaly scan'. Congenital malformations of all organs and systems are detectable. At least 25% of abnormalities can actually be identified earlier, at the time of nuchal translucency assessment (Fig. 18.4). However, particularly with the heart, many remain undiagnosed even at 20 weeks, and this is related to operator experience. In addition, some abnormalities do not become evident until later either because they are not visible or because they develop with gestation. The development of increased

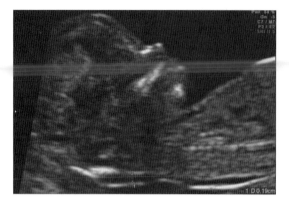

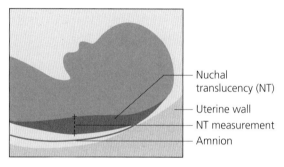

Fig. 18.1 Normal nuchal translucency.

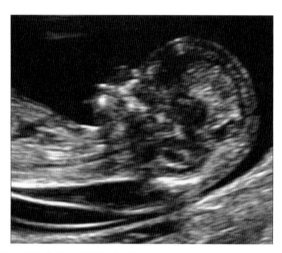

Fig. 18.2 Enlarged nuchal translucency.

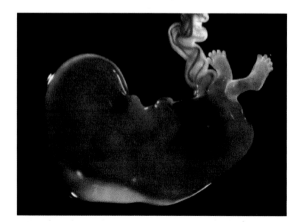

Fig. 18.3 Photograph of enlarged nuchal translucency.

liquor volume, polyhydramnios, in later pregnancy can be the result of a fetal abnormality and warrants a repeat detailed ultrasound examination.

Fetal magnetic resonance imaging

Magnetic resonance imaging (MRI) scanning of the fetus *in utero* is used to aid diagnosis of intracranial lesions and is better at differentiating between different types of soft tissue, e.g. liver and lung. It may also have a role as an alternative to postmortem examination.

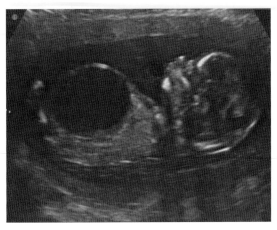

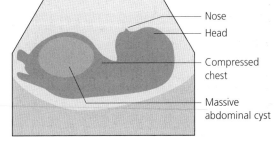

Nose
Head
Compressed chest
Massive abdominal cyst

Fig. 18.4 Abdominal cyst at nuchal scan.

3-D/4-D ultrasound

3-D or real-time 3-D (known as 4-D ultrasound) using a computer-reconstructed 3-D ultrasound image can allow better evaluation of certain abnormalities, and is being intensively used, largely in tertiary referral centres.

Invasive testing

Amniocentesis

This diagnostic test involves removal of amniotic fluid using a fine-gauge needle under ultrasound guidance (Fig. 18.5). It is safest performed from 15 weeks' gestation, and it may be done later. This enables prenatal diagnosis of chromosomal abnormalities, some infections such as cytomegalovirus (CMV) and toxoplasmosis, and inherited disorders such as sickle cell anaemia, thalassaemia and cystic fibrosis. One per cent of women miscarry after an amniocentesis (*Obstet Gynecol* 2006; **108**: 1067), most unrelated to the procedure.

Chorionic villus sampling (CVS)

This diagnostic test involves biopsy of the trophoblast, by passing a fine-gauge needle through the abdominal wall (or cervix) and into the placenta, from 11 weeks. The result is therefore obtained earlier than with amniocentesis and allows an abnormal fetus to be identified at a time when abortion, if requested, is usually performed under general anaesthesia. The miscarriage rate is slightly higher than after amniocentesis, but this is because it is performed earlier, when spontaneous miscarriage is more common, and because it is a more difficult procedure. Its uses are similar to amniocentesis.

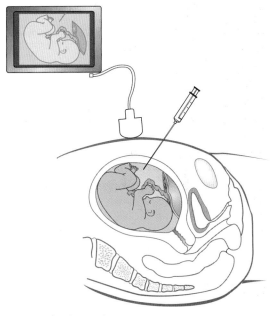

Fig. 18.5 Amniocentesis.

Testing of samples

Fluorescence in situ *hybridization* (FISH) *and polymerase chain reaction* (PCR) can both be used to diagnose the most common abnormalities from chorionic villi or amniotic fluid in less than 48 hours.

Karyotyping involves inspection of the chromosomes by looking down a microscope.

Microarray-CGH: Comparative genomic hybridization (CGH) techniques allow a closer or more 'magnified' inspection of the chromosomes, detecting smaller deletions or abnormalities. This is replacing karyotyping

Preimplantation genetic diagnosis

In vitro fertilization (IVF) allows cell(s) from a developing embryo to be removed for genetic analysis before the embryo is transferred to the uterus. This allows selection, and therefore implantation, only of embryos that will not be affected by the disorder for which it is being tested. The technique is expensive and presents ethical dilemmas, but has been used in prenatal diagnosis of sex-linked disorders, trisomies, and both autosomal dominant and recessive conditions. It does require IVF, even in couples who are fertile.

Chromosomal abnormalities

These affect 6 per 1000 live births, but are much more common in early pregnancy as a cause of miscarriage. Most are trisomies.

Down's syndrome

Trisomy 21 is the most common chromosomal abnormality among live births. It is usually the result of random non-dysjunction at meiosis, although occasionally (6%) it arises as a result of a balanced chromosomal translocation in the parents. It is more common with advancing maternal age (Fig. 18.6). The affected infant has mental handicap, characteristic facies and often (50%) congenital cardiac disease. Other structural abnormalities may also be present. Unless the result of a parental balanced translocation, the recurrence risk is low and determined largely by maternal age.

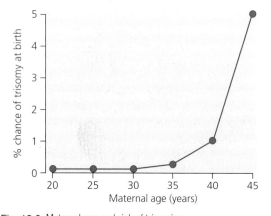

Fig. 18.6 Maternal age and risk of trisomies.

The nuchal scan
Ultrasound component of 'combined test' for aneuploidy
Dates pregnancy, determines chorionicity in multiples
Many structural abnormalities visible

Other chromosomal abnormalities

Trisomy 18 (Edwards' syndrome) and *trisomy 13* (Patau's syndrome) are also more common with advanced maternal age. They are associated with major structural defects, and affected fetuses die *in utero* or after birth. Sex chromosome abnormalities include *Klinefelter's syndrome* (47 XXY). These males have normal intellect, small testes and are infertile. In *Turner's syndrome* (a single X chromosome only: X0), affected individuals are female, infertile but with normal intellect.

Deletions, translocations and 'microarray' abnormalities

Sections of chromosomes can be deleted, duplicated or translocated in an unbalanced fashion. Improved 'magnification' of the chromosomes using comparative genomic hybridization (microarray-CGH) will detect less extensive abnormalities than a traditional karyotype and is commonly performed where a fetus is structurally abnormal. One problem is that the phenotype of many abnormalities is poorly understood and, in the absence of a fetal abnormality, may not always be abnormal.

Risk factors for Down's syndrome	
History	High maternal age
	Previous affected baby (risk increased 1%)
	Balanced parental translocation (rare)
Ultrasound	Thickened nuchal translucency
	Some structural abnormalities
	Absent or shortened nasal bone
	Tricuspid regurgitation
	Severe fetal growth restriction
Blood tests	Low pregnancy-associated plasma protein A (PAPP-A) (1st trimester)
	High human chorionic gonadotrophin beta-subunit (β-hCG) (1st/2nd trimester)
	Low alpha fetoprotein (AFP) (1st/2nd trimester)
	Low oestriol (2nd trimester)
	High inhibin (2nd trimester)

Screening for chromosomal abnormalities

Traditionally, women over the age of about 35 years were considered high risk. However, younger women have more babies and therefore, despite a lower individual risk, account for more Down's syndrome pregnancies. These would go undetected without a screening programme for all consenting women. In the UK, all pregnant women are offered a screening test for trisomies including Down's syndrome, which for the latter has a 75% sensitivity and a 3% false-positive rate, equivalent to calling a risk of 1 in <150 a high risk. This cut-off is probably not sensitive enough; NIPT is often used with risks up to 1 in <1000.

The combined test: This integrates the risk from maternal age, with PAPP-A and β-hCG blood tests, and nuchal translucency measurement by ultrasound at 11–13 + 6 weeks. The performance of this test can be enhanced using other risk factors, e.g. presence or absence of the nasal bone and tricuspid regurgitation.

The quadruple test: Where booking is too late for the nuchal scan or it is technically not possible (e.g. increased body mass index (BMI)), the 'quadruple' test is used. This comprises a blood test, from 14 to 22 weeks, integrating the risk from maternal age with that calculated from AFP, total hCG, inhibin and oestriol.

Other ultrasound abnormalities: Some structural abnormalities (e.g. exomphalos), severe polyhydramnios and severe fetal growth restriction are also associated with chromosomal abnormalities.

Diagnosis of chromosomal abnormalities

Chromosomal abnormalities are diagnosed using amniocentesis or CVS. Increasingly, NIPT is used; the near 100% sensitivity means a negative result is very reassuring, albeit in the absence of a structural abnormality, whilst a positive one should still prompt invasive testing.

Structural abnormalities

The following are some more common structural abnormalities amenable to prenatal diagnosis. Many coexist, as syndromes or associations. Physical or mental handicap may follow, as part of an associated syndrome (e.g. some cases of exomphalos), because of effects on the brain (e.g. spina bifida) or because of postnatal treatment or surgery (e.g. diaphragmatic herniae).

Central nervous system abnormalities

Neural tube defects (NTDs) are the result of failure of closure of the neural tube. Neural tissue is often exposed, allowing degeneration. Less than 1 in 200 pregnancies are affected, and the incidence is declining. The best known examples are *spina bifida* and *anencephaly* (Fig. 18.7); in the former, severe disability is common but not invariable; the latter is incompatible with life. Preconceptual folic acid supplementation for 3 months (0.4 mg/day)

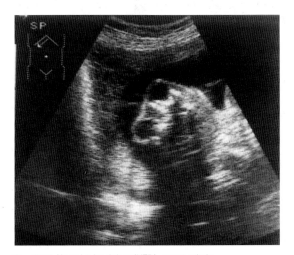

Fig. 18.7 Neural tube defect (NTD): anencephaly.

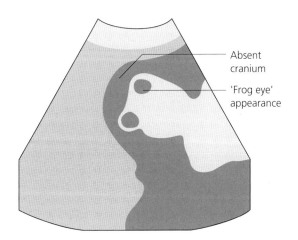

Absent cranium

'Frog eye' appearance

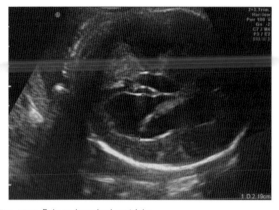

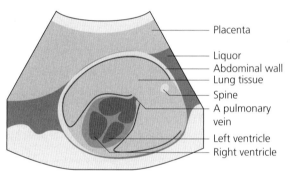

Fig. 18.8 Enlarged cerebral ventricles.

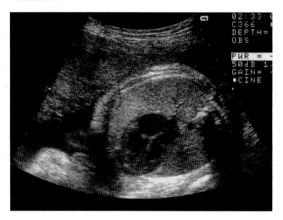

Fig. 18.9 Normal heart: transverse view of chest.

reduces the incidence of NTDs and should be taken by all women considering pregnancy. Screening at the nuchal scan shows promise (*Ultrasound Obstet Gynecol* 2010; **35**: 133), but ultrasound at 20 weeks has a sensitivity of >95%. NTDs recur in 1 in 10 pregnancies, but this risk is greatly reduced by high-dose folic acid (5 mg). Disability from NTDs may be reduced where open surgery is performed *in utero* (*NEJM* 2011; **364**: 993), but involves maternal risk.

Ventriculomegaly, particularly of the lateral ventricle (Fig. 18.8), is common and often due to NTDs, aqueduct stenosis or agenesis of the corpus callosum. The prognosis depends on the severity and the cause. Babies with isolated, mild ventriculomegaly are usually normal.

Akinesia syndromes cause abnormal posture and are often lethal. Polyhydramnios follows impaired swallowing.

Cardiac defects and fetal echocardiography

These occur in 1% of pregnancies. They are more common in women with congenital cardiac disease, diabetes, on antiepileptic medications, when previous offspring have been affected (overall recurrence risk 3%) and where other structural abnormalities or chromosomal disorders are present. In about half of major abnormalities, the nuchal translucency was increased at the 11–14-week scan. Ultrasound in expert hands can be used to diagnose prenatal cardiac disease very accurately (Fig. 18.9). This is usually at 20 weeks, but assessment is often possible at the nuchal scan. In practice, less than one-third of cases are diagnosed prenatally. Most are non-lethal; others may be correctable or partly correctable with surgery after birth. Invasive testing (amniocentesis) is usually offered to check for chromosomal abnormalities, including the 22q11 deletion. *In utero* treatment is possible for arrhythmias (e.g. digoxin, flecainide) and, occasionally, using valvoplasty for critical aortic stenosis.

In utero therapy	
Medical	Steroids to mature lungs (see Chapter 23)
	Antiarrhythmic drugs
	Non-steroidal anti-inflammatory drugs for polyhydramnios
Minimally invasive	Laser treatment for twin–twin transfusion syndrome (TTTS)
	Amnioreduction for polyhydramnios
	Pleuroamniotic shunt for hydrops/effusions
	Vesicoamniotic shunt for urethral valves
	Other shunt/drainage of a cystic lesion
	Blood/platelet transfusion
	Tracheal occlusion (FETO) for diaphragmatic hernia
	Valvoplasty for critical aortic stenosis
	Cord occlusion of monochorionic twins
Open	Neural tube defect surgery

Abdominal wall defects

Exomphalos is characterized by partial extrusion of the abdominal contents in a peritoneal sac. Fifty per cent of affected infants have a chromosomal problem and amniocentesis is offered. Isolated, small defects have a good prognosis after postnatal surgery.

Gastroschisis (Figs 18.10, 18.11) is characterized by free loops of bowel in the amniotic cavity and is rarely associated with other abnormalities. It is more common when the mother is very young. Postnatal surgery is indicated: >90% survive.

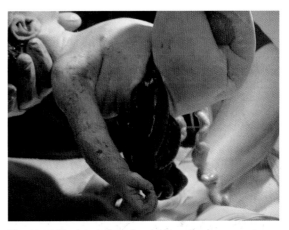

Fig. 18.11 Newborn with gastroschisis.

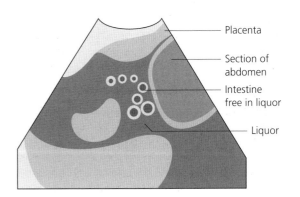

Fig. 18.10 Gastroschisis.

Placenta

Section of abdomen

Intestine free in liquor

Liquor

Chest defects

Diaphragmatic hernias cause the abdominal contents to herniate into the chest, causing pulmonary hypoplasia. Associated anomalies are common. Approximately 60% of babies with isolated defects survive; this may be improved in severe cases with *in utero* tracheal occlusion (FETO) (*Fetal Diagn Ther* 2011; **29**: 6). The trachea is plugged with a balloon that stimulates lung growth. It needs to be removed before or immediately after delivery or asphyxiation will occur.

Pleural effusions may cause pulmonary hyoplasia and hydrops. *In utero* shunting, allowing continuous drainage of accumulated fluid into the amniotic cavity, is useful (*Ultrasound Obstet Gynecol* 2010; **36**: 58).

Congenital cystic adenomatous malformations (CCAM) (Fig. 18.12) and *pulmonary sequestration* are visible as chest masses of varying sizes. *In utero* shunting is possible for large cystic lesions but many regress and the prognosis is usually good.

Gastrointestinal defects

Oesophageal atresia and tracheo-oesophageal fistulae: The stomach is non-visible or small. Other abnormalities commonly coexist. Polyhydramnios is present. Postnatal surgery is required.

Duodenal atresia causes a classic ultrasound appearance of a 'double bubble' of stomach and dilated upper duodenum. Down's syndrome is very common. Polyhydramnios occurs (Fig. 18.13).

Lower gut atresia causes dilated bowel ± polyhydramnios. Meconium ileus due to cystic fibrosis is common.

Urogenital defects

Hydronephrosis can be mild to severe, unilateral or bilateral, and due to obstruction or reflux. Children are prone to infection and therefore renal damage, and postnatal investigation is needed.

Posterior urethal valves obstruct the male urethra, causing oligohydramnios, bladder and renal dilation and damage, ranging from the lethal to renal failure in early adulthood. Treatment with *in utero* shunting is controversial (*Clin Perinatol* 2009; **36**: 377).

Skeletal defects

Skeletal dysplasia syndromes, of which there are very many (e.g. osteogenesis imperfecta), affect the limbs. Abnormalities of the digits, bone length and appearances, and the pattern of other abnormalities aid differentiation. Where lethal, e.g. thanatophoric dysplasia, the chest is frequently small.

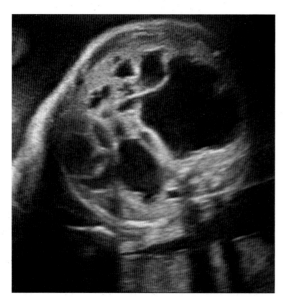
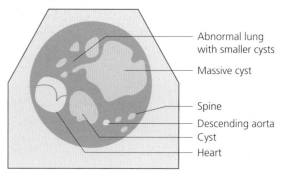

Fig. 18.12 Transverse section of fetal chest containing congenital cystic adenomatous malformation (CCAM).

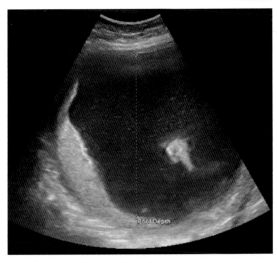

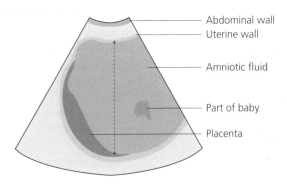

Abdominal wall
Uterine wall
Amniotic fluid
Part of baby
Placenta

Fig. 18.13 Uterus with polyhydramnios.

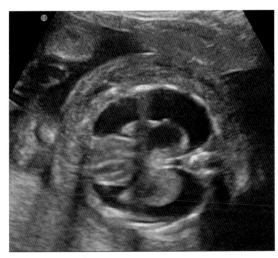

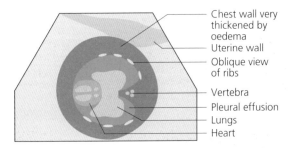

Chest wall very
thickened by
oedema
Uterine wall
Oblique view
of ribs
Vertebra
Pleural effusion
Lungs
Heart

Fig. 18.14 Fetal hydrops: pleural effusions and skin oedema in transverse section of fetal chest.

Isolated limb abnormalities are often due to 'amniotic bands', constriction deformities involving the amnion or vascular occlusion.

Facial abnormalities

Cleft lip is common and may be unilateral, bilateral or central. The palate is variably involved. Other abnormalities may coexist; this is most common with palatal abnormalities without a cleft lip, and with central clefts. Postnatal surgery is required.

Fetal hydrops

This occurs when extra fluid accumulates in two or more areas in the fetus (Figs 18.14, 18.15). It occurs in 1 in 500 pregnancies and, because of its high mortality, is rarer in late pregnancy. It can be '*immune*', due to anaemia and haemolysis as a result of antibodies including Rhesus disease. Or it can be '*non-immune*', secondary to another cause. There are five main categories of non-immune hydrops.

• *Chromosomal abnormalities* such as trisomy 21 are the most common in early pregnancy.

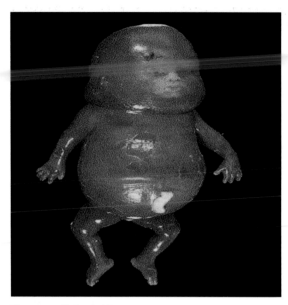

Fig. 18.15 Hydropic fetus.

- *Structural abnormalities* (e.g. pleural effusions) (see Fig. 18.14) can cause hydrops.
- *Cardiac abnormalities* or *arrhythmias* may be present.
- *Anaemia* causing cardiac failure (e.g. parvovirus infection, fetomaternal haemorrhage or fetal alpha thalassaemia major) may also be responsible.
- *Twin–twin transfusion syndrome* in monochorionic twins causes hydrops in severe cases.

Investigation involves ultrasound assessment, including echocardiography and assessment of the middle cerebral artery. Maternal blood is taken for Kleihauer and parvovirus, CMV and toxoplasmosis IgM testing. Fetal blood sampling is performed if anaemia is suspected; it or amniocentesis are performed for karyotyping. Treatment and prognosis depend on the cause: cure is only possible where anaemia (transfusion), or compression by fluid collection such as pleural effusions (vesicoamniotic shunting), or twin–twin transfusion syndrome (laser ablation) have caused hydrops.

Single gene disorders

Autosomal dominant conditions (e.g. neurofibromatosis) affect 1 in 150 live births. One affected parent has a 50% chance of passing on the condition. Many are actually new mutations: neither parent is affected, and the recurrence risk is often about 10%.

Autosomal recessive genes (e.g. cystic fibrosis or sickle cell disease) have different prevalences in different populations. If both parents are carriers, the neonate has a 1 in 4 chance of being affected by the disease, whilst half will be carriers. Detection of carrier status is possible for most cystic fibrosis genes and for haemoglobinopathies. Partners of women who have or are carriers of recessively inherited disease may be tested to see if they too are carriers. Prenatal diagnosis, usually with CVS, may then be offered.

Further reading

www.fetalmedicine.com

www.nsc.nhs.uk

ACOG Committee Opinion 2013. *The Use of Chromosomal Microarray Analysis in Prenatal Diagnosis*. Available at: www.acog.org/Resources-And-Publications/Committee-Opinions/Committee-on-Genetics/The-Use-of-Chromosomal-Microarray-Analysis-in-Prenatal-Diagnosis (accessed 13 July 2016).

Daley R, Hill M, Chitty LS. Non-invasive prenatal diagnosis: progress and potential. *Archives of Diseases in Childhood Fetal Neonatal Edition*. Available at: http://fn.bmj.com/content/early/2014/04/30/archdischild-2013-304828 (accessed 13 July 2016).

Deprest JA, Flake AW, Gratacos E, *et al*. The making of fetal surgery. *Prenatal Diagnosis* 2010; **30**: 653–667.

Manning N, Archer N. *Fetal Cardiology*. Oxford: Oxford University Press, 2009.

NHS Rapid Project. *Introduction to NIPD/NIPT: A Guide for Patients and Healthcare Professionals*. Available at: www.rapid.nhs.uk/guides-to-nipd-nipt/introduction/ (accessed 13 July 2016).

Nicolaides KH. First trimester screening for chromosomal abnormalities. *Seminars in Perinatology* 2005; **29**: 190–194.

Royal College of Obstetricians and Gynaecologists. *Amniocentesis and Chorionic Villus Sampling*. Green-top Guideline 8. Available at: www.rcog.org.uk/en/guidelines-research-services/guidelines/gtg8/ (accessed 13 July 2016).

Ultrasound in pregnancy at a glance

Definition 3.5–9.0 MHz sound waves are passed into the body; the intensity of deflection from different tissues depends on their densities: this can be represented in 2-D form or computer-reconstructed 3-D form

Obstetric First trimester In exclusion of ectopic pregnancy, assessment of pregnancy viability, detection of retained products of conception after miscarriage
Estimation of gestational age (e.g. crown–rump length at 9–12 weeks)
Detection of multiple pregnancy and determination of chorionicity.
Screening for chromosomal abnormalities (nuchal translucency).
Diagnosis of structural abnormalities

Second trimester Diagnosis of structural abnormalities
Help other diagnostic (e.g. amniocentesis) or therapeutic (e.g. transfusion) techniques.
Doppler of uterine arteries for screening for pre-eclampsia/growth restriction
Measurement of cervical length as screening test for preterm delivery

Third trimester Assessment of fetal growth
Doppler, e.g. of umbilical or middle cerebral arteries, for fetal health assessment
Doppler of middle cerebral artery (velocity) for fetal anaemia
Diagnosis of placenta praevia
Determining presentation in difficult cases

Benefits Aids diagnosis in gynaecology and first trimester. Maternal reassurance, screening for and detection of abnormalities. Reduction of perinatal mortality in high-risk pregnancy. Benefit in low-risk pregnancy mainly better diagnosis of abnormalities

Safety Extremely safe. Possible small increase in left-handedness and lower birth weight

Prenatal screening and diagnosis of congenital abnormalities at a glance

Booking Counsel all regarding prenatal diagnosis options
Check rubella immunity to identify need for postnatal immunization
Check hepatitis B to allow immunoglobulin administration to neonate
Check for syphilis infection and HIV status
Arrange genetic counselling ± later chorionic villus sampling (CVS) or amniocentesis if risk of inherited disorder

9–12 weeks Ultrasound scan to date pregnancy and identify twins
Advise regarding screening for chromosomal trisomies, e.g. combined test
Counsel and offer CVS or amniocentesis if the risk is high, or advise regarding non-invasive prenatal testing (NIPT)

18-21 weeks Routine anomaly ultrasound to detect structural abnormalities
Counsel and consider amniocentesis if abnormalities found
Offer cardiac scan if high risk

Later Some abnormalities only visible in later pregnancy: ultrasound if polyhydramnios, breech, suspected fetal intrauterine growth restriction (IUGR)

Polyhydramnios at a glance

Definition	Liquor volume increased. Normal volume varies with gestation, but deepest liquor pool >10cm generally considered abnormal	
Epidemiology	Severe in 1% of pregnancies	
Aetiology	Idiopathic; maternal disorders (established and gestational diabetes, renal failure); twins (particularly twin–twin transfusion syndrome); fetal anomaly (20%) (particularly upper gastrointestinal obstructions or inability to swallow, central nervous system, cardiac or renal chest abnormalities, myotonic dystrophy)	
Clinical features	Maternal discomfort. Large for dates, taut uterus, fetal parts difficult to palpate	
Complications	Preterm labour; maternal discomfort, abnormal lie and malpresentation	
Management	To diagnose fetal anomaly	Detailed ultrasound screening
	To diagnose diabetes	Maternal blood glucose testing
	To reduce liquor	If <34 weeks and severe, amnioreduction, or use of non-steroidal anti-inflammatory drugs (NSAIDS) to reduce fetal urine output
		Consider steroids if <34 weeks
	Delivery	Vaginal unless persistent unstable lie or other obstetric indication

CHAPTER 19
Infections in pregnancy

Infections assume a particular importance in pregnancy in several ways.

- *Maternal illness* may be worse, as with varicella.
- *Maternal complications*, as with pre-eclampsia in HIV-positive women, may be more common.
- *Preterm labour* is also associated with infection.
- *Vertical transmission* of otherwise fairly innocuous infections can cause miscarriage, can be teratogenic (e.g. rubella) or damage already developed organs. Or, as with human immunodeficiency virus (HIV) or hepatitis B, it can cause serious infection in the child. Vertical transmission occurs, or is most damaging, at different times in pregnancy with different infections.
- *Neurological damage* (in addition to the above effects) is more common in the presence of bacterial infection in both preterm and term babies.
- *Antibiotic* usage in pregnancy is occasionally limited by adverse effects to the fetus.

Viruses

Cytomegalovirus

Pathology/epidemiology: Cytomegalovirus (CMV) is a herpesvirus that is transmitted by personal contact. About 35% of women in the UK are immune. Up to 1% of women develop CMV infection, usually subclinical, in pregnancy. CMV is a common cause of childhood handicap and deafness.

Fetal/neonatal effects: Vertical transmission to the fetus occurs in 40%. Approximately 10% of infected neonates are symptomatic at birth, with intrauterine growth restriction (IUGR), pneumonia and thrombocytopenia; most of these will develop severe neurological sequelae such as hearing, visual and mental impairment, or will die. The asymptomatic neonates are at risk (15%) of deafness.

Diagnosis: Ultrasound abnormalities such as intracranial or hepatic calcification are evident in only 20%, and most infections are diagnosed when CMV testing is specifically requested. CMV immunoglobulin M (IgM) remains positive for a long time after infection, which could predate the pregnancy; titres will rise and IgG avidity will be low with a recent infection. If maternal infection is confirmed, amniocentesis at least 6 weeks after maternal infection will confirm or refute vertical transmission.

Management: Most infected neonates are still not seriously affected; close surveillance for ultrasound abnormalities may help determine those at most risk for severe sequelae. There is no prenatal treatment, and termination may be offered. Because most maternal infections do not result in neonatal sequelae and amniocentesis involves risk, routine screening is not advised. Vaccination is not available.

Herpes simplex

Pathology/epidemiology: The type 2 DNA virus is responsible for most genital herpes (Figs 19.1, 19.2). Less than 5% of pregnant women have a history of prior infection, but many more have antibodies.

Fetal/neonatal effects: Herpes simplex is not teratogenic. Neonatal infection is rare, but has a high mortality. Vertical transmission occurs at vaginal delivery, particularly if vesicles are present. This is most likely to follow recent primary maternal infection (risk 40%), because the fetus will not have passive immunity from maternal antibodies.

Obstetrics & Gynaecology, Fifth Edition. Lawrence Impey, Tim Child.
© 2017 John Wiley & Sons, Ltd. Published 2017 by John Wiley & Sons, Ltd.

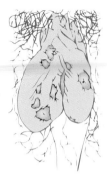

Fig. 19.1 Genital herpes simplex.

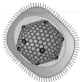

| Herpes simplex virus (HSV) | Cold sores (type 1) Genital herpes (type 2) |
| Cytomegalovirus (CMV) | Cytomegalic inclusion disease in neonates |

Fig. 19.2 Herpesvirus.

Diagnosis: This is usually clear clinically and swabs are of little use in pregnancy.

Management: Referral to a genitourinary clinic is indicated. Caesarean section is recommended for those delivering within 6 weeks of a primary attack, and for those with genital lesions from primary infection at the time of delivery. The risk is very low in women with recurrent herpes who have vesicles present at the time of labour, and caesarean delivery is not recommended. Daily aciclovir in late pregnancy may reduce the frequency of recurrences at term. Exposed neonates are given aciclovir. Screening is of little benefit.

Herpes zoster

Pathology/epidemiology: Primary infection with this DNA herpesvirus causes chickenpox, a common childhood illness; reactivation of latent infection is shingles, which usually affects adults in one or two dermatomes. A woman who is not immune to zoster can develop chickenpox after exposure to chickenpox or shingles. Chickenpox in pregnancy is rare (0.03%), but can cause severe maternal illness.

Fetal/neonatal effects: Teratogenicity is a rare (1–2%) consequence of early pregnancy infection, which is immediately treated with oral aciclovir. Maternal infection in the 4 weeks preceding delivery can cause severe neonatal infection; this is most common (up to 50%) if delivery occurs within 5 days after or 2 days before maternal symptoms.

Management: Immunoglobulin is used to prevent, and aciclovir to treat infection. Therefore, pregnant women exposed to zoster are tested for immunity; immunoglobulin is recommended within 10 days if they are non-immune, and aciclovir if infection occurs. In late pregnancy, neonates delivered 5 days after or 2 days before maternal infection are given immunoglobulin, closely monitored and given aciclovir if infection occurs. Vaccination is possible but not universal.

Infections suitable for screening		
Syphilis		
Hepatitis B		
Rubella		
Probably:	*Chlamydia*	
	Bacterial vaginosis	
	Beta-haemolytic streptococcus	

Teratogenic infections
Cytomegalovirus (CMV)
Rubella
Toxoplasmosis
Syphilis
Herpes zoster (rare)

Rubella

Pathology/epidemiology: The rubella virus usually affects children and causes a mild febrile illness with a macular rash, which is often called 'German measles'. Congenital rubella is very rare in UK women because of widespread immunization: <10 affected neonates are born each year (*BMJ* 1999; **7186**: 769). Immunity is lifelong.

Fetal/neonatal effects: Maternal infection in early pregnancy frequently causes multiple fetal abnormalities, including deafness, cardiac disease, eye problems and mental retardation. The probability and severity of malformation decrease with advancing gestation: at 9 weeks the risk is 90%; after 16 weeks, the risk is very low.

Management/screening: If a non-immune woman develops rubella before 16 weeks' gestation, termination of pregnancy is offered. Screening remains routine at booking to identify those in need of vaccination after the end of pregnancy. Rubella vaccine is live and contraindicated in pregnancy, although harm has not been recorded.

Parvovirus

Epidemiology: The B19 virus infects 0.25% of pregnant women, and more during epidemics; 50% of women are immune. A 'slapped cheek' appearance (erythema infectiosum) is classic but many have arthralgia or are asymptomatic. Infection is usually from children.

Neonatal/fetal effects: The virus suppresses fetal erythropoiesis causing anaemia. Variable degrees of thrombocytopenia also occur. Fetal death occurs in about 10% of pregnancies, usually with infection before 20 weeks' gestation.

Diagnosis: Where maternal exposure or symptoms have occurred, positive maternal IgM testing will prompt fetal surveillance. Anaemia is detectable on ultrasound, initially as increased blood flow velocity in the fetal middle cerebral artery and subsequently as oedema (fetal hydrops) from cardiac failure. Or maternal testing may follow the identification of fetal hydrops. Spontaneous resolution of anaemia and hydrops occurs in about 50%.

Management: Mothers infected are scanned regularly to look for anaemia. Where hydrops is detected, *in utero* transfusion is given if this is severe. Survivors have an excellent prognosis although very severe disease has been associated with neurological damage (*Obstet Gynecol* 2007; **109**: 42).

Hepatitis B

Pathology/epidemiology: This is caused by a small DNA virus, transmitted by blood products or sexual activity. Infection resolves in 90% of adults, but in 10% persistent infection occurs. This infectious state is present in 1% of pregnant women in the West but in up to 25% of women in, or from, parts of Asia and Africa. The degree of infectivity depends on antibody status: individuals with the 'surface' antibody (HBsAb positive) are immunologically cured and of low infectivity to others and their fetus. Those with the surface antigen but not the antibody (HBsAg positive) and those with the E antigen (HBeAg positive) are more infectious.

Neonatal effects: Vertical transmission occurs at delivery. Importantly, 90% of infected neonates become chronic carriers, compared to only 10% of infected adults.

Management/screening: Because high-risk groups encompass only 50% of chronic carriers, maternal screening is routine in the UK. Neonatal immunization (*BMJ* 2006; **332**: 328) reduces the risk of infection by >90% and is given to all positive women. In addition, women with a high viral load are treated with antiviral agents from 32 weeks, with additional passive immunization given postnatally to the neonate. Known carriers should be handled with sensitive precautions to avoid infecting staff.

Hepatitis C

In the UK, about 0.5% of pregnant women are infected, although worldwide the incidence is 3%, and 30% in HIV-positive women. Risk factors are drug abuse and sexual transmission: the latter is the more common route worldwide. Hepatitis C leads to chronic hepatitis in about 80% but most pregnant women are asymptomatic. Vertical transmission of HCV occurs in 3–5% but is higher with higher viral loads and with coexisting HIV infection. Elective caesarean section, avoidance of breast feeding, and administration of immune globulin do not reduce vertical transmission to the neonate. Screening is restricted to high-risk groups, e.g. HIV positive.

Human immunodeficiency virus

Epidemiology: In the UK, approximately 1000 pregnancies a year are infected by the retroviruses (Fig. 19.3) that cause acquired immune deficiency syndrome (AIDS). In parts of Africa and Asia, rates of infection are nearly 40%. Heterosexual transmission is now the most important route with a risk of <1% per episode of sexual intercourse.

Maternal effects: Pregnancy does not hasten progression to AIDS. The incidence of pre-eclampsia is greater in HIV-infected women, and this may be increased by antiretroviral therapy (*Lancet* 2002; **360**: 1152). Gestational diabetes may also be more common.

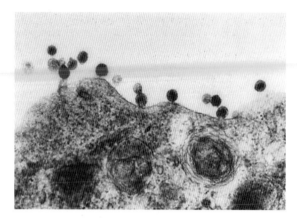

Fig. 19.3 Electron micrograph of HIV virus. Source: Rogstad K. *ABC of STIs*, 6th edn. Reproduced with permission of John Wiley & Sons Ltd.

Neonatal/fetal effects: Stillbirth, pre-eclampsia, growth restriction and prematurity are more common. Congenital abnormalities are not, and antiretrovirals are not teratogenic. The most important risk is of vertical transmission. This is mostly beyond 36 weeks, intrapartum or during breastfeeding. It occurs in 15% in the absence of preventive measures, and in up to 40% of breastfeeding women in Africa, although passively acquired antibodies in the neonate are universal because of transplacental transfer. Transmission is greater with low CD4 counts and high viral load (early and late-stage disease), coexistent infection, premature delivery and during labour, particularly with ruptured membranes for more than 4 hours. Twenty-five per cent of HIV-infected neonates develop AIDS by 1 year and 40% will develop AIDS by 5 years.

Management/screening: Screening in the UK is universal. HIV-positive women should be managed in conjunction with a physician and have regular CD4 and viral load tests. Genital tract infections such as chlamydia should be sought. Prophylaxis against *Pneumocystis carinii* pneumonia (PCP) is given if the CD4 count is low. Drug toxicity is monitored with liver and renal function, haemoglobin and blood glucose testing.

Strategies to prevent vertical transmission unfortunately need to differ according to the social and economic circumstances of the population. This is because of the cost of medication and complications of obstetric intervention, and the benefits of breastfeeding in an under-resourced population. The 'ideal' policy is highly active antiretroviral therapy (HAART), which reduces

viraemia (Fig. 19.4) and maternal disease progression. This is continued throughout pregnancy and delivery, and the neonate is treated for the first 6 weeks. When women are not receiving pre-pregnancy treatment, therapy is started around 28 weeks: Therapy is modified if viraemia is not suppressed. Caesarean section is recommended if the viral load is above 50 copies/mL, and if there is coexistent hepatitis C infection. Breastfeeding is avoided. This 'best' strategy reduces vertical transmission to <1%.

In under-resourced countries, nevirapine, as single doses in labour and to the neonate, greatly reduces vertical transmission in women delivering vaginally. Amniotomy is deferred. Breastfeeding is still advised but should be exclusive, limited to 6 months, and with antiviral prophylaxis. A policy of formula feeding under these conditions, whilst associated with a slightly lower vertical transmission rate than breastfeeding with zidovudine prophylaxis, is associated with a higher mortality (*JAMA* 2006; **296**: 794).

Vertical transmission still occurs, even in resourced countries, and at 20–30% in developing countries, largely because of lack of knowledge of HIV status and poor access to healthcare.

Methods to prevent vertical transmission of HIV
Maternal antiretroviral therapy
Elective caesarean section
Avoidance of breastfeeding
Neonatal antiretroviral therapy

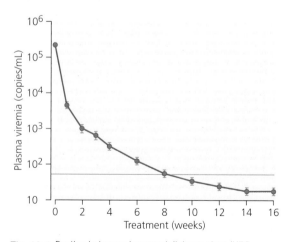

Fig. 19.4 Decline in human immunodeficiency virus (HIV) particles with highly active antiretroviral therapy (HAART).

Influenza

Pathology/epidemiology: In the US and northern Europe, influenza A H3N2 was predominant in the 2014–15 season; influenza A H1N1 the previous season. Influenza B strains are also seen.

Maternal effects: The pandemic influenza A H1N1 ('swine flu') strain particularly affects pregnant women, especially those with comorbidity including obesity: during the 2009–10 pandemic, 12% of pregnancy-related deaths in the US could be attributed to the virus (*Obstet Gynecol* 2015; **126**(3): 486–490); a similar percentage was reported in the UK.

Neonatal effects: There are no known adverse effects. The benefits include improved maternal, and therefore fetal, safety and postnatal passive immunity.

Management/immunization: Where symptoms are present, the diagnosis should be considered, oseltamivir prescribed and admission considered, particularly where there are respiratory symptoms. Seasonal, yearly vaccination with an inactivated vaccine is strongly recommended for pregnant women at any gestation, for healthcare workers and for vulnerable groups. The vaccine must be active against the current strain.

ZIKA

The ZIKA virus was declared a public health emergency of international concern in 2016, following outbreaks in multiple countries including northern South America, particularly Brazil, Africa and South Asia. All cases in northern Europe have been imported. A likely link with fetal central nervous system (CNS) abnormalities, manifest as intracranial calcification, ventriculomegaly and microcephaly, has recently been made with maternal infection, largely in the first and second trimester.

The ZIKA virus is transmitted by the *Aedes* mosquito which, in contrast to the malaria vector, is active in the day and therefore best protected against by repellent rather than nets. Maternal symptoms are mild and include a rash and fever, but also Guillain–Barré syndrome. The virus can be detected by polymerase chain reaction (PCR) but antibody testing is currently unreliable due to cross-reactivity. Pregnant women should be advised not to travel to countries affected by outbreaks. Those returning, particularly with or following suggestive symptoms, should have fetal assessment for CNS abnormalities. As no treatment is currently available, termination can be offered to women with clearly affected fetuses.

Bacteria, parasites and others

Group A streptococcus

This is the bacterium traditionally responsible for puerperal sepsis. In the UK, it is the most common bacterium associated with maternal death, of which sepsis is a leading direct cause. Group A streptococcus, or *Streptococcus pyogenes*, is carried by 5–30% of people; the most common symptom of infection is a sore throat. Infection during, as opposed to after, pregnancy is usually from children, with maternal hand to perineal contamination. Chorioamnionitis with abdominal pain, diarrhoea and severe sepsis may occur. The infected fetus often dies *in utero* and labour will usually then ensue. Early recognition, cultures and high-dose antibiotics ± intensive care in severe cases are required. The management of severe sepsis is covered in the Obstetric management section.

Group B streptococcus

Pathology/epidemiology: The bacterium *Streptococcus agalactiae* (Fig. 19.5) is carried, without symptoms, by about 25% of pregnant women.

Neonatal effects: The fetus can be infected, normally during labour after the membranes have ruptured. This is most common with preterm labours, if labour is prolonged or there is a maternal fever. Early-onset neonatal group B streptococcus (GBS) sepsis occurs in 0.35/1000 neonates in the UK. It causes severe illness and has a mortality of 6% in term infants and 18% in preterm infants.

Management/screening: Vertical transmission can be mostly prevented by high–dose intravenous penicillin

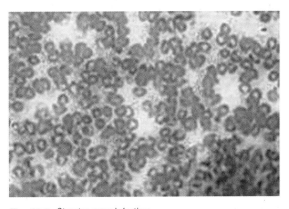

Fig. 19.5 *Streptococcus* infection.

throughout labour. Policies differ in different countries: in the US (Strategy 2) universal screening is recommended; in the UK, currently, it is not. In the UK, treatment is used merely if risk factors for vertical transmission of GBS are present, or if GBS is found incidentally (Strategy 1).

• *Strategy 1*: in the UK, screening is not recommended because of fears of anaphylaxis, and the relatively low incidence of disease in the UK. Treatment is restricted to those with risk factors: a previous affected neonate, positive urinary culture for GBS, preterm labour, rupture of the membranes for >18 hours and a maternal fever in labour. In addition, treatment is usual for incidental GBS carriage. An unfortunate result of UK policy is greatly increased prophylactic administration of antibiotics to newborns.

• *Strategy 2*: screening is the most effective practice, reducing early-onset neonatal GBS sepsis by about 80%. Cultures from both vagina and anus are taken at 35–37 weeks. Antibiotics are given to culture-positive women and to those who have had a positive urine culture for GBS, those with an infant previously affected by GBS, and those who develop clinical risk factors (see below) for GBS disease.

Prevention of vertical transmission of group B streptococcus	
Strategy 1: risk factors	No screening
	Treat with intravenous penicillin in labour if:
	Previous history
	Intrapartum fever >38°C
	Current preterm labour
	Rupture of the membranes >18 h
Strategy 2: screening	Vaginal and rectal swab at 35–37 weeks
	Treat with intravenous penicillin in labour if swabs positive or risk factors present

Syphilis

This sexually transmitted infection due to *Treponema pallidum* is rare (0.02%) in pregnant women in the UK,

although endemic in developing countries. Active disease in pregnancy usually causes miscarriage, severe congenital disease or stillbirth. Prompt treatment with benzylpenicillin is safe and will prevent, but not reverse, fetal damage. Therefore screening tests, such as the Venereal Disease Research Laboratories (VDRL) test, which are cheap and accurate, are still in routine use. False positives occur particularly with autoimmune disease and the diagnosis should be confirmed using *Treponema*-specific tests.

Toxoplasmosis

Pathology/epidemiology: This is due to the protozoan parasite *Toxoplasma gondii*. It follows contact with cat faeces or soil, or eating infected meat. In the UK, 20% of adults have antibodies; infection in pregnancy occurs in 0.2% of women in the UK, but it is more common in mainland Europe.

Fetal/neonatal effects: Fetal infection follows in about 30%; this is more common as pregnancy progresses, but earlier infection is more likely to result in severe sequelae. These include mental handicap, convulsions, spasticities and visual impairment (<10 per year in the UK).

Diagnosis: Ultrasound may show hydrocephalus, but maternal infection is usually diagnosed after maternal testing for IgM is performed because of exposure or anxiety. False positives and negatives are common. Vertical transmission is diagnosed or excluded using amniocentesis performed after 20 weeks.

Management: Health education, for example washing hands after contact with soil or cat litter, reduces the risk of maternal infection. Spiramycin is started as soon as maternal toxoplasmosis is diagnosed. If vertical transmission is subsequently confirmed, additional combination therapy of pyrimethamine and sulfadiazine with folinic acid is used, though termination may be requested. Whilst this protocol probably improves the prognosis for the neonate, this remains debated. Screening is not recommended where the prevalence is low.

Mycobacterium tuberculosis

Worldwide, tuberculosis (TB) is very common, and its incidence in the UK is increasing because of immigration, HIV infection and travel. Tuberculin testing is safe; Bacille bilié de Calmette–Guérin (BCG) vaccination is live and contraindicated. Diagnosis in late pregnancy is associated with prematurity and intrauterine growth retardation (IUGR), and TB is a significant cause of maternal mortality in the developing world. Treatment with first-line drugs and additional vitamin B6 is safe in pregnancy, but streptomycin is contraindicated. Congenital TB is very rare in the UK.

Malaria

Although rare in the UK, malaria infection is very common in developing countries: in sub-Saharan Africa 8% of infant mortality is attributed to it. Maternal complications, including severe anaemia, are more frequent in pregnancy, and IUGR and stillbirth are more common. Congenital malaria complicates 1% of affected pregnancies. Drug usage is dictated by local sensitivity, but most falciparum malaria is resistant to chloroquine or mefloquine, and artemisin combination therapy (ACT) is increasingly used and appears safe (*Mal J* 2007; **6**: 15). Following the diagnosis, surveillance of growth restriction is required. Prevention of maternal and neonatal effects involves intermittent preventive treatment (IPT) of two doses at least a month apart, insecticide-impregnated mosquito nets and appropriate drug treatment.

Listeriosis

Listeria monocytogenes, a Gram-positive bacillus, infection can follow consumption of pâtés, soft cheeses and prepacked meals, and causes a non-specific febrile illness. If bacteraemia occurs in pregnancy (0.01% of women), potentially fatal infection of the fetus may follow. The diagnosis is established from blood cultures. Screening is impractical. Prevention involves the widely publicized avoidance of high-risk foods in pregnancy.

Chlamydia and gonorrhoea

Chlamydia trachomatis infection in pregnancy in the UK occurs in about 5% of women and *Neisseria gonorrhoeae* in 0.1%. Most women are asymptomatic. Although best known as causes of pelvic inflammatory disease and subfertility, both have been associated with preterm labour and with neonatal conjunctivitis. Chlamydia is treated with azithromycin or erythromycin; tetracyclines cause fetal tooth discoloration.

Gonorrhoea is treated with cephalosporins as resistance to penicillin is common. Screening and treatment are worthwhile in developing countries, before termination of pregnancy and in women with a history of preterm labour: treatment may reduce the incidence of preterm birth.

Bacterial vaginosis

This common overgrowth of normal vaginal lactobacilli by anaerobes such as *Gardnerella vaginalis* and *Mycoplasma hominis* can be asymptomatic or cause an offensive vaginal discharge in women. Preterm labour and late miscarriage are more common. Screening and treatment (best with oral clindamycin) reduce the risk of preterm birth if used before 20 weeks (*Cochrane* 2007; CD 000262) in women with a history of preterm birth.

Other obstetric infections

Urinary tract infections and pyelonephritis (see Chapters 8 and 20).
Endometritis (see Chapter 10).
Chorioamnionitis (see Chapter 23).

Further reading

ACOG Committee Opinion No. 485. Prevention of early-onset group B streptococcal disease in newborns. *Obstetrics and Gynecology* 2011; **117**(4): 1019–1027. Available at: www.ncbi.nlm.nih.gov/pubmed/21422882 (accessed 15 July 2016).

British HIV Association. *British HIV Association Guidelines for the Management of HIV Infection in Pregnant Women 2012 (2014 Interim Review)*. Available at: www.bhiva.org/documents/Guidelines/Pregnancy/2012/BHIVA-Pregnancy-guidelines-update-2014.pdf (accessed 15 July 2016).

Dellinger P, Levy MM, Rhodes A, et al. Surviving Sepsis Campaign: International Guidelines for Management of Severe Sepsis and Septic Shock. *Available at:* www.sccm.org/Documents/SSC-Guidelines.pdf *(accessed 15 July 2016).*

Lamberth J, Reddy S, Pan J, Dasher K. Chronic hepatitis B infection in pregnancy. *World Journal of Hepatology* 2015; **7**(9): 1233–1237.

Lamont RF, Sobel JD, Vaisbuch E, et al. Parvovirus B19 infection in human pregnancy. *BJOG* 2011; **118**: 175–186.

MBRRACE-UK. *Saving Lives, Improving Mothers' Care.* Available at: www.npeu.ox.ac.uk/mbrrace-uk/reports (accessed 15 July 2016).

Mnyani CN, McIntyre JA. Tuberculosis in pregnancy. *BJOG* 2011; **118**: 226–231.

Royal College of Obstetricians and Gynaecologists. *Chickenpox in Pregnancy.* Green-top Guideline No. 13. Available at: www.rcog.org.uk/globalassets/documents/guidelines/gtg13.pdf (accessed 15 July 2016).

Royal College of Obstetricians and Gynaecologists. *The Prevention of Early-onset Neonatal Group B Streptococcal Disease*, 2nd edn. Green-top Guideline No. 36. Available at: www.rcog.org.uk/globalassets/documents/guidelines/gtg_36.pdf (accessed 15 July 2016).

Royal College of Obstetricians and Gynaecologists. *The Diagnosis and Treatment of Malaria in Pregnancy.* Green-Top Guideline 54B. Available at: www.rcog.org.uk/globalassets/documents/guidelines/gtg-54bdiagnosistreatmentmalariapregnancy0810.pdf (accessed 15 July 2016).

Royal College of Obstetricians and Gynaecologists/BASSH. *Management of Genital Herpes in Pregnancy.* Available at: www.rcog.org.uk/globalassets/documents/guidelines/genitalherpesotherguideline.pdf (accessed 15 July 2016).

Society of Obstetricians and Gynaecologists of Canada. *Toxoplasmosis in Pregnancy: Prevention, Screening, and Treatment. Clinical Practice Guideline No. 285.* Available at:http://sogc.org/wp-content/uploads/2013/02/gui285CPG1301E-Toxoplasmosis.pdf (accessed 15 July 2016).

Yinon Y, Farine D, Yudin M. Screening, diagnosis, and management of cytomegalovirus infection in pregnancy. *Obstetrics and Gynecology Survey* 2010; **65**(11): 736–743.

HIV in pregnancy at a glance

Epidemiology	Approx. 1000 pregnancies/year in UK; >10 million worldwide
Maternal effects	Pre-eclampsia. Disease progression not faster
Fetal effects	Prematurity, intrauterine growth restriction (IUGR), stillbirth
	Vertical transmission: <1% with best prophylaxis, 15% with none, up to 40% if under-resourced area and breastfeeding. Increased by early/late disease, high CD4 or low viral load, prematurity, other infection, labour, long rupture of membranes, breastfeeding
Management	If resources available: combination therapy (continue or start at 28 weeks), elective caesarean section if viral load not very low, avoid breastfeeding, treat neonate for 6 weeks. Screen for other infections
	If poor resources: nevirapine during labour and for breastfeeding

Infections in pregnancy at a glance

Cytomegalovirus (CMV)	1% maternal infection rate, 40% vertical transmission. Maternal diagnosis from IgM, IgG avidity. Fetal diagnosis from amniocentesis at 20+ weeks. 10% of infected fetuses severely affected, deafness common. No treatment, screening or vaccination
Rubella	Most women immune, so rare. High percentage of fetuses affected if <16 weeks: termination of pregnancy (TOP) offered. Screening identifies those in need of postnatal immunization

(Continued)

Infections in pregnancy at a glance (Continued)

Toxoplasmosis	0.2% maternal infection rate (UK). Low percentage of fetuses permanently affected. Screening not routine in the UK. Maternal diagnosis from IgM; fetal from amniocentesis at 20+ weeks. Proven infection treated with spiramycin; fetal toxoplasmosis treated with combination therapy
Syphilis	Rare. Screening routine because treatment prevents congenital syphilis
Herpes simplex virus (HSV)	Common. Neonatal infection is rare but serious. High risk of neonatal herpes (therefore caesarean is indicated) if primary infection <6 weeks of delivery. Aciclovir used
Group B streptococcus	25% maternal carrier rate; major cause of severe neonatal illness. Treatment with intrapartum penicillin of high-risk groups ± positive third trimester screen greatly reduces neonatal infection
Group A streptococcus	Common cause of sore throat, occasionally causes: (1) severe illness in pregnancy with chorioamnionitis or (2) puerperal sepsis. Treatment with antibiotics ± supportive therapy
Herpes zoster	Many immune. Severe maternal illness in pregnancy. Infection <20 weeks occasionally teratogenic. Infection around delivery can cause severe neonatal infection, so IgG given to neonate
Hepatitis B	Carriage common in high-risk women. High transmission rate, high chronic disease rate and mortality in neonate. Universal screening identifies neonates in need of immunoglobulin
Hepatitis C	Mostly in high-risk (e.g. human immunodeficiency virus [HIV]) women: 6% vertical transmission
Chlamydia	5% in pregnancy. Neonatal conjunctivitis and preterm labour. Antibiotics may prevent latter, so screening probably worthwhile
Influenza	Major recent cause (approx. 10%) of maternal mortality, so seasonal vaccination essential
Bacterial vaginosis	Common. Associated with preterm labour. Screening and treatment if previous preterm labour
Parvovirus	0.25%, more in epidemics. 10% excess fetal death, most with infection pre-20 weeks. Fetus develops anaemia and subsequent hydrops. If IgM positive, surveillance for anaemia with middle cerebral artery Doppler and ultrasound. In utero transfusion if anaemia very severe

CHAPTER 20

Hypertensive disorders in pregnancy

Normal blood pressure changes in pregnancy

Blood pressure is dependent on systemic vascular resistance and cardiac output. It normally falls to a minimum level in the second trimester, by about 30/15 mmHg, because of reduced vascular resistance. This occurs in both normotensive and chronically hypertensive women. By term, the blood pressure again rises to pre-pregnant levels (Fig. 20.1). Hypertension due to pre-eclampsia is largely caused by an increase in systemic vascular resistance. Protein excretion in normal pregnancy is increased, but in the absence of underlying renal disease is less than 0.3 g/24 h.

Classification of hypertensive disorders in pregnancy

Pregnancy-induced hypertension

This is when the blood pressure rises above 140/90 mmHg after 20 weeks. It can be due to either pre-eclampsia or transient hypertension. *Pre-eclampsia* is a disorder in which hypertension and proteinuria (>0.3 g/24 h) appear in the second half of pregnancy, often with oedema. Eclampsia, or the occurrence of epileptiform seizures, is simply the most dramatic complication of many. Occasionally, proteinuria is absent, for example in early disease, when it is not always distinguishable from *gestational hypertension*, which is new hypertension presenting after 20 weeks without proteinuria.

Pre-existing or chronic hypertension

This is present when the blood pressure is more than 140/90 mmHg before pregnancy or before 20 weeks' gestation, or the woman is already on antihypertensive medication. This may be *primary hypertension*, or it may be *secondary* to renal or other disease. There may also be pre-existing proteinuria because of renal disease. Patients with underlying hypertension are at an increased risk (sixfold) of 'superimposed' pre-eclampsia.

Classification of hypertension	
Pregnancy induced	Pre-eclampsia
	Gestational
Pre-existing	Primary
	Secondary

Pre-eclampsia

Definitions and classification

Pre-eclampsia is a multisystem syndrome that is usually manifest as new hypertension after 20 weeks with significant proteinuria. It is peculiar to pregnancy, of placental origin and cured only by delivery. Blood vessel endothelial cell damage leads to vasospasm, increased capillary permeability and clotting dysfunction. Both the fetus and mother are at risk, although the clinical manifestations vary considerably. Hypertension is just a sign rather than the disease itself; both it and

Obstetrics & Gynaecology, Fifth Edition. Lawrence Impey, Tim Child.
© 2017 John Wiley & Sons, Ltd. Published 2017 by John Wiley & Sons, Ltd.

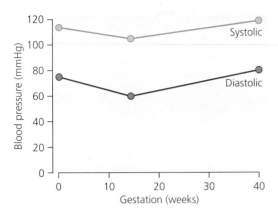

Fig. 20.1 Blood pressure changes in pregnancy.

proteinuria can be, despite the presence of other manifestations. absent until late stages; proteinuria can be absent in early disease. Although traditionally central to *establishing* the diagnosis, one or other or even both of these features may nevertheless initially be absent in a woman who clearly has the pathological process of pre-eclampsia.

Two indistinct phenotypes exist.

- *'Early-onset'* pre-eclampsia is that which causes complications before 34 weeks. Typically the fetus is growth restricted.

- *'Late-onset'* pre-eclampsia, manifest at any later gestation, is not usually associated with growth restriction, although fetal death or damage may also occur.

Pathophysiology

The mechanism is incompletely understood but has two principal steps.

The first step comprises poor placental perfusion. In normal pregnancy, trophoblastic invasion of spiral arterioles leads to vasodilatation of vessel walls to allow adequate placental perfusion (Fig. 20.2). In early-onset pre-eclampsia, this is incomplete, causing oxidative stress. The effects of this process can be detected as a high-resistance flow in uterine arteries. In late-onset pre-eclampsia, as growth of an apparently normal placental reaches its limits, intervillous perfusion may reduce, perhaps because terminals become overcrowded, also causing oxidative stress (*Placenta* 2014; **35** Suppl: S20–25).

The second step: Both mechanisms cause the oxidatively stressed placenta to oversecrete proteins that regulate angiogenic balance. This can be detected as increased soluble fms-like tyrosine kinase (sFlt-1) and reduced placental growth factor (PlGF) levels in maternal blood. Widespread endothelial cell damage

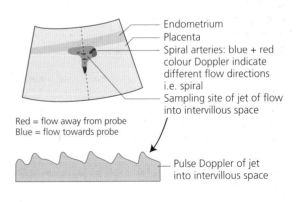

Fig. 20.2 Ultrasound of the maternal–placental interface. Red: flow away from probe; blue: flow towards probe.

may follow, causing vasoconstriction, increased vascular permeability and clotting dysfunction. These cause the clinical manifestations of the disease.

Classification and degrees of pre-eclampsia

Pre-eclampsia is new hypertension presenting after 20 weeks with significant proteinuria.

Severe pre-eclampsia is pre-eclampsia with severe hypertension and/or with symptoms, and/or biochemical and/or haematological impairment.

Hypertension is classified as mild (140/90–149/99 mmHg), moderate (150/100–159/109 mmHg) or severe (160/110+ mmHg)	
Classifications of pre-eclampsia vary: the ones below encompass the principles and diversity of the disease	
Classification based on manifestations (NICE 2010)	
Mild or moderate	Pre-eclampsia without severe hypertension and no symptoms and no biochemical or haematological impairment
Severe	Pre-eclampsia with severe hypertension and/or with symptoms, and/or biochemical and/or haematological impairment.
Classification based on timing of manifestations	
Early	<34 weeks
Late	>34 weeks

Epidemiology

Pre-eclampsia variably affects 6% of nulliparous women. It is less common in multiparous women unless additional risk factors are present. There is an approximately 15% recurrence rate; this is up to 50% if there has been severe pre-eclampsia before 28 weeks.

Risk factors and indications for low-dose aspirin from early pregnancy
High risk: aspirin if any of:
• hypertensive disease during a previous pregnancy
• chronic kidney disease
• autoimmune disease such as systemic lupus erythematosus or antiphospholipid syndrome
• type I or II diabetes
• chronic hypertension

Moderate risk: aspirin if >1 of:
• nulliparous
• age ≥40 years
• pregnancy interval of more than 10 years
• body mass index (BMI) of >35 at booking
• family history of pre-eclampsia
• multiple pregnancy

Aetiology

Predisposing factors include nulliparity, a previous or family history of pre-eclampsia, long interpregnancy interval, obesity, extremes of maternal age (particularly >40 years), disorders characterized by microvascular disease (chronic hypertension, chronic renal disease, sickle cell disease, diabetes, autoimmune disease, particularly antiphospholipid syndrome) and pregnancies with a large placenta (twins, fetal hydrops, molar pregnancy).

Assessment of urinary protein		
Dipsticks (bedside)	Trace	Seldom significant
	1+	Possible significant proteinuria: quantify
	≥2+	Significant proteinuria likely: quantify
Protein:creatinine ratio (PCR)	>30 mg/nmol	Confirmed significant proteinuria
24 h collection	>0.3 g/24 h	Confirmed significant proteinuria

HELLP syndrome	
1 H (haemolysis)	Dark urine, raised lactic dehydrogenase (LDH), anaemia
2 EL (elevated liver enzymes)	Epigastric pain, liver failure, abnormal clotting
3 LP (low platelets)	Normally self-limiting

Clinical features

History: Pre-eclampsia is usually asymptomatic, but headache, drowsiness, visual disturbances, nausea/vomiting or epigastric pain may occur at a late stage.

Examination: Hypertension is usually the first sign, but it is occasionally absent until the late stages. Oedema is found in most pregnancies but in pre-eclampsia may be massive, not postural or of sudden onset.

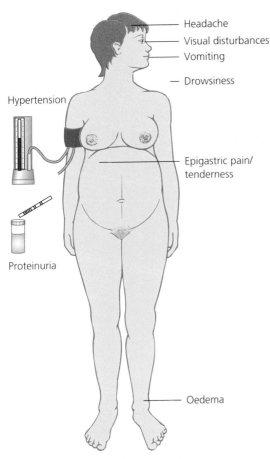

Headache
Visual disturbances
Vomiting
Drowsiness
Hypertension
Epigastric pain/
tenderness
Proteinuria
Oedema

Fig. 20.3 Clinical features of pre-eclampsia.

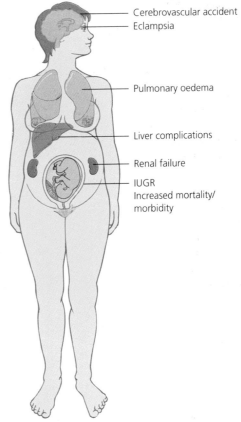

Cerebrovascular accident
Eclampsia
Pulmonary oedema
Liver complications
Renal failure
IUGR
Increased mortality/
morbidity

Fig. 20.4 Complications of pre-eclampsia. IUGR, intrauterine growth retardation.

The presence of epigastric tenderness is suggestive of impending complications. Urine dipstick testing for protein should be considered part of the clinical examination (Fig. 20.3).

Complications of pre-eclampsia (Fig. 20.4)

Maternal

Early-onset disease is often more severe. The occurrence of any of the following complications, which may occur together, is an indication for delivery whatever the gestation. They may also occur postpartum as it takes at least 24 hours for delivery to 'cure' the disease. *Eclampsia* is grand mal seizures (0.03% of all pregnancies in UK), probably resulting from cerebrovascular vasospasm. Mortality can result from hypoxia and concomitant complications of severe disease. Treatment is

with magnesium sulphate and intensive surveillance for other complications.

Cerebrovascular haemorrhage (Fig. 20.5) results from a failure of cerebral blood flow autoregulation at mean arterial pressures above 140 mmHg. Treatment of hypertension should prevent this.

Liver and coagulation problems: HELLP syndrome consists of haemolysis (H), elevated liver enzymes (EL) and low platelet count (LP). Disseminated intravascular coagulation (DIC), liver failure and liver rupture may also occur. The woman typically experiences severe epigastric pain; occasionally this is the presenting feature of pre-eclampsia, and it may occur postnatally in a hitherto well woman. Haemolysis turns the urine dark. Treatment is supportive and includes magnesium sulphate prophylaxis against eclampsia. Liver infarction or subcapsular haemorrhage may occur. Intensive care therapy is required in severe cases.

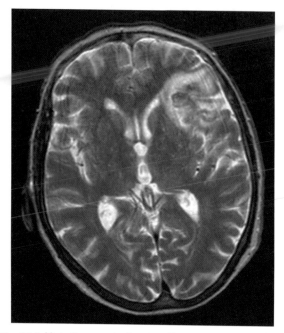

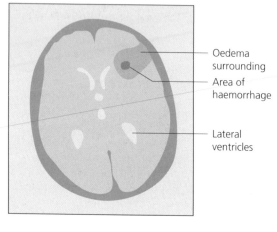

Oedema surrounding

Area of haemorrhage

Lateral ventricles

Fig. 20.5 Magnetic resonance imaging of haemorrhagic stroke.

Renal failure is identified by careful fluid balance monitoring and creatinine measurement. Haemodialysis is required in severe cases.

Pulmonary oedema: The severe pre-eclamptic is particularly vulnerable to fluid overload. Pulmonary oedema is treated with oxygen and furosemide; assisted ventilation may be required. Adult respiratory distress syndrome (ARDS) may develop.

Complications of pre-eclampsia	
Maternal (can cause maternal death)	Eclampsia Cerebrovascular accident (CVA) Haemolysis, elevated liver enzymes and low platelet count (HELLP) Disseminated intravascular coagulation (DIC) Liver failure Renal failure Pulmonary oedema
Fetal (can cause fetal death)	Intrauterine growth restriction (IUGR) Preterm birth Placental abruption Hypoxia

Fetal

Perinatal mortality and morbidity of the fetus are increased: pre-eclampsia accounts for about 5% of stillbirths and up to 10% of preterm deliveries.

In early-onset pre-eclampsia, the principal problem is growth restriction (Fig. 20.6). Preterm delivery is often required, although spontaneous preterm labour is also more common.

At term, pre-eclampsia affects fetal growth less but is nevertheless also associated with an increased morbidity and mortality. At all gestations there is an increased risk of placental abruption.

Investigations

To confirm the diagnosis: If bedside dipstick urinalysis is positive, the protein is quantified. Traditionally, a 24-hour urine collection was performed. Nearly as good, and faster and cheaper, the protein:creatinine ratio (PCR) on a single sample can also be used. A level of 30 mg/nmol is roughly equivalent to approximately 0.3 g/24 h protein excretion. Proteinuria may be absent in early disease and testing for proteinuria is repeated.

To monitor maternal complications: Blood tests often show elevation of the uric acid; the haemoglobin is often

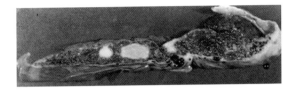

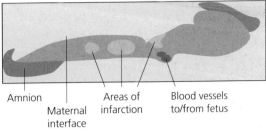

Amnion Areas of Blood vessels
Maternal infarction to/from fetus
interface

Fig. 20.6 Section through infarcted placenta.

high. A rapid fall in platelets due to platelet aggregation on damaged endothelium indicates impending HELLP. A rise in liver function tests (alanine aminotransferase, ALT) suggests impending liver damage or HELLP; LDH levels rise with liver disease and haemolysis. Renal function is often mildly impaired; a rapidly rising creatinine suggests severe complications and renal failure. *To monitor fetal complications*: An ultrasound scan helps estimate fetal weight at early gestations and is used to assess fetal growth. Umbilical artery Doppler and cardiotocography (CTG) are required to evaluate fetal well-being. The short-term variability (STV) from computerized CTG analysis is the best form of daily monitoring.

Screening and prevention

Early prediction: The most commonly used screening test is *uterine artery Doppler* at 20 weeks' gestation, although its routine usage is not recommended in the UK. The sensitivity for pre-eclampsia at any stage in pregnancy is about 40% for a 5% screen-positive rate; for early-onset pre-eclampsia, the figures are much better. Integration of uterine artery Doppler at the time of a nuchal scan, with other risk factors such as blood pressure and angiogenic factors, yields a higher sensitivity but is also not yet in common usage.

Later prediction: the ratio of sFlt-1 to PlGF in maternal blood in later pregnancy, particularly in women with mild hypertension, is useful in determining who will actually develop pre-eclampsia (*Circulation* 2013; **128**: 2121) and will become widely used.

Prevention: Low-dose aspirin (75 mg) starting before 16 weeks, and preferably in the evening, modestly reduces the risk of pre-eclampsia, and is now recommended by NICE in women at risk. High-dose vitamin D with calcium supplementation might also be effective.

Management

Assessment

Women with new hypertension greater than 140/90 mmHg are assessed in a day assessment unit, where blood pressure is rechecked and investigations are performed. SFlt-1:PlGF ratio assays may determine who is at highest risk. Patients without proteinuria and with mild or moderate hypertension (i.e. <160/110 mmHg) are usually managed as outpatients. Their blood pressure and urinalysis are repeated twice weekly and ultrasound is performed every 2–4 weeks unless suggestive of fetal compromise.

Criteria for admission in pre-eclampsia or suspected pre-eclampsia

Symptoms
Proteinuria with PCR >30, or >0.3 g/24 h on 24-h collection
Severe hypertension: blood pressure ≥160/110 mmHg
Growth restriction with abnormal umbilical artery Doppler or abnormal CTG
Abnormal sFlt-1/PlGF assay

Admission

This is necessary with severe hypertension and where there is proteinuria. In the absence of hypertension, women with new proteinuria of 1+ or more should have the protein quantified (PCR or 24-hour testing) and admitted if the PCR is ≥ 30 or there is >0.3 g/24 h. Assessment using a sFlt-1/PlGF assay may determine which women with mild hypertension or proteinuria are at most risk and should be admitted.

Drugs in pre-eclampsia

Antihypertensives are given if the blood pressure reaches 150/100 mmHg and are urgently required at 160/110 mmHg. Labetalol maintenance is recommended. Oral nifedipine is used for initial control, with intravenous labetalol as second line with severe hypertension. The aim is a pressure of about 140/90 mmHg. Antihypertensives do not change the course of pre-eclampsia, but increase safety for the mother, reduce hospitalization and, provided monitoring remains intense, may allow prolongation of a pregnancy affected preterm.

Magnesium sulphate is used both for the treatment, and in severe disease, prevention of eclampsia (*Cochrane* 2010; CD000025). An intravenous loading dose is followed by an intravenous infusion. This drug is not an anticonvulsant but, by increasing cerebral perfusion, probably treats the underlying pathology of eclampsia. Toxicity is severe, resulting in respiratory depression and hypotension, but is preceded by loss of patellar reflexes, which are tested regularly. The dose is reduced or even stopped if renal impairment or anuria develops. If magnesium is required, delivery is indicated.

Steroids are used to promote fetal pulmonary maturity if the gestation is <34 weeks.

Timing of delivery

Pre-eclampsia is progressive, unpredictable and cured only by delivery. Women with pre-eclampsia should be delivered by 36 weeks; diagnosis after this time should prompt delivery. Conservative management before 36 weeks is appropriate (if <28 weeks in a specialist unit with full neonatal care facilities), but the possible benefits of increasing fetal maturity must be weighed against the risks of disease complications. Steroids are given prophylactically, hypertension is treated and there is intensive maternal and fetal surveillance involving daily clinical assessment, CTG and fluid balance, and frequent blood testing. Clinical deterioration or maternal complications or reduced STV on computerized CTG monitoring, will prompt delivery, which can therefore sometimes be extremely preterm. As a general rule, one or more fetal or maternal complications are likely to occur within 2 weeks of the onset of proteinuria.

Gestational hypertension (i.e. no proteinuria) without fetal compromise is monitored for deterioration; delivery by 40 weeks is usual.

Conduct of delivery

Before 34 weeks, or if there is severe growth restriction or an abnormal CTG, caesarean section is usual. After 34 weeks, labour can usually be induced with prostaglandins. Epidural analgesia helps reduce the blood pressure. The fetus is continuously monitored by CTG and the blood pressure and fluid balance are closely observed. Antihypertensives are used in labour. Maternal pushing should be avoided if the blood pressure reaches 160/110 mmHg in the second stage, as it raises intracranial pressure and risks cerebral haemorrhage. Oxytocin rather than ergometrine is used for the third stage as the latter can increase the blood pressure.

Pitfalls in managing pre-eclampsia
Pre-eclampsia is unpredictable
Hypertension may be absent: beware of proteinuria
Epigastric pain is ominous and liver function testing is mandatory
Severe hypertension must be treated
Treatment of hypertension may disguise pre-eclampsia
Excessive fluid administration causes pulmonary oedema
Complications commonly arise after delivery

Postnatal care of the pre-eclamptic patient

Whilst delivery is the only cure for pre-eclampsia, it often takes at least 24 hours for severe disease to improve and it may worsen during this time.

Blood investigations: Liver function tests, platelets and renal function are still monitored closely. Low platelet levels usually return to normal within a few days.

Fluid balance monitoring is essential; pulmonary oedema and respiratory failure may follow uncontrolled administration of intravenous fluid, which is restricted to 80 mL/h plus losses. If the urine output is persistently low, central venous pressure (CVP) monitoring will guide management. If the CVP is high (suggesting overload), furosemide is given. If it is low, fluid but not albumin is given. If it is normal and oliguria persists, renal failure is likely, and a rising potassium level may dictate the need for dialysis.

The blood pressure is maintained at around 140/90 mmHg. The highest level tends to be reached 4–5 days after birth. Postnatal treatment is usually with a beta-blocker; second-line drugs include nifedipine and angiotensin-converting enzyme (ACE) inhibitors. Treatment may be needed for several weeks.

Long-term management: Communication with the GP and community midwives is essential to blood pressure monitoring after discharge. At 6 weeks, women with persistent proteinuria or hypertension should be referred to a renal or hypertension clinic respectively.

Pre-existing hypertension in pregnancy

Definitions and epidemiology

This is diagnosed when the blood pressure is already treated or exceeds 140/90 mmHg before 20 weeks. Underlying hypertension is present in about 5% of pregnancies. It is more common in older and obese women, and in women with a positive family history or who developed hypertension taking the combined oral contraceptive. Patients with pregnancy-induced hypertension also have an underlying predisposition to hypertension and may need treatment later in life.

Aetiology

Primary or 'idiopathic' hypertension is the most common cause. Secondary hypertension is commonly associated with obesity, diabetes or renal disease such as polycystic disease, renal artery stenosis or chronic pyelonephritis. Rarer causes include phaeochromocytoma, Cushing's syndrome, cardiac disease and coarctation of the aorta.

Clinical features

Hypertension increases in late pregnancy. Symptoms are usually absent, although fundal changes, renal bruits and radiofemoral delay should be excluded in all hypertensives. Proteinuria in patients with renal disease is usually present at booking.

Complications

The principal risks are worsening hypertension and pre-eclampsia, the risk of which is increased sixfold; in the absence of these, perinatal mortality is only marginally increased.

Investigations

To identify secondary hypertension: In severe cases, phaeochromocytoma is excluded by performing at least two 24-hour urine collections for vanillylmandelic acid (VMA). This is worthwhile because the maternal mortality of this condition is very high.

To look for coexistent disease: Renal function is assessed and a renal ultrasound is performed.

To identify pre-eclampsia (see below): Quantification of any proteinuria at booking and a uric acid level allow for comparison in later pregnancy.

Management

Hypertension: Ideally, medication will be changed before pregnancy. ACE inhibitors are teratogenic and affect fetal urine production. Labetalol is normally used, with nifedpine as a second-line agent. Medication may not be required in the second trimester because of the physiological fall in blood pressure.

Risk of pre-eclampsia: The pregnancy is treated as 'high risk'. Low-dose aspirin is advised. Screening using uterine artery Doppler and additional antenatal visits are usual. Pre-eclampsia is suggested by worsening hypertension and confirmed by the finding of significant proteinuria for the first time after 20 weeks.

Delivery is usually undertaken at 38-40 weeks, although the benefits of this are debated.

Further reading

For information on pre-eclampsia: www.apec.org.uk.

Czeizel AE, Bánhidy F. Chronic hypertension in pregnancy. *Current Opinion in Obstetrics and Gynecology* 2011; **23**: 76–81.

Duhig KE, Shennan AH. Recent advances in the diagnosis and management of pre-eclampsia. *F1000Prime Reports* 2015; **7**: 24.

Duley L, Gülmezoglu AM, Henderson-Smart DJ, Chou D. Magnesium sulphate and other anticonvulsants for women with pre-eclampsia. *Cochrane Database of Systematic Reviews* 2010; **11**: CD000025.

National Institute for Health and Care Excellence. *Hypertension in Pregnancy: The Management of Hypertensive Disorders During Pregnancy*. Clinical Guideline No. 107. Available at: www.nice.org.uk/nicemedia/live/13098/50418/50418.pdf (accessed 18 July 2016).

Redman CW, Sargent IL, Staff AC. IFPA Senior Award Lecture: making sense of pre-eclampsia – two placental causes of preeclampsia? *Placenta* 2014; **35**(Suppl): S20–25.

Pre-eclampsia at a glance

Definition	Multisystem disease unique to pregnancy that usually manifests as hypertension (blood pressure [BP] >140/90 mmHg) after 20 weeks with proteinuria that is due to:	
Pathology	Endothelial cell damage and vasospasm, which can affect the fetus and almost all maternal organs. It is of placental origin and cured only by delivery	
Degrees	Mild	Proteinuria and mild-to-moderate hypertension
	Moderate	Proteinuria and severe (160/110+ mmHg) hypertension
	Severe	Proteinuria and any hypertension before 34 weeks, or with maternal complications
Classification	Early: manifestations <34 weeks	
	Late: manifestations >34 weeks	
Epidemiology	6%	
Aetiology	Nulliparity, previous/family history, older age, obesity, pre-existing hypertension, diabetes, autoimmune disease, multiple pregnancy	
Features	None until late stage, then headache, epigastric pain, visual disturbances	
Complications	Maternal	Eclampsia, cerebrovascular accidents (CVAs), liver/renal failure, haemolysis, elevated liver enzymes and low platelet count (HELLP), pulmonary oedema
	Fetal	Fetal growth restriction (FGR), abruption, fetal morbidity and mortality
Investigations	To confirm diagnosis	Urine protein measurement (PCR or 24-h collection); sFlt-1:PlGF ratio assay
	To monitor	Watch BP, serial full blood count (FBC), uric acid, urea and electrolytes (U&E), liver function tests (LFTs) and fetal surveillance
Screening	Regular BP and urinalysis checks	
	Early: Integrated tests including uterine artery Doppler under development	
	Later: sFlt-1:PlGF ratio	
Prevention	Aspirin 75 mg from <16 weeks if pregnancy at increased risk	
Management	Investigate if:	BP >140/90 mmHg or 1+ proteinuria
	Admit if:	Confirmed pre-eclampsia (e.g. PCR >30 or 24-h collection>0.3 g/24 h)
		BP 160/110+ mmHg
	Antihypertensives if:	BP reaches 150/100 mmHg, urgently if 160/110 mmHg
	Steroids if:	<34 weeks
	Delivery	All by 36 weeks
		If maternal complications whatever the gestation
	Magnesium sulphate if:	Eclampsia; consider prophylactic use in severe disease. Always deliver
	Postnatally	Watch BP, urine output, blood tests: FBC, U&E, LFTs
		Ensure adequate follow-up

CHAPTER 21

Other medical disorders in pregnancy

Diabetes and gestational diabetes

Physiology

Glucose tolerance decreases in pregnancy due to altered carbohydrate metabolism and the antagonistic effects of human placental lactogen, progesterone and cortisol. Pregnancy is 'diabetogenic': women without diabetes but with impaired or potentially impaired glucose tolerance often 'deteriorate' enough to be classified as diabetic in pregnancy (Fig. 21.1), to become 'gestational diabetics'. Even slightly increased glucose levels have adverse pregnancy effects: these are reduced by treatment, so the definition and diagnosis are driven by the levels at which treatment is beneficial.

The kidneys of non-pregnant women start to excrete glucose at a threshold level of 11 mmol/L. In pregnancy, this varies more but often decreases, so glycosuria may occur at physiological blood glucose concentrations, so urinalysis for glycosuria is not a useful diagnostic test. Raised fetal blood glucose levels induce fetal hyperinsulinaemia, causing fetal fat deposition and excessive growth (macrosomia).

Definition and epidemiology

Pre-existing diabetes (whether type I or II) affects at least 1% of pregnant women. In those on insulin, increasing amounts will be required in these pregnancies to maintain normoglycaemia.

Gestational diabetes is 'carbohydrate intolerance which is diagnosed in pregnancy and may or may not resolve after pregnancy' (NICE 2015). It is becoming more common, largely because of the increasing prevalence of obesity and varying diagnostic thresholds. NICE stipulates a fasting glucose level ≥ 5.6 mmol/L or >7.8 mmol 2 hours after a 75 g glucose load (glucose tolerance test: GTT) to diagnose gestational diabetes. Depending on the criteria used for diagnosis, up to 16% of pregnant women will develop gestational diabetes.

Types of diabetes in pregnancy	
Pre-existing diabetes	Insulin/oral hypogly-
Type I: 5% of diabetes	caemic requirements
Type II: 7.5% of diabetes	increase in pregnancy
Gestational diabetes: 87.5%	Glucose levels rise
	temporarily to diabetic
	level (definitions vary)

Fetal complications (Fig. 21.2)

Complications are related to glucose levels, so women with gestational diabetes (and generally better control) are less affected. Women with type I and II diabetes are similarly affected.

Congenital abnormalities (particularly neural tube and cardiac defects) are 3–4 times more common in women with established diabetes, and are related to periconceptual glucose control. Preterm labour, natural or induced, occurs in >10% of women with established diabetes, and *fetal lung maturity* at any given gestation is less than with non-diabetic pregnancies. *Birthweight* is increased as fetal pancreatic islet cell hyperplasia

---

Obstetrics & Gynaecology, Fifth Edition. Lawrence Impey, Tim Child.
© 2017 John Wiley & Sons, Ltd. Published 2017 by John Wiley & Sons, Ltd.

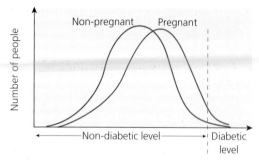

Fig. 21.1 Distribution of glucose tolerance in the non-pregnant and pregnant population.

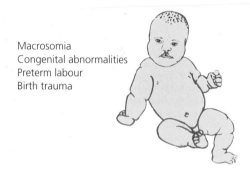

Macrosomia
Congenital abnormalities
Preterm labour
Birth trauma

Fig. 21.2 Fetal complications of diabetes.

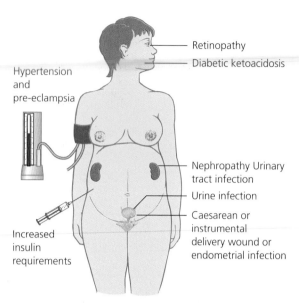

Fig. 21.3 Maternal complications of diabetes.

leads to hyperinsulinaemia and fat deposition. This leads to increased urine output and *polyhydramnios* (increased liquor) is common. As the fetus tends to be larger, *dystocia* and *birth trauma* (particularly shoulder dystocia) are more common. *Fetal compromise, fetal distress* in labour and *sudden fetal death* are more common, and related particularly to poor third trimester glucose control.

Maternal complications (Fig. 21.3)

Complications are related to glucose levels, so women with gestational diabetes (and generally better control) are less affected. *Insulin requirements* increase by up to 300% by the end of pregnancy. *Ketoacidosis* is rare, but *hypoglycaemia* may result from attempts to achieve optimum glucose control. *Urinary tract infection* and *wound or endometrial infection* after delivery are more common. Pre-existing *hypertension* is detected in up to 25% of women with diabetes and *pre-eclampsia* is more common. Pre-existing *ischaemic heart disease* often

worsens. *Caesarean* or *instrumental delivery* is more likely because of fetal compromise and increased fetal size. Diabetic *nephropathy* (5–10%) is associated with poorer fetal outcomes and can lead to massive proteinuria and deterioration in maternal renal function. Diabetic *retinopathy* often deteriorates in pregnancy and may need to be treated. This is counterintuitively due to rapid control of blood glucose.

Management of pre-existing diabetes in pregnancy

Precise glucose control and fetal monitoring for evidence of compromise are the cornerstones of management. Antenatal care is consultant based, with delivery in a unit with neonatal facilities. A multidisciplinary approach involving an obstetrician, midwife, GP, dietician and a physician is necessary (Fig. 21.4). The key member, however, is the woman, who has day-to-day control of her diabetes and needs to be educated about optimizing control. If she is not motivated, normoglycaemia will not be achieved.

Preconceptual care for pre-existing diabetics

Glucose levels: Optimal control reduces the risk of congenital abnormalities and preterm labour. Ideally,

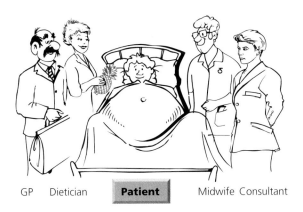

GP   Dietician   **Patient**   Midwife Consultant

Fig. 21.4 The multidisciplinary approach to diabetes in pregnancy.

monthly glycosylated haemoglobin (HbA1c) assessment is offered: a level of <6.5% is best and pregnancy not advised if >10%. Fasting glucose levels should be 4–7 mmol/L if achievable without hypoglycaemia. Metformin and insulin are appropriate; other hypoglycaemic drugs are stopped.

Other: 5 mg of folic acid is given, any statins are stopped and if needed, antihypertensives suitable for pregnancy (usually labetalol or methyldopa) are substituted. Renal function (creatinine should be <120 μmol/L), blood pressure and retinae are assessed.

Monitoring and treating the diabetes

HbA1c levels reflect prior control: the level is checked at booking. Glucose levels are checked on a home glucometer fasted in the morning, before meals, 1 hour after meals and at bedtime. If achievable without hypoglycaemia, the aim is for a fasting level of <5.3 mmol/L, and 1-hour level <7.8 mmol/L. Direct or electronic contact with healthcare professionals should be no less than fortnightly. Metformin or insulin (rapid-acting analogues are best) are used; doses will usually need to be progressively increased as the pregnancy advances and metformin may need to be supplemented with insulin in women with type II diabetes. In those requiring insulin, a combination of once- or twice-daily long/intermediate-acting, usually with three preprandial short-acting insulin injections, is used. Pumps are only advised if control is poor. The fasting level should be >4 mmol/L and glucagon should be prescribed. Advice on exercise and diet is essential.

Monitoring or treating the complications of diabetes

The renal function should be checked and the retinae screened for retinopathy and, if abnormal, this will need to be repeated in each trimester. Aspirin, 75 mg daily from 12 weeks, is advised to reduce the risk of pre-eclampsia. Diabetic acidosis, usually ketotic, is a medical emergency and should be treated appropriately.

Monitoring the fetus

In addition to the usual pregnancy scans, fetal echocardiography is indicated. Ultrasound is used to monitor fetal growth and liquor volume at 32 and 36 weeks. Even where glucose control has been good, macrosomia and polyhydramnios can occur (Fig. 21.5). Umbilical artery Doppler is not useful unless pre-eclampsia or intrauterine growth restriction (IUGR) develops.

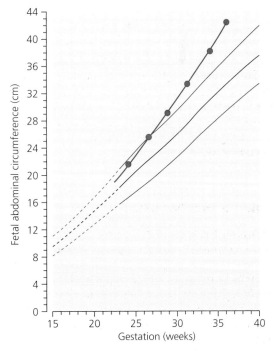

Fig. 21.5 Accelerated fetal growth of a fetus with a diabetic mother.

Timing and mode of delivery

Delivery at 37–39 weeks is advised. Birth trauma is more likely and although ultrasound prediction is imprecise, elective caesarean section is often used where the estimated fetal weight exceeds 4 kg. During labour, glucose levels are maintained with a 'sliding scale' of insulin and a dextrose infusion.

The neonate and puerperium

The neonate commonly develops hypoglycaemia because it has become 'accustomed to' hyperglycaemia and its insulin levels are high. Respiratory distress syndrome occasionally occurs, even after 38 weeks. Breastfeeding is strongly advised. The mother's dose of insulin can be rapidly changed to pre-pregnancy doses: less than 70% of the pre-pregnancy dose is often needed, especially if breastfeeding. Early and regular feeding is advised; neonatal blood glucoses should be checked within 4 hours of birth.

Management of diabetes
Preconceptual glucose control
Assessment of maternal diabetic complications
Patient education and team involvement
Glucose monitoring and insulin adjustment
Anomaly and cardiac ultrasound and fetal surveillance
Delivery by 39 weeks

Detection of and screening for gestational diabetes

Screening using pre-existing risk factors: A previous large baby (>4.5 kg) or unexplained stillbirth, a first-degree relative with diabetes, a body mass index (BMI) >30 kg/m2 or being of a minority ethnic family origin with a high prevalence of diabetes (e.g. South Asian, black Caribbean or Middle Eastern) increase the risk. In the UK, these women are screened using a GTT (75 g load) at 24–28 weeks. Those with previous gestational diabetes are also screened early, following booking.
Screening using pregnancy risk factors: Where there is polyhydramnios or persistent glycosuria, a GTT is also indicated.
Universal screening: In practice, screening is often missed, and universal screening is probably worthwhile.

Screening and treatment of gestational diabetes	
Step 1a	**Universal screening** Perform 75 g glucose tolerance test (GTT) at 24–28 weeks (if previous history of gestational diabetes, do at 18 weeks). If fasting >5.6 or 2 h >7.8, go to step 2
Step 1b	OR … **Risk-based screening** (UK practice) If 1+ risk factors, perform GTT at 28 weeks. If fasting >5.6, or 2 h >7.8, go to step 2
Step 2	**Initial treatment** Give glucometer Advise re diet and exercise Check HbA1c to identify pre-existing diabetes If fasting >7, go to step 4 If fasting <7 but after 2 weeks, levels >5.3 before meals, or >7.8 h 1 h after meals, go to Step 3
Step 3	**Metformin** If after 2 weeks, levels >5.3 before meals, or >7.8 1 h after meals, go to Step 4
Step 4	**Insulin** Treat as pre-existing diabetic

Risk factors for gestational diabetes
Previous history of gestational diabetes
Previous fetus >4.5 kg
Previous unexplained stillbirth
First-degree relative with diabetes
Body mass index (BMI) >30
Racial origin
Polyhydramnios
Persistent glycosuria

Management of gestational diabetes

Monitoring and treating the diabetes

The HbA1c is checked to identify pre-existing diabetes. Target glucose levels and principles are the same as for women with pre-existing diabetes.

Diet: Initially, women with an abnormal GTT should be given dietary and exercise advice and will monitor their glucose levels at home on at least 2 days a week. If adequate control is not achieved, metformin and/or insulin are used. If the fasting level is >7 mmol/L, diet will be inadequate and metformin or insulin is usually started immediately.

Oral hypoglycaemic agents such as metformin are increasingly used.

Insulin will be required in the rest. Management is as for women with pre-existing diabetes.

Antenatal care and delivery

Women should be managed as for pre-existing diabetes, although with well-controlled gestational diabetes delivery need not be before 41 weeks.

The neonate and puerperium

Treatment can be discontinued postnatally, but a fasting glucose should be measured at about 6 weeks postnatal, because of the increased risk of type II diabetes in later life. More than 50% will become diabetic within the next 10 years.

Cardiac disease

In pregnancy there is a 40% increase in cardiac output, due to both an increase in stroke volume and heart rate, and a 40% increase in blood volume. There is also a 50% reduction in systemic vascular resistance: blood pressure often drops in the second trimester, but is usually normal by term. The increased blood flow produces a flow (ejection systolic) murmur in 90% of pregnant women. The electrocardiogram (ECG) is altered during pregnancy: a left axis shift and inverted T-waves are common.

Epidemiology

Cardiac disease affects 0.3% of pregnant women. The incidence is increasing in the UK, because of immigration, and because more women with congenital disease are reaching reproductive age. The maternal risk is dependent on the cardiac status and most encounter no problems. However, cardiac disease is the leading cause of maternal death in the UK (49 of 214 maternal deaths in 2011–13; MBRRACE-UK 2015) and a major cause of maternal morbidity. Increased cardiac output acts as an 'exercise test' with which the heart may be unable to cope. This usually manifests after 28 weeks or soon after labour, with decompensation particularly in association with blood loss or fluid overload. The latter can occur in the early puerperium, as uterine involution 'squeezes' a large 'fluid load' into the circulation.

Principles of management

Patients with significant disease are preferably assessed before pregnancy. Some drugs, such as warfarin and angiotensin-converting enzyme (ACE) inhibitors, are contraindicated. Those with severe decompensated disease are advised against pregnancy. *Cardiac assessment*, particularly echocardiography, is needed. Fetal cardiac anomalies are more common (3%) and are best detected on *ultrasound* at 20 weeks' gestation. *Hypertension* should be treated. Women who have conceived on contraindicated *drugs* will need to have these altered: care needs to be individualized but beta-blockers are often used for hypertension. *Thromboprophylaxis* needs to be continued, usually with low molecular weight heparin (LMWH). Regular checks for anaemia are made. In labour, attention is paid to *fluid balance; elective epidural analgesia* reduces afterload. *Elective forceps* delivery helps avoid the additional stress of pushing in severe cases. Elective caesarean is rarely required but is usual with a severely dilated ascending aorta and in those with moderate-to-severe left ventricular failure. *Antibiotic* prophylaxis against endocarditis is recommended as in non-pregnant women and not routinely in all in labour.

Types of cardiac disease and their management

Mild abnormalities such as mitral valve prolapse, patent ductus arteriosus (PDA), uncomplicated ventricular septal defects (VSD) or uncomplicated atrial septal defects (ASD) do not usually cause complications.

Pulmonary hypertension (e.g. Eisenmenger's syndrome): Because of a high maternal mortality (20%) rate, pregnancy is contraindicated and termination is offered.

Cyanotic heart disease without pulmonary hypertension: Although usually corrected, the particular risk is of paradoxical embolism and anticoagulation is therefore advised.

Aortic stenosis: Severe disease (e.g. small valve area or large gradient) causes an inability to increase cardiac output when required and should be corrected before pregnancy. Beta-blockade is often used. Epidural analgesia is contraindicated in the most severe cases. Anticoagulation is required for mechanical aortic valves.

Mitral valve disease: This should be treated before pregnancy. In the rare, severe cases of stenosis, heart failure may develop late in the pregnancy; beta-blockade is used. Artificial metal valves are particularly prone to thrombosis therefore anticoagulation with meticulous monitoring is required.

Myocardial infarction is unusual but becoming more frequent in women of reproductive age; mortality is greater at later gestations.

Peripartum cardiomyopathy is a rare (1 in 3000) cause of heart failure, specific to pregnancy. It develops in the last month or first 6 months after pregnancy and in the absence of a recognizable cause. It is frequently diagnosed late. It is a cause of maternal death (risk 15%) and in more than 50% of cases leads to permanent left ventricular dysfunction. Treatment is supportive, with diuretics and ACE inhibitors. There is a significant recurrence rate in subsequent pregnancies.

Respiratory disease

Tidal volume increases by 40% in pregnancy, although there is no change in respiratory rate. Asthma is common in pregnancy. Pregnancy has a variable effect on the disease; drugs should not be withheld, because they are generally safe and because a severe asthma attack is potentially lethal to mother and fetus. Well-controlled asthma has little detrimental effect on perinatal outcome. Women on long-term steroids require an increased dose in labour because the chronically suppressed adrenal cortex is unable to produce adequate steroids for the stress of labour.

Epilepsy

Epilepsy affects 0.5% of pregnant women. Seizure control can deteriorate in pregnancy, and particularly in labour. Epilepsy is a significant cause of maternal death and antiepileptic treatment should be continued. However, the risk of congenital abnormalities (e.g. neural tube defects (NTDs)) is increased (4% overall), and this is largely due to drug therapy. The risks are dose dependent, higher with multiple drug usage and higher with certain drugs (e.g. sodium valproate). The newborn has a 3% risk of developing epilepsy.

Management of epilepsy in pregnancy

Preconceptual assessment is ideal: Management involves seizure control with as few drugs as possible at the lowest dose, together with folic acid (5 mg/day) supplementation. Ideally, sodium valproate should be avoided because it is associated with a higher rate of congenital abnormalities and with lower intelligence in children. Therefore, all women of reproductive age are best managed as if they are contemplating pregnancy. Carbamazepine and lamotrigine are safest. Lamotrigine and to a lesser extent levetiracetam plasma levels fall in pregnancy and dose increases are commonly required but the benefits of routine drug level monitoring remain debated. Folic acid 5 mg is continued throughout pregnancy and from 36 weeks, 10 mg vitamin K is given orally for women on enzyme-inducing antiepileptics. The 20-week scan and fetal echocardiography are important to exclude fetal abnormalities.

Thyroid disease in pregnancy

Thyroid status does not alter in pregnancy, although iodine clearance is increased. Goitre is more common (Fig. 21.6). Fetal thyroxine production starts at

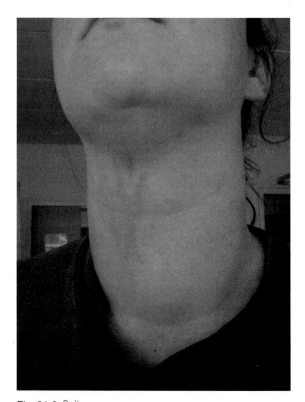

Fig. 21.6 Goitre.

12 weeks; before, it is dependent on maternal thyroxine. Maternal thyroid-stimulating hormone (TSH) is increased in early pregnancy.

Hypothyroidism

This affects 1% of pregnant women. In the UK, most cases of hypothyroidism are due to Hashimoto's thyroiditis or thyroid surgery, but hypothyroidism is common where dietary iodine is deficient. Untreated disease is rare as anovulation is usual but is associated with a high perinatal mortality. Even subclinical hypothyroidism has been associated with miscarriage, preterm delivery and intellectual impairment in childhood. Hypothyroidism is also associated with a slightly increased risk of pre-eclampsia, particularly if antithyroid antibodies are present. Replacement with thyroxine is important and TSH levels are monitored 6-weekly: in normal pregnancy the TSH is lowered, so the dose may need to be increased until delivery.

Hyperthyroidism

This affects 0.2% of pregnant women and is usually due to Graves' disease. Untreated disease is rare as anovulation is usual. Inadequately treated disease increases perinatal mortality. Antithyroid antibodies also cross the placenta; rarely, this causes neonatal thyrotoxicosis and goitre. For the mother, thyrotoxicosis may improve in late pregnancy but poorly controlled disease risks a 'thyroid storm' whereby the mother gets acute symptoms and heart failure. Symptoms may be confused with those of pregnancy. Hyperthyroidism is treated with propylthiouracil (PTU) in the first trimester, rather than carbimazole. PTU crosses the placenta and can occasionally cause neonatal hypothyroidism; the lowest possible dose is used and thyroid function is tested monthly. Graves' disease often worsens postpartum.

Postpartum thyroiditis

This is common (5–10%) and can be a cause of postnatal depression. Risk factors include antithyroid antibodies and type I diabetes. In affected patients, there is a transient and usually subclinical hyperthyroidism, usually about 3 months postpartum, followed after about 4 months by hypothyroidism. This is permanent in 20%.

Liver disease

Acute fatty liver

This is a very rare (1 in 9000) but serious condition that may be part of the spectrum of pre-eclampsia. Acute hepatorenal failure, disseminated intravascular coagulation (DIC) and hypoglycaemia lead to a high maternal and fetal mortality. There is extensive fatty change in the liver. Malaise, vomiting, jaundice and vague epigastric pain are early features, while thirst may occur weeks earlier. Early diagnosis and prompt delivery are essential, although correction of clotting defects and hypoglycaemia are needed first. Treatment is then supportive, with further dextrose, blood products, careful fluid balance and, occasionally, dialysis. The recurrence rate is low.

Intrahepatic cholestasis of pregnancy

This is a multifactorial condition characterized by otherwise unexplained pruritus and abnormal liver function tests (LFTs) and/or raised bile acids in pregnancy, which resolves after delivery. It is due to abnormal sensitivity to the cholestatic effects of oestrogens. It occurs in 0.7% of pregnant women in the West, is familial and tends to recur (50%). It is traditionally associated with an increased risk of sudden stillbirth, meconium passage and postpartum haemorrhage. The risk of stillbirth is difficult to estimate, is commonly overestimated by pregnant women but is probably <1%. It is thought to be due to the toxic effects of bile salts, and is vaguely related to the bile acid levels.

Ultrasound and cardiotocography predict adverse outcomes poorly and are unhelpful, although liver function and bile acid levels are usually checked at least fortnightly following diagnosis. Ursodeoxycholic acid (UDCA) helps relieve itching and may reduce the obstetric risks by reducing bile acid levels. Because there is an increased maternal and fetal tendency to haemorrhage, vitamin K 10 mg/day is given from 36 weeks. Induction of labour is often offered, a policy that will reduce stillbirth anyway, but this remains controversial and may cause prematurity as well as increased maternal morbidity through intervention. No clear guidance exists and a practical compromise is induction by 40 weeks, and by 38 weeks if bile acid levels are very high. Six-week follow-up is indicated to ensure liver function returns to normal.

Renal disease

In pregnancy, the glomerular filtration rate increases 40%, causing urea and creatinine levels to decrease.

Chronic kidney disease

This affects 0.2% of pregnant women. Fetal and maternal complications are dependent on the degree of hypertension and renal impairment; pregnancy is considered very high risk if the creatinine level is >200 mmol/L. Renal function often deteriorates late in the pregnancy; this is more common in severe disease and can lead to a permanent deterioration. Rejection of renal transplants is not more common; immunosuppressive therapy, e.g. tacrolimus, must continue, and levels must be checked regularly, as an increased dosage is usually required. Proteinuria can cause diagnostic confusion with pre-eclampsia, which is more common, but will usually have been present before 20 weeks. Fetal complications include pre-eclampsia, IUGR, polyhydramnios and preterm delivery. Management involves ultrasound for fetal growth, measurement of renal function, screening for urinary infection (which may exacerbate renal disease) and control of hypertension. In severe cases dialysis is indicated. Vaginal delivery is usually appropriate.

Urinary infection

Urine infection is associated with preterm labour, anaemia and increased perinatal morbidity and mortality. *Asymptomatic bacteriuria* affects 5% of women, but in pregnancy is more likely (20%) to lead to pyelonephritis (Fig. 21.7). The urine should be cultured at the booking visit, and asymptomatic bacteriuria is treated. Subsequently, culture is performed if nitrites are detected on routine urinalysis. *Pyelonephritis* affects 1–2% of women, causing loin pain, rigors, vomiting and a fever. This requires treatment with intravenous antibiotics. *Escherichia coli* accounts for 75% and is often resistant to amoxicillin.

Thrombophilias and the antiphospholipid syndrome

Antiphospholipid syndrome (APS)

This is when the lupus anticoagulant and/or anticardiolipin antibodies (ACA) occur (measured on two occasions at least 3 months apart) in association with

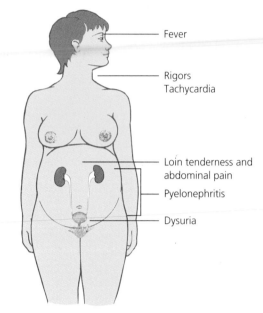

Fig. 21.7 Clinical features of pyelonephritis.

— Fever

— Rigors
Tachycardia

— Loin tenderness and abdominal pain

— Pyelonephritis

— Dysuria

adverse pregnancy complications or thrombotic events. Because of placental thrombosis, recurrent miscarriage, IUGR and early pre-eclampsia are common, and the fetal loss rate is high. Low levels of these antibodies are also present in nearly 2% of all pregnant women but treatment, normally with aspirin and LMWH (*Rheumatology* 2010; **49**: 281), should be restricted to those with the *syndrome*. The pregnancy is managed as 'high risk', with serial ultrasound and elective induction of labour at least by term. Postnatal anticoagulation is recommended to prevent venous thromboembolism.

Diagnosis of antiphospholipid syndrome	
1+ clinical criteria	Vascular thrombosis 1+ death of fetus >10 weeks Pre-eclampsia or intrauterine growth retardation requiring delivery <34 weeks 3+ fetal losses <10 weeks, otherwise unexplained
With Laboratory criteria	Lupus anticoagulant or high ACAs or anti-β_2-glycoprotein I antibody (measured twice >3 months apart)

Other prothrombotic disorders

Other prothrombotic conditions, such as *anti-thrombin deficiency, protein S and C deficiency* and, to a lesser extent, the *prothrombin gene mutation and factor V Leiden* heterozygosity, also cause increased risk of pregnancy complications, as well as venous thromboembolism. The risk is greater where these conditions coexist and if there have been previous complications.

Hyperhomocysteinaemia is also associated with increased pregnancy loss and pre-eclampsia; treatment is usually with high-dose folic acid. Women with prothrombotic tendencies and an adverse pregnancy history are usually treated as for antiphospholipid syndrome, although the effectiveness of this is not proven. Postnatal anticoagulation is recommended.

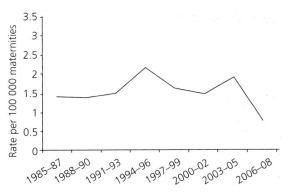

UK Deaths from thrombocmbolim

Fig. 21.8 UK deaths from thromboembolism. Source: Centre for Child and Maternal Enquiries (CMACE) *BJOG* 2011; **118**(Suppl. 1): 1–203. Reproduced with permission of John Wiley & Sons Ltd.

Systemic lupus erythematosus

Systemic lupus erythematosus (SLE) affects 0.1–0.2% of pregnant women. In the absence of lupus anticoagulant or anticardiolipin antibodies (see above), the risks to the pregnancy are largely confined to those with active disease or associated hypertension, renal or cerebral disease. Maternal symptoms often relapse after delivery.

Venous thromboembolic disease

Pregnancy is prothrombotic and the incidence of venous thromboembolism (VTE) is increased sixfold. Blood clotting factors are increased, fibrinolytic activity is reduced and blood flow is altered by mechanical obstruction and immobility. Women with inherited prothrombotic conditions and those with a family or personal history are particularly prone to thromboses; other risks are outlined below. Of the 48 maternal deaths in 2009–13 in the UK, half were antenatal; of these. half were in the first trimester.

Pulmonary embolus is the leading 'direct' cause of maternal death in the UK (Fig. 21.8). Embolism occurs in <0.3%, with a mortality of 3.5% (Fig. 21.9). Chest pain and dyspnoea are common; key signs are a tachycardia, raised respiratory rate and jugular venous pressure (JVP), and chest abnormalities. Diagnosis is as in the non-pregnant woman using a chest X-ray, arterial blood gas analysis and computed tomography (CT)

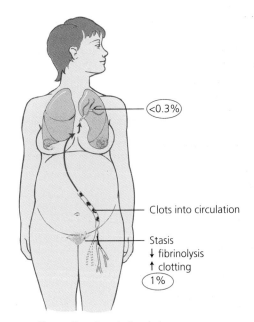

Fig. 21.9 Venous thromboembolism in pregnancy.

(Fig. 21.10) or with perfusion ± ventilation (VQ) scanning. The ECG changes of normal pregnancy can mimic a pulmonary embolus.

Deep vein thrombosis (DVT) occurs in about 0.1% of pregnant women. Thromboses are more often iliofemoral and on the left. Doppler examination and occasionally

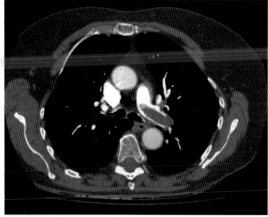

Fig. 21.10 CT angiogram of pulmonary embolus.

a venogram or pelvic magnetic resonance imaging (MRI) is used.

Cerebral venous thrombosis occurs in 1 in 10 000 pregnancies, particularly during the puerperium, and presents as headache and or stroke. Imaging with MRI is best.

Management of VTE in pregnancy

A thrombophilia screen is performed before treatment with subcutaneous LMWH. Dosing is weight based and can be adjusted according to the anti-Factor Xa level; more is needed than in non-pregnant women as clearance is more rapid. If possible, treatment is stopped shortly before labour, but is restarted and continued into the puerperium. Warfarin is teratogenic, may cause fetal bleeding and is seldom used antenatally. Both LMWH and warfarin may be used in breastfeeding women.

Thromboprophylaxis

Because of the importance of pulmonary embolism as a cause of maternal death, thromboprophylaxis is used frequently. Every woman requires an early antenatal risk assessment, which is reviewed according to subsequent events, such as caesarean delivery or hospitalization. Algorithms are complex: an attempt at simplification of the current UK recommendations in the 2015 RCOG Green-top Guideline is presented in the box below.

Non-pharmacological

General measures are required for all: mobilization and maintenance of hydration.

Compression stockings are useful for those where LMWH is contraindicated (e.g. during/ immediately post surgery).

Prophylaxis with low molecular weight heparin

Maternal weight determines dosage; it is essential this is weight adjusted.

Antenatal prophylaxis (see box below) is restricted to women at very high risk, such as a previous thrombosis, particularly if unprovoked or with a thrombophilia, or those with intermediate risk factors such as medical comorbidities, or if there are 3–4 more minor risk factors (see box below).

Postpartum prophylaxis (see box below) is more frequently used. If it has been used antenatally it is continued. If there is a major or intermediate risk factor, or two or more minor risk factors, LMWH is prescribed for at least 10 days. LMWH can usually be given within 12 hours of caesarean section or vaginal delivery.

Thromboprophylaxis simplified

Risk factors for venous thromboembolism (VTE)		*Recommended prophylaxis*	
Major	Any previous VTE (unless single post surgery)	Antenatal:	Low molecular weight heparin (LMWH)
		Postnatal:	LMWH for 6 weeks
	High-risk thrombophilia	Antenatal:	Consider LMWH
	Low-risk thrombophilia with family history	Postnatal:	LMWH for 6 weeks
Intermediate	Morbid obesity (body mass index (BMI) ≥40)	Antenatal:	Consider LMWH
	Readmission or prolonged admission (≥ 3 days)	Postnatal:	LMWH for 10 days
	Surgical procedure (except perineal repair)		
	Major medical comorbidity		
	Caesarean section in labour	Postnatal:	LMWH for 10 days
Minor	Age >35 years	Antenatal:	LMWH if 3–4 risks
	Any obesity (BMI ≥30)	Postnatal:	LMWH if 2+, for 10 days
	Parity ≥3		
	Smoker		
	Elective caesarean section		
	Family history of VTE		
	Low-risk thrombophilia		
	Gross varicose veins		
	Current systemic infection		
	Immobility		
	Current pre-eclampsia		
	Multiple pregnancy		
	Preterm delivery in this pregnancy (<37 + 0 weeks)		
	Stillbirth in this pregnancy		
	Mid-cavity rotational or operative delivery		
	Prolonged labour (>24 hours)		
	Postpartum haemorrhage >1 litre or blood transfusion		
	Assisted reproduction technology used		

Note: risk factors combined for simplicity. Some risk factors, e.g. elective lower segment caesarean section, not applicable antenatally.

Obesity in pregnancy

Up to 20% of pregnant women now have a BMI >30. Most risks are linearly related to the BMI.

Risks in pregnancy

Maternal: Obese women have a higher risk of thromboembolism, pre-eclampsia and diabetes, caesarean section, wound infections, difficult surgery, postpartum haemorrhage and maternal death.
Fetal: A higher rate of congenital abnormalities (e.g. NTDs), diabetes and pre-eclampsia contributes to a 2–3-fold increase in perinatal mortality. Ultrasound is less accurate.

Management of obesity in pregnancy

Preconceptual weight advice is ideal; high-dose (5 mg) preconceptual folic acid supplementation is recommended, as is vitamin D. Weight is best maintained; loss in pregnancy is impractical and may cause malnutrition. The pregnancy should be considered as high risk, particularly if the BMI is ≥35; screening for gestational diabetes (if BMI >30) and closer blood pressure surveillance with an appropriately sized cuff are required. A formal anaesthetic risk assessment and antenatal thromboprophylaxis are recommended if the BMI is ≥40. There is an increasing and probably undesirable trend towards elective caesarean in very obese women.

Classification of obesity	
BMI 30–34.9	moderate
BMI 35–39.9	severe
BMI 40+	morbid

Mental illness in pregnancy

The early postnatal period represents the highest risk period for women developing new-onset mental illness. Indeed, mental illness in pregnancy and the postnatal period is recognized as a major risk factor for maternal suicide, with 23% of women who died between 6 weeks and 1 year postnatal dying from psychiatric causes (MBRRACE-UK 2015). There is robust evidence of detrimental effects on the long-term physical and psychological health of children. In the UK difficulties identifying women at risk of mental illness, and accessing specialist services, are major obstacles to successful treatment.

'Red flag signs' requiring urgent senior psychiatric assessment are a recent significant change in mental state or emergence of new symptoms, new thoughts or acts of violent self-harm, or new and persistent expressions of incompetency as a mother or estrangement from the infant.

Criteria for considering admission to a mother and baby unit
Rapidly changing mental state
Suicidal ideation (particularly of a violent nature)
Pervasive guilt or hopelessness
Significant estrangement from the infant
New or persistent beliefs of inadequacy as a mother
Evidence of psychosis

Bipolar affective disorder

The lifetime risk is up to 1%; onset is most commonly during child-bearing age. A family history is common. It is characterized by episodes of depression or mania, each persisting for several weeks at a time, sometimes with psychotic symptoms. Delivery can precipitate relapse in women with bipolar disorder, and the condition is a major risk factor for postpartum psychosis.

The mainstay of treatment is mood stabilizers; antipsychotics, anticonvulsants or lithium. Anticonvulsants, especially valproate and carbamazepine, are teratogenic

and lithium is associated with cardiac defects. Treatment decisions must weigh the risks to the fetus against the increased risk of relapse or postpartum psychosis if medication is stopped.

Postpartum psychosis

This is a severe mental illness which can affects 1–2/1000 women. It is a psychiatric emergency, presenting suddenly in the early postnatal period with psychotic and severe mood symptoms, There may be acute risk of suicide, self-harm or neglect, and neglect of the baby. Intentional harm to the baby is rare.

Depression

Depression is common, affecting 10–15% pregnant and postnatal women. The incidence of severe depression in women is highest in the postnatal period, affecting around 3% of mothers. Symptoms are similar to those in non-pregnant women. The term 'postnatal depression' does not represent a distinct clinical entity and should not distract from the significance of depression in the antenatal period.

Treatment of depression in pregnant and postnatal women broadly follows the same guidelines as depression in the general population. Cognitive behavioural therapy should be sought as first line in mild-to-moderate depression. Antidepressants are effective, especially for severe depressive illness. Antidepressants are not thought to be teratogenic; selective serotonin reuptake inhibitors (SSRIs) and tricyclics are used. However, adverse effects in the child have been documented and include short-term side effects and withdrawal responses in the neonate and possibly longer-term neurodevelopmental effects, but absolute risks appear to be low. Up to 3% of women conceive while taking antidepressants (*BJOG* 2007; **114**: 1055).

Anxiety disorders

These include generalized anxiety disorder, panic disorder, phobias, obsessive compulsive disorder (OCD) and post-traumatic stress disorder (PTSD). Anxiety disorders are common in the perinatal period and anxiety may also be the prominent symptom in depression. Prevalence rates are similar to the general population. The incidence of OCD may increase in the perinatal period; the content of the obsessive thoughts may involve the baby but are not usually associated with risk of intentional harm. PTSD may be triggered by traumatic experiences during delivery, particularly instrumental delivery. 'Tokophobia', fear of childbirth, can cause great distress to pregnant women and in severe cases may constitute an indication for elective caesarean section.

As with depression, treatment guidelines broadly follow those for the general population, with psychological therapies recommended as first line. Medications should be reserved for more severe cases. Antidepressants are the mainstay of pharmacological treatment. Benzodiazepines are not recommended in pregnancy due to risks of dependency, neonatal withdrawal and oversedation.

Schizophrenia

This affects up to 1% of women over the course of a lifetime, and most commonly during child-bearing age. The majority of people with schizophrenia require long-term treatment with antipsychotics. Antipsychotics have not been shown to be teratogenic, and for this reason they are the mood stabilizer of choice in women with bipolar disorder. Second-generation antipsychotics such as olanzapine and quetiapine are associated with weight gain and therefore gestational diabetes. Treatment is usually continued due to the high risks of relapse if medication is stopped prematurely. Relapse of schizophrenia in the perinatal period is associated with poor outcomes for the mother and child.

'Recreational' drugs in pregnancy

Illegal drugs

Women abusing drugs in pregnancy are often vulnerable personally and socially. They are at increased risk of other illnesses such as sexually transmitted infections (STIs), HIV and hepatitis C. Substance abuse is a major cause of maternal (MBRRACE-UK 2015). Pregnancy care should be multidisciplinary and include social support. The newborn may be the subject of a care order. Depending on the drugs taken, the fetus may be at increased risk of congenital abnormalities; the pregnancy should be considered high risk, particularly for IUGR and preterm delivery.

Opiates: These are not teratogenic, but their use is associated with preterm delivery, IUGR, stillbirth, developmental delay and sudden infant death syndrome (SIDS). Methadone maintenance, without use of street drugs, is advised; withdrawal of methadone is not. Some neonates experience severe withdrawal symptoms and convulsions.

Cocaine is probably teratogenic and can cause childhood intellectual impairment, but is particularly associated with IUGR and placental abruption, as well as preterm delivery, stillbirth and SIDS. Proper counselling concerning risks, social support and pregnancy monitoring is required.

Ecstasy is teratogenic, with an increased risk of cardiac defects and probably gastroschisis. Pregnancy complications are probably similar to cocaine and counselling and social support are required.

Benzodiazepines have been associated with facial clefts, and cause neonatal hypotonia as well as withdrawal symptoms.

Cannabis: Abuse of other drugs makes attribution of risk difficult but cannabis may cause IUGR and affect later childhood development.

Legal drugs

Alcohol

In the West, about 50% of women drink no alcohol at all in pregnancy; about 10% admit to drinking more than three units per week. Below this level, there is no consistent evidence of harm, although there is conflicting evidence regarding childhood development and best advice is to avoid alcohol altogether, particularly in the first 12 weeks when it may cause miscarriage. At higher levels, the incidence of IUGR and birth defects increases.

Alcohol abuse in pregnancy greatly increases these risks and is associated with the fetal alcohol syndrome. The incidence in North America is 0.6 per 1000, and affected individuals have facial abnormalities, growth restriction, a small or abnormal brain and developmental delay, in conjunction with confirmed alcohol exposure (>18 units per day). *Alcohol spectrum disorders* (incidence 9 per 1000) encompass lesser variants of the syndrome. Advice and social support are required; ultrasound may not detect the syndrome, but is used to monitor fetal growth.

Tobacco

Smoking in pregnancy is related to social class: approximately one-third of women smoke during pregnancy and one-tenth of pregnancies are exposed to environmental smoke. Smoking is probably not teratogenic but is associated, in a dose–response manner, with an increased risk of miscarriage, IUGR, preterm birth, placental abruption, stillbirth and SIDS. It is also associated with a wide variety of childhood illnesses. Pre-eclampsia is less common but more severe if it occurs. Women should be encouraged to stop or at least cut down their smoking; nicotine replacement therapy is effective and is preferable to smoking. The pregnancy should be considered higher risk.

Anaemias

The 40% increase in blood volume in pregnancy is relatively greater than the increase in red cell mass. The result is a net fall in haemoglobin concentration, such that the lower limit of normal is 11.0 g/dL. Iron and folic acid requirements increase, and iron absorption increases threefold (Fig. 21.11). A high haemoglobin level is actually associated with an increased risk of pregnancy complications such as preterm delivery and IUGR (*AJOG* 2005; **193**: 220), possibly because it reflects low blood volume, as found in pre-eclampsia, and because of its association with smoking.

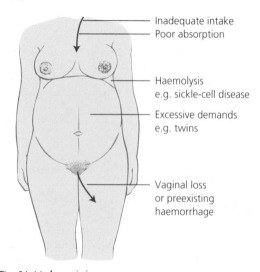

Fig. 21.11 Anaemia in pregnancy.

Inadequate intake
Poor absorption

Haemolysis
e.g. sickle-cell disease

Excessive demands
e.g. twins

Vaginal loss
or preexisting
haemorrhage

Iron deficiency anaemia

This affects >10% of pregnant women, although 80% of women not receiving iron have depleted stores by term. Folic acid deficiency may coexist. Symptoms are usually absent unless the haemoglobin is <9 g/dL. The mean cell volume (MCV) reduces (Fig. 21.12), but is often initially normal; ferritin levels are reduced. Treatment with oral iron, achieving an increase of up to 0.8 g/dL per week, can cause gastrointestinal upset. In severe cases, intravenous iron is quicker and may prevent the need for blood transfusion; intramuscular iron is painful.

Folic acid and vitamin B12 deficiency anaemia

Folic acid deficiency is more common than that of vitamin B12. The MCV is usually increased. Red cell folic acid or vitamin B12 levels are low. Folic acid deficiency should always be considered if anaemia is present without marked microcytosis. Treatment is with oral folic acid or vitamin B12.

Prophylaxis against anaemia

Routine iron supplements reduce the incidence of anaemia without affecting perinatal outcome (*Cochrane* 2007; CD003094). Nevertheless, postnatal blood transfusion is required less frequently. Further, fetal and neonatal anaemia have adverse outcomes although their relationship to maternal iron stores is unknown. Iron is often poorly tolerated, and routine supplementation is not universal: all women are given dietary advice, and the haemoglobin is checked at booking and at 28 and 34 weeks. Iron ± folic acid are given if the haemoglobin (Hb) is <11.0 g/dL in the first and third trimesters and if <10.5 g/dL in the second trimester. Because routine preconceptual and first-trimester folic acid supplements (0.4 mg) reduce the incidence of NTDs, these

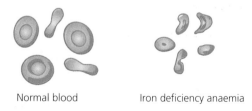

Normal blood   Iron deficiency anaemia

Fig. 21.12 Picture of blood film of iron deficiency anaemia.

are recommended to all women. In those with epilepsy, diabetes, obesity or a previous history of an NTD, a higher dose (5 mg) is used.

Dietary advice to avoid anaemia	
Food rich in iron	Meat, particularly kidney and liver, eggs, green vegetables
Food rich in folic acid	Lightly cooked or raw green vegetables, fish
Guinness is not recommended in pregnancy	

Influenza

Influenza accounted for 10% of all maternal deaths in the UK and US during the 2009–10 swine flu (H1N1) pandemic; in 2011–13 in the UK it accounted for 4%. Pregnancy, particularly with comorbidity, increases susceptibility to severe disease. Presentation is typical; the diagnosis must be considered and early use of Relenza (zanamivir) is recommended. With more severe disease or in these pre-existing chest disease, Tamiflu (oseltamivir) is recommended. Intensive care unit admission, and even extracorporeal membrane oxygenation (ECMO) may be required. The best management is prevention: vaccination of pregnant women, at any stage of pregnancy, is to be strongly advised during winter months. Healthcare workers should similarly be vaccinated. Pregnancy vaccination has no known adverse fetal effects and will reduce both maternal and fetal mortality.

Haemoglobinopathies

The adult haemoglobin molecule (HbA) is made of two alpha chains and two beta chains, bound together in a tetramer. Fetal haemoglobin (HbF), which is normally gradually replaced by the adult type after birth, is made of two alpha chains and two gamma chains.

Sickle cell disease

Pathology and epidemiology

This recessive disorder is due to abnormal beta-chain formation (called an S chain) in the haemoglobin molecule. The result is an abnormal haemoglobin molecule made of two alpha chains bound to two S chains. A further variant of the beta-chain (C) is found. Sickle

S is found in people with Afro-Caribbean ancestry. In the UK, there are 100–200 pregnancies in homozygotic individuals every year, but 300 000 affected individuals are born worldwide every year.

Heterozygotes (sickle minor) have 35% HbS and usually have no problems; *homozygotes* (sickle major) have only HbS, or HbSC. Haemoglobin electrophoresis is now performed in the UK on all pregnant women.

Complications of sickle cell disease

Homozygous individuals have often been affected with 'crises' of bony pain and pulmonary symptoms, and have chronic haemolytic anaemia all their life. Pulmonary hypertension and proliferative retinopathy may occur.

Maternal complications in pregnancy include acute painful crises (35%), pre-eclampsia and thrombosis.

Fetal complications are miscarriage, IUGR, preterm labour and death.

Following routine haemoglobinopathy screening, the partners of heterozygotes are also tested: if positive, prenatal diagnosis for homozygosity is offered.

Management of sickle cell disease

Management should be in conjunction with a haemoglobinopathy specialist. Advice on avoiding dehydration and seeking early help is given. Hydroxycarbamide is probably teratogenic and is stopped. Penicillin V is continued, high-dose (5 mg) folic acid supplements are given, aspirin is advised for prophylaxis against pre-eclampsia and LMWH is often indicated. Monthly urine culture is advised. Iron is avoided because of overload. Routine transfusion is not warranted but exchange transfusions may be required for crises and have been used in recurrent pregnancy loss in uncontrolled studies. These crises are managed with hydration, analgesia, and often antibtiotics and anticoagulation. Ultrasound is used 4 weekly for fetal growth and delivery is normally indicated by 38 weeks.

Thalassaemias

Pathology and epidemiology

Alpha thalassaemia results from impaired synthesis of the alpha chain in the haemoglobin molecule. It occurs largely in people of South-East Asian origin. Four genes are responsible for a chain synthesis. Individuals with four gene deletions die *in utero*. Those with three gene deletions (HbH disease, rare) have a lifelong requirement for transfusions. Those with one or two gene deletions are carriers, and are usually well but mildly anaemic.

Beta thalassaemia results from impaired beta-chain synthesis. It occurs largely in people of South-East Asian and Mediterranean ancestry. It is a recessive disorder and the heterozygous state of one defective chain (beta thalassaemia minor) causes little illness, although a chronic anaemia which can worsen during pregnancy. Homozygous beta thalassaemia (major) in pregnancy is rare in the UK, but 70 000 affected individuals are born worldwide every year.

Complications of beta thalassaemia major

A chronic haemolytic anaemia is present and multiple transfusions cause iron overload and therefore hepatic and cardiac dysfunction, and endocrine disease, particularly of the thyroid and parathyroid, and diabetes. Monitoring for effects of iron overload and use of chelation therapy have been key to reducing mortality.

Maternal complications: Fertility is reduced, liver disease, cardiac failure and diabetes are common.

Fetal complications: Growth restriction and fetal demise are more common. Prenatal diagnosis is offered if the partner is heterozygous for either the beta or alpha form.

Management of beta thalassaemia major

Preconceptual planning is crucial, not least because chelation therapy is probably teratogenic and is avoided in the first trimester. Desferrioxamine can be used after this time. Care is multidisciplinary with endocrinology and cardiac input particularly. Ultrasound is used 4 weekly.

Female genital mutilation (FGM)

Also known as 'female circumcision', this practice involves partial or total removal of the external female genitalia, or other injury to the female genital organs for non-medical reasons. It is classified into four types.

- Type 1: Clitoridectomy: partial or total removal of the clitoris, or of the prepuce.
- Type 2: Excision: partial or total removal of the clitoris and the labia minora, ± the labia majora.
- Type 3: Infibulation: narrowing of the vaginal opening by cutting and repositioning the labia, with or without removal of the clitoris.
- Type 4: Other: all other non-medical procedures to the female genitalia for non-medical purposes.

Female genital mutilation is practised in many countries in Africa and the Middle East and in Malaysia and Indonesia. Communities practise FGM for different reasons, including ideas of preservation of virginity, promoting hygiene, adherence to cultural norms, and religion. FGM is not condoned in the Bible or Koran. FGM is performed from infancy to 15 years, depending on the country and culture. Tools used include knives, scissors, scalpels, pieces of glass and razor blades, usually without septic technique or anaesthesia. FGM is a violation of human rights, is child abuse and has no health benefits.

Complications include pain, bleeding, infection, urinary retention, damage to pelvic organs and death. Longer-term complications include failure to heal, urinary tract infections, difficulty urinating or menstruating, chronic pelvic infection, vulval pain due to cysts and neuromas, pain during sex, infertility, fistula and severe perineal trauma during childbirth. Psychological complications are common.

FGM and the law: In the UK it is illegal to perform FGM, including reinstatement after vaginal birth, or to arrange for FGM to happen. It is also illegal to take or arrange for a girl to be taken to another country for FGM, even if it is legal in that country. Female children may be at risk of FGM and healthcare workers have a statutory duty to safeguard them.

Further reading

CMACE/RCOG Joint Guideline. *Management of Women with Obesity in Pregnancy. Available at*: www.rcog.org.uk/globalassets/documents/guidelines/cmacercogjointguidelinemanagementwomenobesitypregnancya.pdf (accessed 18 July 2016).

de Groot L, Abalovich M, Alexander E, *et al. Management of Thyroid Dysfunction during Pregnancy and Postpartum: An Endocrine Society Clinical Practice Guideline.* Available at: *http://press.endocrine.org/doi/abs/10.1210/jc.2011-2803* (accessed 18 July 2016).

Mackillop L, Williamson C. Liver disease in pregnancy. *Postgraduate Medical Journal* 2010; **86**: 160–164.

MBRRACE-UK. Saving Lives, Improving Mothers' Care. Lessons learned to inform future maternity care from the UK and Ireland Confidential Enquiries into Maternal Deaths and Morbidity 2009–2012. Available at: www.npeu.ox.ac.uk/downloads/files/mbrrace-uk/reports/Saving%20Lives%20Improving%20Mothers%20Care%20report%202014%20Full.pdf (accessed 18 July 2016).

Myers B, Pavord S. Diagnosis and management of antiphospholipid syndrome in pregnancy. *Obstetrician and Gynaecologist* 2011; **13**: 15–21.

National Institute for Health and Care Excellence. Domestic Violence and Abuse: Multi-Agency Working. Available at: *www.nice.org.uk/guidance/ph50* (accessed 18 July 2016).

National Institute for Health and Care Excellence. Antenatal and Postnatal Mental Health: Clinical Management and Service Guidance. Clinical Guideline No. 192. Available at: *www.nice.org.uk/guidance/cg192/chapter/1-recommendations* (accessed 18 July 2016).

National Institute for Health and Care Excellence. Diabetes in Pregnancy: Management of Diabetes and Its Complications from Preconception to the Postnatal Period. Available at: *www.nice.org.uk/guidance/ng3/evidence/full-guideline-3784285* (accessed 18 July 2016).

Patra J, Bakker R, Irving H, Jaddoe V, Malini S, Rehm J. Dose–response relationship between alcohol consumption before and during pregnancy and the risks of low birthweight, preterm birth and small for gestational age (SGA) – a systematic review and meta-analyses. *BJOG* 2011; **118**: 1411–1421.

Royal College of Obstetricians and Gynaecologists. Obstetric Cholestasis. Green-top Guideline 43. Available at: www.rcog.org.uk/globalassets/documents/guidelines/gtg_43.pdf (accessed 18 July 2016).

Royal College of Obstetricians and Gynaecologists. Reducing the Risk of Venous Thromboembolism during Pregnancy and the Puerperium. Green-top Guideline No. 37a. Available at: *www.rcog.org.uk/globalassets/documents/guidelines/gtg-37a.pdf* (accessed 18 July 2016).

Royal College of Obstetricians and Gynaecologists. Management of Sickle Cell Disease in Pregnancy. Green-top Guideline No. 61. Available at: *www.rcog.org.uk/globalassets/documents/guidelines/gtg_61.pdf* (accessed 18 July 2016).

Royal College of Obstetricians and Gynaecologists. Management of Beta Thalassaemia in Pregnancy. Green-top Guideline No. 66. Available at: www.rcog.org.uk/globalassets/documents/guidelines/gtg_66_thalassaemia.pdf

SIGN 141. British Guideline on the Management of Asthma. Available at: *www.brit-thoracic.org.uk/document-library/clinical-information/asthma/bts-sign-asthma-guideline-2014/* (accessed 18 July 2016).

Stratta P, Canavese C, Quaglia M. Pregnancy in patients with kidney disease. *Journal of Nephrology* 2006; **19**: 135–143.

Taskforce on the Management of Cardiovascular Diseases during Pregnancy of the European Society of Cardiology. ESC guidelines on the management of cardiovascular diseases during pregnancy. *European Heart Journal* 2011; **32**: 3147–3197. Available at: http://eurheartj.oxfordjournals.org/content/ehj/32/24/3147.full.pdf (accessed 18 July 2016).

Walker SP, Permezel M, Berkovic SF. The management of epilepsy in pregnancy. *British Journal of Obstetrics and Gynaecology* 2009; **116**: 758.

Diabetes in pregnancy at a glance

Definitions	Pre-existing (T1 or T2) diabetes: 1%
Complications	Maternal: increased insulin requirements, hypoglycaemia, worsening retinopathy, pre-eclampsia, infections, operative delivery, rarely ketoacidosis Fetal: congenital abnormalities, preterm labour, macrosomia, birth trauma, fetal death
Management	
Preconceptual	Optimize glucose (HbA1c <6.5 and fasting glucose <7) Review drugs; check renal function and eyes 5 mg folic acid
Glucose levels	Check with glucometer, aim for tight control (<5.3 fasting, <7.8 1 h after food) Use insulin ± metformin; give glucagon Reduce doses post delivery
Monitoring	Monitor renal function and eyes if affected
Other	Aspirin 75 mg for pre-eclampsia
Fetus	Cardiac scan, growth scans at 32 and 36 weeks Induction at 37–39 weeks; caesarean if >4–4.5 kg Beware neonatal hypoglycaemia

Gestational diabetes at a glance

Definitions	Impaired glucose tolerance in pregnancy: 16%
Epidemiology	Abnormal glucose tolerance test (GTT): fasting level >5.6; 2 h after 75 g glucose >7.8
Screening	GTT at 24–28 weeks if family history of diabetes mellitus (DM), at-risk ethnic group, body mass index(BMI) >30, previous large baby or stillbirth, persistent glycosuria or polyhydramnios GTT also after booking if previous gestational diabetes
Management	Baseline HbA1c Glucometer monitoring, aim for similar glucose levels to pre-existing diabetics Initially diet and exercise advice, then metformin, then insulin Fetal monitoring as for pre-existing diabetics Induction by 41 weeks, caesarean if >3–4.5 kg
Postnatally	Do fasting blood glucose at 6 weeks

Thrombophilia in pregnancy at a glance

High-risk types	Antiphospholipid syndrome, protein S and C deficiency, activated protein C resistance and antithrombin III deficiency
Lower risk	Factor V Leiden heterozygosity, prothrombin gene variant, hyperhomocysteinaemia, antiphospholipid Ab with no syndrome
Complications	Venous thromboembolism Miscarriage, preterm delivery, pre-eclampsia, placental abruption, intrauterine growth restriction (IUGR), fetal death largely limited to high-risk types
Management	Individualized. Increased maternal and fetal surveillance Aspirin as pre-eclampsia prophylaxis Low molecular weight heparin (LMWH) for postnatal ± antenatal thromboprophylaxis Antenatal LMWH if previous pregnancy loss or complication High-dose folic acid if hyperhomocysteinaemia

Venous thromboembolism at a glance

Deep vein thrombosis (DVT)	0.1% Usually left leg swelling and pain Diagnosed with ultrasound or venogram Anticoagulate with low molecular weight heparin (LMWH)
Pulmonary embolism	Collapse, chest pain, dyspnoea, tachycardia Diagnosed with computed tomography pulmonary angiogram or VQ scan Anticoagulate with LMWH
Thromboprophylaxis	Risk assessment scores used for prevention of venous thromboembolism High risk, e.g. previous DVT: antenatal LMWH LMWH given antenatally and frequently postnatally on basis of number of risk factors and severity

Anaemia and haemoglobinopathy in pregnancy at a glance

Iron deficiency	>10% of women Mean cell volume (MCV), mean cell haemoglobin concentration (MCHC) and ferritin reduced Prophylaxis: disputed. Treat if haemoglobin (Hb) <11.0 g/dL Oral iron poorly tolerated; intravenous for rapid response/severe anaemia
Folate deficiency	Rarer MCV raised or normal; red cell folate reduced Prophylaxis: routine (0.4 mg) in early pregnancy and preconceptually. High (5 mg) dose if woman has epilepsy, diabetes, body mass index >30, malabsorption syndromes, previous deficiency, sickle cell disease, hyperhomocysteinaemia or previous neural tube defect
Sickle cell	Major: homozygous HbSS or SC. Heterozygotes common Maternal complications: crises, thrombosis, pre-eclampsia Fetal complications: intrauterine growth retardation increased perinatal mortality Management: folic acid, aspirin, penicillin V; avoid precipitating factors for crises ± low molecular weight heparin and exchange transfusions Test partner (including if heterozygote) ± prenatal diagnosis

Other medical disorders at a glance

Influenza
Major cause of mortality
Vaccinate in winter
Recognize symptoms and treat early

Cholestasis
Pruritus without rash with elevated liver enzymes/bile acids
Increased but often overestimated risk of stillbirth
Monitor liver function, give vitamin K late pregnancy
Discuss induction from 38 weeks

Obesity
Body mass index >30, 20% incidence
Increased risk of most maternal and fetal complications
High-dose folate, aspirin, screen for gestational diabetes
Thromboprophylaxis according to individual risk

Cardiac disease
Major cause of maternal mortality
Preconceptual review essential if severe. Manage with cardiologist
Anticoagulation depending on type
Fetal echo as increased risk

Renal disease
Major risks pre-eclampsia, polyhydramnios and preterm delivery
If immunosuppressed (transplant), monitor levels
Assess renal function: may deteriorate

Hyperthyroidism
Use propylthiouracil

Hypothyroidism
Common, often dose increases, maintain thyroid-stimulating hormone <2.5

Female genital mutilation
Illegal to perform or repair in the UK
Identification difficult but key to safe delivery and prevention of FGM in child

Epilepsy
Common
Preconceptual change to non-teratogenic drugs ideal
High-dose folate, fetal echo, vitamin K late pregnancy
May need drug level increase/monitoring

Depression
Very common, particularly postpartum. Important cause of maternal death
Screen using questionnaire
Cognitive behavioural therapy ± antidepressants
Discuss safety issues with selective serotonin reuptake inhibitors
Early referral if severe/suicidal

CHAPTER 22
Red blood cell isoimmunization

Definition

Red blood cell isoimmunization occurs when the mother mounts an immune response against antigens on fetal red cells that enter her circulation. The resulting antibodies then cross the placenta and cause fetal red blood cell destruction.

Pathophysiology

Blood groups

Blood is classified according to its ABO and Rhesus genotype. The Rhesus system consists of three linked gene pairs; one allele of each pair is dominant to the other: *C/c*, *D/d* and *E/e*. An individual inherits one allele of each pair from each parent in a Mendelian fashion. The most significant in isoimmunization is the *D* gene. As *D* is dominant to *d*, only individuals who are *DD* or *Dd* (i.e. homozygous or heterozygous) express the D antigen and are 'D Rhesus positive' (Fig. 22.1). Individuals homozygous for the recessive *d* (*dd*) are 'D Rhesus negative' and their immune system will recognize the D antigen as foreign if they are exposed to it.

Sensitization

Small amounts of fetal blood cross the placenta and enter the maternal circulation during uncomplicated pregnancies and particularly at sensitizing events, such as delivery. If the fetus is D Rhesus positive and the mother is D Rhesus negative, the mother will mount an immune response (sensitization), creating anti-D antibodies.

Haemolysis

Immunity is permanent, and if the mother's immune system is again exposed to the antigen (e.g. a subsequent pregnancy), large numbers of antibodies are rapidly created. They can cross the placenta and bind to fetal red blood cells, which are then destroyed in the fetal reticuloendothelial system (Fig. 22.2). This can cause haemolytic anaemia and ultimately death, and is called Rhesus haemolytic disease. A similar immune response can be mounted against other red blood cell antigens; the principal antibodies affecting the fetus are anti-c, anti-E and anti-Kell (a non-Rhesus antibody).

Potentially sensitizing events
Termination of pregnancy or evacuation of retained products of conception (ERPC) after miscarriage
Ectopic pregnancy
Vaginal bleeding >12 weeks, or <12 weeks if heavy
External cephalic version
Invasive uterine procedure, e.g. amniocentesis or chorionic villus sampling (CVS)
Intrauterine death
Delivery

Prevention: using anti-D

Production of maternal anti-D can be prevented by the administration of exogenous anti-D to the mother. This 'mops up' fetal red cells that have crossed the placenta, by binding to their antigens, thereby preventing recognition by the mother's immune system. If both parents are known to be D Rhesus negative, the fetus

Obstetrics & Gynaecology, Fifth Edition. Lawrence Impey, Tim Child.
© 2017 John Wiley & Sons, Ltd. Published 2017 by John Wiley & Sons, Ltd.

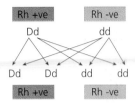

Fig. 22.1 Mendelian inheritance of *D/d* gene pair.

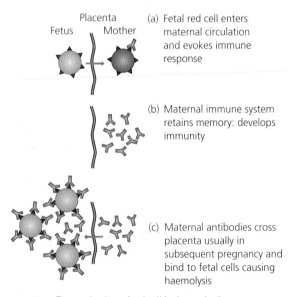

(a) Fetal red cell enters maternal circulation and evokes immune response

(b) Maternal immune system retains memory: develops immunity

(c) Maternal antibodies cross placenta usually in subsequent pregnancy and bind to fetal cells causing haemolysis

Fig. 22.2 The mechanism of red cell isoimmunization.

must also be Rhesus negative and therefore will be unaffected. Routine *non-invasive prenatal testing* (NIPT) for fetal Rhesus type, using maternal blood, is now recommended in the UK to determine whether anti-D is necessary. Anti-D is pointless if maternal anti-D is already present, as sensitization has already occurred.

Antenatal: Anti-D (1500 IU) should be given to all women who are Rhesus negative if fetal status is unknown or the baby is Rhesus positive, at 28 weeks; this alone will reduce the rate of isoimmunization in a first pregnancy from 1.5% to 0.2%. Anti-D is also given to such women within 72 hours of any sensitizing event, although some benefit is gained within 10 days. These include a miscarriage or threatened miscarriage after 12 weeks, or before if the uterus is instrumented (e.g. ERPC), termination of pregnancy and ectopic pregnancy. Anti-D is also given

after *in utero* procedures such as amniocentesis and after external cephalic version, fetal death or antepartum haemorrhage.

Postnatal: The neonate's blood group is checked and if Rhesus positive, anti-D is given to the mother within 72 hours of delivery. A Kleihauer test, to assess the number of fetal cells in the maternal circulation, is also performed within 2 hours of birth to detect occasional larger fetomaternal haemorrhages that require larger doses of anti-D to 'mop up'. Anti-D is unnecessary if the neonate is Rhesus negative.

Prevention of rhesus disease	
Booking and 28 weeks	Check all women for antibodies
Rhesus-negative women with baby unknown Rh status or Rh+	Give anti-D 1500 IU at 28 weeks, after any bleeding or potentially sensitizing event and after delivery if neonate is Rhesus positive

Epidemiology

Fifteen per cent of Caucasian women, but fewer African or Asian women, are D Rhesus negative. The use of anti-D, smaller family size and good management of isoimmunization has resulted in perinatal deaths attributable to Rhesus disease becoming extremely rare. Currently about 1% of D Rhesus-negative women have been sensitized in the UK, mostly as a result of omitted or inadequate anti-D. Anti-c, anti-E and anti-Kell now account for as many cases of fetal anaemia, largely because of the decline in anti-D Rhesus disease. Many other, rare, antibodies can cause mild fetal anaemia and postnatal jaundice.

Manifestations of Rhesus disease

As antibody levels rise in a sensitized woman, the antibodies will cross the placenta and cause haemolysis. In mild disease, this may lead to *neonatal jaundice* only. Or there may be sufficient haemolysis to cause neonatal anaemia (haemolytic disease of the newborn). More

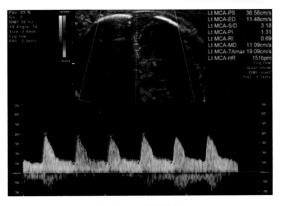

Fig. 22.3 Middle cerebral artery (MCA) Doppler.

severe disease causes *in utero* anaemia and, as this worsens, cardiac failure, ascites and oedema (hydrops) and fetal death follow. Rhesus disease usually worsens with successive pregnancies as maternal antibody production increases.

Management of isoimmunization

The management of rhesus isoimmunization varies widely but comprises:
- identification of women at risk of fetal haemolysis and anaemia
- assessing if/how severely the fetus is anaemic
- blood transfusion *in utero* or delivery for affected fetuses.

Identification

Fetal rhesus status: Unsensitized women are screened for antibodies at booking and at 28 weeks' gestation. If antibodies are found, the fetal genotype needs to be determined. If the father is homozygous (i.e. DD), the fetus will be Rh positive (Dd) and at risk. If the father is heterozygous (i.e. Dd), or cannot be tested, maternal blood is sampled for free fetal DNA to assess fetal Rh status. If the fetus is D negative (dd), it is not at risk. Routine antibody testing only, as with a normal pregnancy, is performed.

Maternal antibody level: If anti-D levels are <10IU/mL, and there is no previous history of an affected baby, a significant fetal problem is very unlikely and levels are subsequently checked every 2–4 weeks. When anti-D levels are above 4IU/mL (for anti-c, threshold is 7.5), the fetus is investigated for anaemia using ultrasound. If there is a previous history of fetal effects, antibody levels are less predictive. Equally, anti-Kell antibody levels are less predictive of disease severity so ultrasound is used earlier.

Assessing severity of fetal anaemia

Pregnancies at risk of fetal anaemia are assessed using ultrasound. Doppler ultrasound of the peak velocity in systole (PSV) of the fetal middle cerebral artery (MCA) (Fig. 22.3) has a high sensitivity for significant anaemia (*NEJM* 2000; **342**: 9), at least before 36 weeks. It is therefore used at least fortnightly in at-risk pregnancies. Very severe anaemia (e.g. <5g/dL) is detectable as fetal hydrops or excessive fetal fluid. If anaemia is suspected, fetal blood sampling is performed under ultrasound guidance, using a needle in the umbilical vein at the cord insertion in the placenta, or in the intrahepatic vein. The risk of fetal loss is 1%, and after 28 weeks it should be performed with facilities for immediate delivery if complications arise.

Treatment of fetal anaemia: *in utero* transfusion

Fetal blood sampling is performed with Rh-negative, high haematocrit, cytomegalovirus-negative blood ready, which can be injected into the umbilical vein if anaemia is confirmed. This process of quantification of anaemia and transfusion will need to be repeated at longer intervals (as more of the fetal blood is donor and therefore not subject to haemolysis) until about 36 weeks, after which time delivery is undertaken. Blood can be administered to the neonate; both top-up (for anaemia) and exchange (for hyperbilirubinaemia as a result of haemolysis) transfusions may be required.

All neonates born to Rh-negative women should have the blood group checked; a full blood count (FBC), blood film and bilirubin may detect mild degrees of isoimmunization. A Coombs' test is no longer advised.

Further reading

Qureshi H, Massey E, Kirwan D, *et al.* BCSH guideline for the use of anti-D immunoglobulin for the prevention of haemolytic disease of the fetus and newborn. *Transfusion Medicine* 2014; **24** (1): 8–20. Available at: http://onlinelibrary.wiley.com/doi/10.1111/tme.12091/full (accessed 18 July 2016).

Royal College of Obstetricians and Gynaecologists. *The Management of Women with Red Cell Antibodies during Pregnancy*. Green-top Guideline No. 65. Available at: www.rcog.org.uk/globalassets/documents/guidelines/rbc_gtg65.pdf (accessed 18 July 2016).

Rhesus isoimmunization at a glance

Definition	Maternal antibody response against fetal red cell antigen entering her circulation; passage of antibodies into fetus leads to haemolysis	
Aetiology	Anti-D still prevalent because of inadequate/failed prophylaxis	
	Other major antibodies: anti-c, anti-E and anti-Kell	
Epidemiology	15% of Caucasian women are Rh negative; anti-D responses in 1%	
Pathology	Haemolysis causes anaemia; hydrops and fetal death if severe Neonatal jaundice ± anaemia if less severe	
Prevention	Administer anti-D to Rh-negative women with unknown Rh status or Rh+ fetus, at 28 weeks, and after potentially sensitizing events	
Management	Identification	Determine fetal genotype using paternal blood ± free fetal DNA Antibody testing fortnightly and past obstetric history
	Assess severity	Doppler of fetal middle cerebral artery fortnightly Fetal blood sampling if anaemia likely
	Treat	Transfuse blood if fetus anaemic, deliver if >36 weeks
	Postnatally	Check full blood count (FBC), bilirubin, Rhesus group

CHAPTER 23
Delivery before term

Definitions and epidemiology

Preterm delivery occurs between 24 and 37 weeks' gestation. However, it is most important before 34 weeks because that is when the neonatal risks are greater. Before 24 weeks, labour is tantamount to a miscarriage, although exceptionally fetal survival occurs at 23 weeks.

Some 5–8% of deliveries are preterm. A further 6% of deliveries present preterm with contractions but deliver at term. Preterm delivery can be the result of *spontaneous* labour or, usually at later gestations, can be *iatrogenic*. This is where delivery is expedited by the obstetrician because the fetal or maternal risks of continuation justify exposing the fetus to the risks of preterm delivery. As these risks lessen with increasing gestation, the threshold for such intervention changes. The most common example is pre-eclampsia, where delivery is the only cure, and a pregnancy affected at, say, 28 weeks would have a high risk of both maternal and fetal death if it continued to term.

Late miscarriage occurs between 16 and 23 + 6 weeks with, in reality, an overlap with preterm delivery where the fetus is born alive. The aetiology and management of a subsequent pregnancy overlap with preterm labour although the management of the affected pregnancy (at least before 23 weeks) is different because the chances of survival are almost nil.

Complications

Neonatal: Prematurity accounts for 80% of neonatal intensive care occupancy, 20% of perinatal mortality and up to 50% of cerebral palsy (Fig. 23.1). Other long-term morbidity, including chronic lung disease, blindness and minor disability, is common (Fig. 23.2). The earlier the gestation, the greater the risks to the fetus: at 24 weeks, approximately one-third of babies will be handicapped and one-third will die; by 32 weeks both these risks are less than 5%. Even between 34 and 37 weeks there is increased respiratory distress, infant mortality and an increased risk of subtle cognitive and behavioural problems. Preterm delivery is the most important and possibly least understood area of pregnancy.

Maternal: Infection is frequently associated with preterm labour and can occasionally cause severe maternal illness and death. Caesarean section is more commonly used.

Aetiology of spontaneous preterm labour
(Fig. 23.3)

Risk factors

These are multiple and include a previous history, lower socioeconomic class, extremes of maternal age, a short interpregnancy interval, maternal medical disease such as renal failure, diabetes and thyroid disease, pregnancy complications such as pre-eclampsia or intrauterine growth restriction (IUGR), male fetal gender, a high haemoglobin, sexually transmitted infections (STIs) and vaginal infection (such as bacterial vaginosis), previous cervical surgery, multiple pregnancy, uterine abnormalities and fibroids, urinary infection, polyhydramnios, congenital fetal abnormalities and antepartum haemorrhage.

Mechanisms

To rationalize these disparate risks, the uterus can be thought of as a castle, with the cervix as the castle wall holding the 'defenders' in (see Fig. 23.3). Three groups

Obstetrics & Gynaecology, Fifth Edition. Lawrence Impey, Tim Child.
© 2017 John Wiley & Sons, Ltd. Published 2017 by John Wiley & Sons, Ltd.

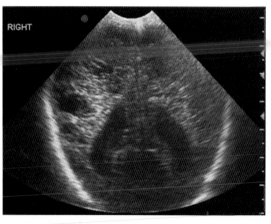
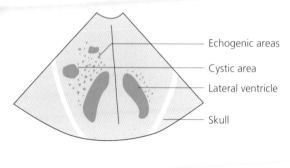

Fig. 23.1 Postnatal ultrasound of cystic periventricular leucomalacia, a precursor to cerebral palsy.

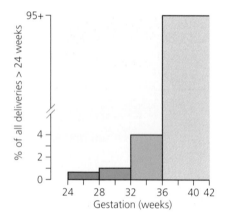

Fig. 23.2 Incidence of preterm delivery. Source: Oxford data.

of mechanisms, affecting the defenders, the castle walls or the enemy, lead to the wall being breached.

Too many defenders: Multiple pregnancy is an increasing contributor because of assisted conception. Delivery before 34 weeks occurs in 20% of twins and is the mean time for delivery of triplets. Excess liquor, polyhydramnios, has the same effect, probably largely mediated by increased stretch.

The defenders 'give up': The 'fetal survival' response. Spontaneous preterm labour is more common where the fetus is at risk, e.g. pre-eclampsia and IUGR, or if there is infection. Likewise, a placental abruption will often be followed by labour. Iatrogenic preterm delivery attempts to improve upon this mechanism.

The castle design is poor: Uterine abnormalities such as fibroids or congenital (Müllerian duct) abnormalities.

The wall is weak: The phrase 'cervical incompetence' unhelpfully describes the painless cervical dilatation that precedes some preterm deliveries. Some follow cervical surgery including treatments for cervical intraepithelial neoplasia (CIN) or cervical cancer, or multiple dilatations of the cervix, but in many no risk factors are known.

The enemy knock down the walls: Infection is implicated in about 60% of preterm deliveries, and is often subclinical. Chorioamnionitis, offensive liquor, neonatal sepsis and endometritis after delivery are all manifestations. Bacterial vaginosis is a well-known risk factor, but many bacteria, including group B streptococcus (GBS), *Trichomonas*, *Chlamydia* and even commensals, have been implicated. The effects of infection are partly dependent on the cervix: whether a castle wall falls down depends on both its strength and that of the enemy. In practice, therefore, a cervical component and infection often coexist.

The enemy get around the walls: Urinary tract infection and poor dental health (*J Periodontol* 2005; **76**: 2144) are risk factors.

Prediction of preterm labour

History: Those at increased risk (see above), particularly those with a previous history of late miscarriage or preterm labour, may undergo investigations and attempts to prevent preterm delivery. Nevertheless, most women who deliver preterm are not identified as high risk on history alone.

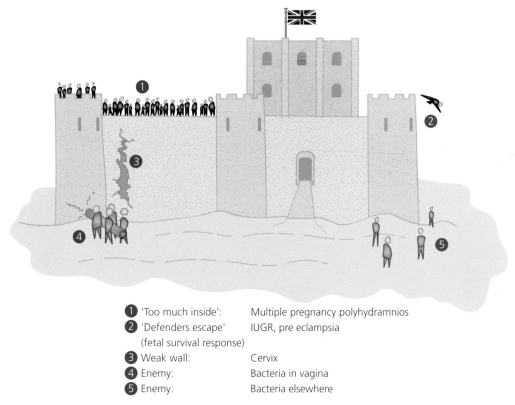

1. 'Too much inside':   Multiple pregnancy polyhydramnios
2. 'Defenders escape'   IUGR, pre eclampsia
   (fetal survival response)
3. Weak wall: Cervix
4. Enemy: Bacteria in vagina
5. Enemy: Bacteria elsewhere

Fig. 23.3 Risk factors for preterm delivery.

Investigations: Even in women apparently at low risk for preterm delivery, the *cervical length* on transvaginal sonography (TVS) (Figs 23.4, 23.5) is both sensitive and specific. Prediction is, however, not the same as prevention.

Prevention of preterm labour

Preventive strategies are usually limited to women at high risk; frequently these are women who have previously delivered between 16 and 34 weeks. It is unclear

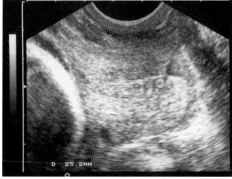

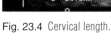

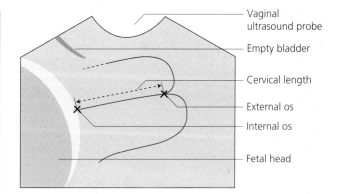

Vaginal ultrasound probe

Empty bladder

Cervical length

External os

Internal os

Fetal head

Fig. 23.4 Cervical length.

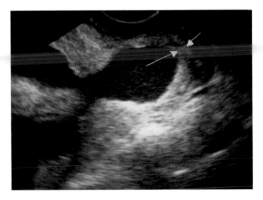

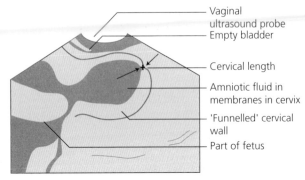

- Vaginal ultrasound probe
- Empty bladder
- Cervical length
- Amniotic fluid in membranes in cervix
- 'Funnelled' cervical wall
- Part of fetus

Fig. 23.5 Abnormal cervical length.

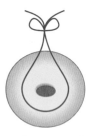

Fig. 23.6 Cervical suture. Transverse section of the cervix.

if universal screening of all women with a cervical scan could lead to an overall reduction in the incidence of preterm labour. In women at high risk, because preterm labour is usually the culmination of events initiated many weeks earlier, strategies should begin by 12 weeks.

The cervix

Cervical cerclage is the insertion of one or more sutures in the cervix to strengthen it and keep it closed (Fig. 23.6). It is commonly used although its effectiveness in isolation is disputed. The vaginal route is usual, but it can be placed abdominally if the cervix is very short or scarred, or if previous vaginal cerclage has failed. This is usually pre-pregnancy and can be laparoscopic.

Cerclage is used in one of three situations. It can be elective, at 12–14 weeks. Or the cervix can be scanned regularly and only sutured if there is significant shortening. This is the most usual policy. Finally, it can be used as a 'rescue suture' that will, in expert hands and in the absence of infection or contractions, prevent delivery even when the cervix is widely dilated in up to 50% of suitable women (*J Mat Fet Neonatal Med* 2010; **23**:670–674).

Progesterone supplementation

Suppositories from early pregnancy reduce the risk of preterm labour in women at high risk. The data suggest even low-risk women with a short cervix (<25 mm) on ultrasound may benefit, meaning that universal screening may indeed be worthwhile (*UOG* 2011; **38**: 18). This is currently not recommended.

Infection

Although infection is common, it is likely that some bacteria are beneficial. In practice, screening and treatment of sexually transmitted disease, urinary tract infections (UTIs) and *bacterial vaginosis* (if before 16 weeks) are beneficial, although the role of antibiotics for other bacteria is disputed.

Fetal reduction

Reduction of higher order multiples is offered at 10–14 weeks.

Treatment of polyhydramnios

Very high amniotic fluid volumes, usually as a result of a fetal abnormality, can be treated by needle aspiration (amnioreduction) or, providing fetal surveillance is intensive, non-steroidal anti-inflammatory drugs (NSAIDs). These reduce fetal urine output, and occasionally cause (reversible) premature closure of the fetal ductus arteriosus.

Treatment of medical disease

The prevention of placental disease associated with autoimmune disease reduces the risk of preterm delivery. Women with thyroid antibodies may also benefit from thyroxine (*BMJ* 2011; **342**: d2616).

Clinical features

History: Typically, women present with painful contractions. In over half of such women, however, the contractions will stop spontaneously and labour will not ensue until term. With 'cervical incompetence', painless cervical dilatation may occur or the woman may experience only a dull suprapubic ache or increased discharge. Antepartum haemorrhage and fluid loss are common: the latter suggests ruptured membranes.

Examination: Fever may occur and severe sepsis may be present. The lie and presentation of the fetus are checked (Fig. 23.7). Digital vaginal examination is performed unless the membranes have ruptured. A dilated cervix confirms the diagnosis, but preterm labour is unpredictable and may be extremely rapid or very slow.

Investigations

To assess the likelihood of delivery if the cervix is uneffaced, 'point of care' testing (e.g. fetal fibronectin assay) is used: a negative result means preterm delivery within the next week is unlikely. TVS of cervical length is also predictive: delivery is unlikely if the cervix is >15 mm long.

To assess fetal state, cardiotocography (CTG) and ultrasound are used.

To look for infection, vaginal swabs should be taken, using a sterile speculum if the membranes have ruptured. The maternal C-reactive protein (CRP) usually rises with chorioamnionitis; white cell count estimation is useful but steroids will cause it to rise.

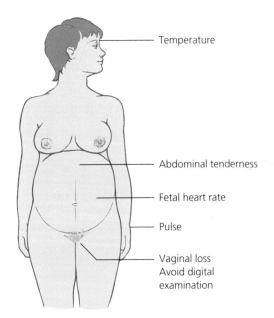

Fig. 23.7 Monitoring the patient with preterm prelabour rupture of the membranes.

Labels: Temperature; Abdominal tenderness; Fetal heart rate; Pulse; Vaginal loss Avoid digital examination

Management

Steroids and tocolysis

Steroids are given between 23 and 34 weeks. In women presenting only with contractions, they can be restricted to those who are fibronectin positive or have a short cervix. Steroids reduce perinatal morbidity and mortality by promoting pulmonary maturity. They do not increase the risk of infection, but additional insulin is often needed in diabetic patients. As they take 24 hours to act, delivery is often artificially delayed using tocolysis. Long-term follow-up has confirmed the safety of one course (*BMJ* 2005; **331**: 665), but repeated doses are not advised.

Tocolysis: Nifedipine or oxytocin receptor antagonists (e.g. atosiban) can be given to allow steroids time to act or to allow *in utero* transfer to a unit with neonatal intensive care facilities. These delay rather than stop preterm labour and should not be used for more than 24 hours or in the presence of infection.

Detection and prevention of infection

The presence of infection within the uterus is life threatening for the mother and worsens the outlook for the neonate. Sepsis requires full rapid evaluation and treatment. This may occur even where the membranes have not ruptured: chorioamnionitis warrants intravenous antibiotics and immediate delivery, whatever the gestation. However, antibiotics should not be administered to non-infected women simply in threatened preterm labour, as long-term cognitive impairment is increased (*Lancet* 2008; **372**: 1319).

Magnesium sulphate

This is neuroprotective for the neonate if given <12 hours prior to anticipated or planned preterm delivery (*NEJM* 2008; **359**: 895). A single dose of 4g by slow IV injection is used prior to delivery between 23 and 34 weeks. Care is required because it is toxic in overdose.

Transfer

Extremely preterm (<27 weeks) or small (<800g) babies have better survival rates if born in unit with intensive neonatal care (Level 3 in UK) facilities. The effect is probably a result of both improved antenatal and postnatal care (*Arch Dis Child Fetal Neonatal Edn* 2014; **99**(3): F181–F188). If delivery is not imminent or the mother unstable, urgent *in utero* transfer should be arranged.

Delivery

Mode of delivery: Vaginal delivery reduces the incidence of neonatal respiratory distress syndrome and caesarean section is undertaken only for the usual obstetric indications. Breech presentation is more common in preterm labour; most preterm breeches now undergo caesarean section.

Conduct of delivery: Paediatric facilities are mobilized. The membranes are not ruptured in labour, at least up to 32 weeks: labour may be slow, allowing steroids more time to act, and the membranes might cushion the delicate preterm fetus against trauma. Forceps, rather than a ventouse, are used only for the usual obstetric indications. Unless immediate neonatal resuscitation is required, the cord should not be clamped for 45 seconds (*Paediatrics* 2006; **117**: 1235), to reduce neonatal morbidity.

Antibiotics for delivery are recommended for women in actual, as opposed to threatened, preterm labour, because of the increased risk and morbidity of GBS.

Preterm prelabour rupture of the membranes

Definition

The membranes rupture before labour at <37 weeks. Often the cause is unknown, but all the causes of preterm labour may be implicated. It occurs before one-third of preterm deliveries.

Complications

Preterm delivery is the principal complication and follows within 48 hours in >50% of cases.

Infection of the fetus or placenta (chorioamnionitis) or cord (funisitis) is common. This may occur before, and therefore be the cause of the membranes rupture, or it may follow membrane rupture. The earlier the gestation at membrane rupture, the higher the risk of pre-existing infection.

Prolapse of the umbilical cord may occur rarely. Absence of liquor (usually before 22 weeks) can result in *pulmonary hypoplasia* and postural deformities.

Clinical features

History: A gush of clear fluid is normal, followed by further leaking.

Examination: The lie and presentation are checked. A pool of fluid in the posterior fornix on speculum examination is diagnostic, but this is not invariable. Digital examination is best avoided for fear of introducing infection. Chorioamnionitis is characterized by contractions or abdominal pain, fever or hypothermia, tachycardia, uterine tenderness and coloured or offensive liquor, although clinical signs often appear late.

Investigations

To confirm the diagnosis in doubtful cases, 'point of care' tests (e.g. Actim Partus) are available but not entirely reliable. Ultrasound may reveal reduced liquor, but the volume can also be normal as fetal urine production continues.

To look for infection, a high vaginal swab (HVS), full blood count (FBC) and CRP are taken. Lactate assesses severity of sepsis. *Fetal well-being* is assessed by CTG. A persistent fetal tachycardia is suggestive of infection.

Management

The risk of preterm delivery must be balanced against the risk of infection, which, if present, increases neonatal mortality and long-term morbidity. The woman is admitted, at least for 48 hours, and given steroids. Close maternal (signs of infection) and fetal surveillance is performed, and if the gestation reaches 34–36 weeks, delivery is normally undertaken.

Identification and management of infection

Chorioamnionitis may produce few signs. Sepsis requires full rapid evaluation and treatment. If there is evidence of uterine infection, intravenous antibiotics are given immediately and the fetus is delivered whatever the gestation: antibiotics alone will not eliminate chorioamnionitis.

Prevention of infection

The prophylactic use of erythromycin in women even without clinical evidence of infection is usual (*Cochrane* 2010; CD001058.2003). Co-amoxiclav is contraindicated, as the neonate is more prone to necrotizing enterocolitis (NEC).

Further reading

Chang E. Preterm birth and the role of neuroprotection. *BMJ* 2015; **350**: g6661. Available at: www.bmj.com/content/350/bmj.g6661 (accessed 19 July 2016).

Clark EA, Varner M. Impact of preterm PROM and its complications on long-term infant outcomes. *Clinical Obstetrics and Gynecology* 2011; **54**: 358–369.

Piso P, Zechmeister-Koss I, Winkler R. Antenatal interventions to reduce preterm birth: an overview of Cochrane systematic reviews. *BMC Research Notes* 2014; 7: 265. Available at: www.biomedcentral.com/1756-0500/7/265 (accessed 19 July 2016).

Royal College of Obstetricians and Gynaecologists. *Cervical Cerclage*. Green-top Guideline No. 60. Available at: www.rcog.org.uk/en/guidelines-research-services/guidelines/gtg60/ (accessed 19 July 2016).

Preterm delivery at a glance

Definition	Delivery >24 weeks and <37 weeks
Epidemiology	8% of deliveries, 20% of perinatal mortality
Aetiology	Subclinical infection, cervical 'incompetence', multiple pregnancy, antepartum haemorrhage, diabetes, polyhydramnios, fetal compromise, uterine abnormalities, idiopathic Iatrogenic
Complications	Neonatal morbidity (approx 50% of all cerebral palsy) and mortality, worse at earlier gestations
Prediction	History; serial ultrasound (transvaginal) of cervical length
Prevention	Antibiotics if bacterial vaginosis, urinary tract infection (UTI), sexually transmitted infection (STI) Vaginal cervical suture if cervix shortens on ultrasound Elective suture only if repeated preterm deliveries/miscarriage Elective suture can be abdominal or vaginal Progesterone pessaries: either from 12 weeks of if cervix shortens Specific strategies, e.g. fetal reduction, amnioreduction

(Continued)

Preterm delivery at a glance (Continued)

Features	Abdominal pain, antepartum haemorrhage, ruptured membranes, sepsis. 'Cervical incompetence' silent
Investigations	Fibronectin assay or cervical scan to rule out false diagnosis. High vaginal swab (HVS), cardiotocography (CTG), CRP, ultrasound
Management	Steroids if <34 weeks, tocolysis for max. 24 h Magnesium if 23–32 weeks Transfer to neonatal intensive care unit if appropriate Antibiotics if in confirmed labour only Caesarean for normal indications Inform neonatologists

CHAPTER 24
Antepartum haemorrhage

Antepartum haemorrhage (APH) is bleeding from the genital tract after 24 weeks' gestation. This is the time at which neonatal survival is better than anecdotal.

Causes of antepartum haemorrhage (APH)	
Common	Undetermined origin
	Placental abruption
	Placenta praevia
Rarer	Incidental genital tract pathology
	Uterine rupture
	Vasa praevia
	Placenta praevia

Placenta praevia

Definitions and epidemiology

Placenta praevia occurs when the placenta is implanted in the lower segment of the uterus. It complicates 0.4% of pregnancies at term. At 20 weeks the placenta is 'low-lying' in many more pregnancies, but appears to 'move' upwards as the pregnancy continues. This is because of the formation of the lower segment of the uterus in the third trimester: it is the myometrium where the placenta implants that moves away from the internal cervical os. Therefore, only 1 in 10 apparently low-lying placentas will be praevia at term.

Classification of placenta praevia	
Marginal (previously types I–II)	Placenta in lower segment, not over os (Fig. 24.1a)
Major (previously types III–IV)	Placenta completely or partially covering os (Fig. 24.1b)

Classification

Placenta praevia is classified according to the proximity of the placenta to the internal os of the cervix. It may be predominantly on the anterior or posterior uterine wall.

Aetiology

This is unknown, but placenta praevia is slightly more common with twins, in women of high parity and age, and if the uterus is scarred (e.g. previous caesarean) (*J Matern Fetal Neonatal Med* 2003; 13: 175).

Complications

The placenta in the lower segment obstructs engagement of the head. Except for some marginal praevias, this necessitates *caesarean section* and may also cause the lie to be *transverse*. *Haemorrhage* can be severe and may continue during and after delivery as the lower segment is less able to contract and constrict the maternal blood supply. If a placenta implants in a previous caesarean section scar, it may be so deep as to prevent placental separation (placenta accreta) or even penetrate through the uterine wall into surrounding structures such as the bladder (placenta percreta). Placenta accreta occurs in 10% of women who have both a placenta praevia and a single previous caesarean scar. This may provoke massive haemorrhage at delivery, often requiring *hysterectomy*.

Clinical features

History: Typically, there are intermittent painless bleeds, which increase in frequency and intensity over several weeks. Such bleeding may be severe.

Obstetrics & Gynaecology, Fifth Edition. Lawrence Impey, Tim Child.
© 2017 John Wiley & Sons, Ltd. Published 2017 by John Wiley & Sons, Ltd.

One-third of women, however, have not experienced bleeding before delivery.

Examination: Breech presentation and transverse lie are common. The fetal head is not engaged and high. Vaginal examination can provoke massive bleeding and is *never* performed in a woman who is bleeding vaginally unless placenta praevia has been excluded.

Presentation of placenta praevia

Incidental finding on ultrasound scan
Vaginal bleeding
Abnormal lie, breech presentation

Investigations

To make the diagnosis, ultrasound is used (Fig. 24.2). Most placenta praevias are now diagnosed prior to any bleeding. If a low-lying placenta has been diagnosed at a second-trimester ultrasound, this is repeated, vaginally if the placenta is posterior, at 32 weeks to exclude placenta praevia. A placenta <2 cm from the internal os is likely to be praevia at term. If the placenta is anterior, and under a caesarean section scar, 3-D power ultrasound (Fig. 24.3) is best to determine if there is placenta accreta (*Obstet Gynecol* 2015; **126**(3): 645–653) and how severe it is. Magnetic resonance imaging (MRI) is also useful. This is to be prepared for haemorrhage at delivery.

To assess fetal and maternal well-being: Where presentation is with bleeding, cardiotocography (CTG), a full blood count (FBC), clotting studies and cross-match are needed. Fetal distress is uncommon.

Management

Admission

This is necessary for all women with bleeding from a placenta praevia. Blood is kept available; anti-D is administered to Rhesus-negative women; intravenous access is maintained; steroids are administered if the gestation is <34 weeks. In women with asymptomatic placenta praevia, admission can be delayed until delivery, provided they can get to hospital easily.

Delivery

This is by elective caesarean section at 39 weeks by the most senior person available. Intraoperative and postpartum haemorrhage are common because the lower segment does not contract well after delivery, or the placenta is accreta. Earlier, emergency delivery is needed if bleeding is severe before this time. Very preterm, pregnancy can often be prolonged with observation and, if necessary, blood transfusion.

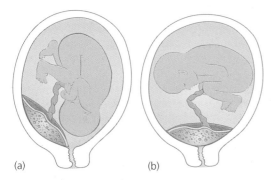

(a)   (b)

Fig. 24.1 (a) Marginal placenta praevia. (b) Major placenta praevia (abnormal lie and malpresentation are common).

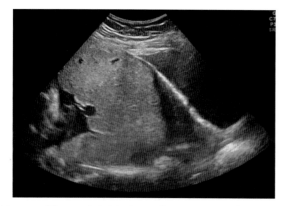

Fig. 24.2 Ultrasound of placenta praevia.

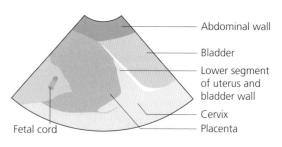

Abdominal wall
Bladder
Lower segment of uterus and bladder wall
Cervix
Placenta
Fetal cord

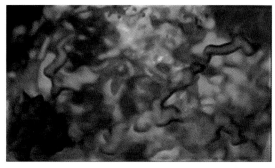

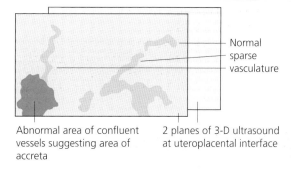

| Abnormal area of confluent vessels suggesting area of accreta | 2 planes of 3-D ultrasound at uteroplacental interface |

Fig. 24.3 3-D power Doppler ultrasound of placenta accreta.

Placenta accreta or percreta should have been anticipated, and a clear plan made for elective delivery with interventional radiology and expert surgical and anaesthetic support. The uterine incision is made away from the placenta, which can be left *in situ* or removed with the entire uterus. Partial separation or transection of the placenta by the uterine incision may provoke massive haemorrhage. Treatment involves compression of the inside of the scar after removal of the placenta with an inflatable (e.g. Rusch) balloon, excision of the affected uterine segment or, frequently, total hysterectomy.

Differentiation between placental abruption and placenta praevia		
	Abruption	*Placenta praevia*
Shock	Inconsistent with external loss	Consistent with external loss
Pain	Common, often severe	No. Contractions occasionally
	Constant with exacerbations	
Bleeding	May be absent	Red and often profuse
	Often dark	Often smaller previous antepartum haemorrhage (APHs)
Tenderness	Usual, often severe	Rare
	Uterus may be hard	
Fetus	Lie normal, often engaged	Lie often abnormal/ head high
	May be dead or distressed	Heart rate usually normal
Ultrasound	Often normal, placenta not low	Placenta low

Placental abruption

Definition

Placental abruption is when part (or all) of the placenta separates before delivery of the fetus. It occurs in 1% of pregnancies. However, it is likely that many antepartum haemorrhages of 'undetermined origin' are in fact small placental abruptions and that this figure is therefore higher.

Pathology

When part of the placenta separates, considerable maternal bleeding may occur behind it. This can have several consequences. Further placental separation and acute fetal distress may follow. Blood usually also tracks down between the membranes and the myometrium to be revealed as APH. It may also enter the liquor. Or it may simply enter the myometrium; visible haemorrhage is absent in 20% (Fig. 24.4).

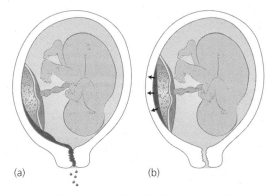

Fig. 24.4 (a) Revealed abruption. (b) Concealed abruption.

Complications

Fetal death is common (30% of proven abruptions). Haemorrhage often necessitates blood transfusion; this, disseminated intravascular coagulation (DIC) and renal failure may rarely lead to maternal death.

Aetiology

Many affected women have no risk factors. However, intrauterine growth restriction (IUGR), pre-eclampsia, autoimmune disease, maternal smoking, cocaine usage, a previous history of placental abruption (risk 6%), multiple pregnancy and high maternal parity all predispose to abruption. It has also been occasionally associated with trauma or a sudden reduction in uterine volume (e.g. rupture of the membranes in a woman with polyhydramnios).

Major risk factors for placental abruption
Intrauterine growth restriction (IUGR)
Pre-eclampsia
Pre-existing hypertension
Maternal smoking
Previous abruption

Clinical features (Fig. 24.5)

History: Classically, there is painful bleeding. The pain is due to blood behind the placenta and in the myometrium, and is usually constant with exacerbations; the blood is often dark. The degree of vaginal bleeding does not reflect the severity of the abruption because some may not escape from the uterus. Indeed, pain or bleeding may occur alone. If pain occurs alone, the abruption is 'concealed'. If vaginal bleeding is evident, it is 'revealed'.

Examination: Tachycardia suggests profound blood loss, which may be out of proportion to the vaginal loss because of 'concealed' loss. Hypotension only occurs after massive blood loss. The uterus is tender and often contracting: labour often ensues. In severe cases, the uterus is 'woody' hard and the fetus is very difficult to feel. Fetal heart tones are often abnormal or even absent.

Investigations

The diagnosis is usually made on clinical grounds. Investigations help to establish the severity of the abruption,

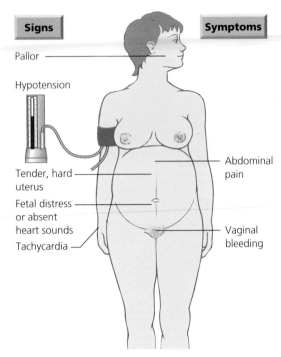

Signs | Symptoms

Pallor
Hypotension
Tender, hard uterus
Fetal distress or absent heart sounds
Tachycardia
Abdominal pain
Vaginal bleeding

Fig. 24.5 Clinical features of placental abruption.

to plan appropriate resuscitation, and whether and how to deliver the fetus.

To establish fetal well-being, CTG is performed. In addition to fetal distress, very frequent uterine activity may be evident on the tocograph (Fig. 24.6). Ultrasound can be used to estimate fetal weight at preterm gestations and will exclude placenta praevia, but a placental abruption may not be visible.

To establish maternal well-being, FBC, coagulation screen and cross-match are performed. Catheterization with hourly urine output, regular FBC, coagulation, and urea and creatinine (U&E) estimations and even intensive care unit care, are required in severe cases.

Features of major placental abruption
Maternal collapse
Coagulopathy
Fetal distress or demise
'Woody' hard uterus
Poor urine output or renal failure
N.B. Degree of vaginal loss is often unhelpful

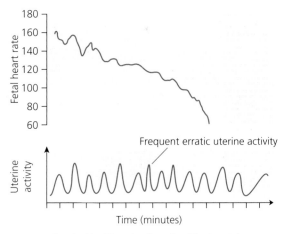

Fig. 24.6 Terminal fetal heart bradycardia with placental abruption.

Management

Assessment and resuscitation

Admission is required, even without vaginal bleeding if there is pain and uterine tenderness. Resuscitation may be required. Intravenous fluid is given, with steroids if the gestation is <34 weeks. Opiate analgesia may be required; anti-D is given to Rhesus-negative women.

Delivery

This depends on the fetal state and gestation. The mother must be stabilized first.
If there is fetal distress, urgent delivery by caesarean section is required.
If there is no fetal distress, but the gestation is 37 weeks or more, induction of labour with amniotomy is performed. The fetal heart is monitored continuously, maternal condition is closely observed and caesarean section is performed if fetal distress ensues.
If the fetus is dead, coagulopathy is also likely. Blood products are given and labour is induced.

Conservative management

If there is no fetal distress, the pregnancy is preterm and the degree of abruption appears to be minor, steroids are given (if <34 weeks) and the patient is closely monitored on the antenatal ward. If all symptoms settle, she may be discharged, but the pregnancy is now 'high risk': ultrasound scans for fetal growth are performed.

Postpartum management

Whatever the mode of delivery, postpartum haemorrhage is a major risk.

Principles of management of major placental abruption
Fetal condition: cardiotocography (CTG)
Maternal condition: fluid balance, renal function, full blood count (FBC) and clotting
Replace fluid loss
Early delivery
Transfusion of blood ± blood products

Other causes of antepartum haemorrhage

Bleeding of undetermined origin

When APH is small and painless but the placenta is not praevia, it may be impossible to find a cause. Ultrasound is of little diagnostic use. Many episodes are likely to be minor degrees of placental abruption: there is no such thing as a 'heavy show' (a show is the occasionally slightly blood-stained mucus plug that usually drops from the cervix around the time that labour begins). This and indeed the 'recurrent show' are likely to be minor abruptions, and patients should be managed as such.

Ruptured vasa praevia

Vasa praevia occurs when a fetal blood vessel runs in the membranes in front of the presenting part. These vessels usually result from the umbilical cord being attached to the membranes rather than the placenta (velamentous insertion) (Figs 24.7, 24.8a) or where the placenta is in parts. This occurs in about 1% of pregnancies and can be, but seldom is, diagnosed on ultrasound. Rupture, usually when the membranes rupture, is more likely with vessels closer to the cervix (i.e. praevia) and occurs in 1 in 5000 pregnancies. Massive fetal bleeding

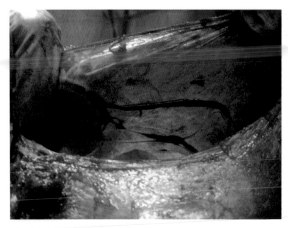

Fig. 24.7 Vasa praevia.

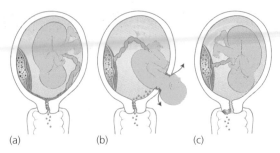

Fig. 24.8 Other causes of antepartum haemorrhage (APH). (a) Vasa praevia. (b) Ruptured uterus (intra-abdominal loss usually predominates). (c) Cervical carcinoma.

follows. The typical presentation is painless, moderate vaginal bleeding at rupture of the membranes, which is accompanied by severe fetal distress. Caesarean section is often not fast enough to save the fetus.

Uterine rupture

Significant antenatal rupture of a lower segment caesarean scar is very rare. However, very occasionally rupture occurs before labour in women with other uterine scars or a congenitally abnormal uterus (Fig. 24.8b).

Bleeding of gynaecological origin

Cervical carcinoma can present in pregnancy (Fig. 24.8c). If a cervical smear is overdue, the woman with small recurrent or postcoital haemorrhage should undergo speculum examination and colposcopy. Cervical polyps, ectropions and vaginal lacerations may also be evident but bleeding should not usually be attributed to them.

Further reading

Special Issue: Abnormally invasive placenta – AIP. *Acta Obstetricia et Gynecologica Scandinavica* 2013; **92**(4): 367–487. Available at: http://onlinelibrary .wiley.com/doi/10.1111/aogs.2013.92.issue-4/issuetoc (accessed 19 July 2016).

Royal College of Obstetricians and Gynaecologists. *Placenta Praevia, Placenta Praevia Accreta and Vasa Praevia: Diagnosis and Management.* Greentop Guideline No. 27. Available at: www.rcog.org .uk/globalassets/documents/guidelines/gtg_27.pdf (accessed 19 July 2016).

Placenta praevia at a glance

Definition	Placenta implanted in uterine lower segment. 'Low-lying' refers to placental site before lower segment formation	
Types	Marginal praevia	Near/adjacent to cervical os
	Major praevia	Over/partly covering cervical os
Epidemiology	0.4% of pregnancies. Low-lying placenta in early pregnancy 5%	
Aetiology	Usually idiopathic. Large placenta, scarred uterus, high parity/age	
Complications	Haemorrhage. Need for preterm or caesarean delivery. If previous lower segment caesarean section (LSCS), risk of placenta accreta	
Features	Painless antepartum haemorrhage (APH), often multiple and increasing in frequency and severity	
	Also abnormal lie, incidental ultrasound finding	
Investigations	Ultrasound to locate the placenta. Full blood count (FBC) and cross-match if bleeding	
Management	If low-lying placenta on early ultrasound, repeat at 32 weeks	
	If previous caesarean	Investigate for placenta accreta if placenta anterior
	Bleeding	Admit whatever gestation. Have blood ready. Steroids if <34 weeks. Blood transfusion if necessary
	Delivery	Caesarean at 39 weeks; before if bleeding heavy

Placental abruption at a glance

Definition	Separation of part/all of placenta before delivery; after 24 weeks	
Epidemiology	1% of pregnancies	
Aetiology	Idiopathic; common associations: intrauterine growth restriction (IUGR), pre-eclampsia, autoimmune disease, smoking, previous abruption	
Complications	Fetal death, massive haemorrhage causing disseminated intravascular coagulation (DIC), renal failure, maternal death	
Features	Painful antepartum haemorrhage (APH), but pain or bleeding can be in isolation. Uterine tenderness and contractions: if major, absent fetal heart, 'woody' uterus, maternal collapse, coagulopathy	
Investigations	Cardiotocography (CTG) to assess fetus. Full blood count (FBC), clotting to assess maternal state	
	Ultrasound scan excludes placenta praevia if diagnosis in doubt. If severe, intensive maternal monitoring (renal and liver function, urine output)	
Management	Admit	If severe, resuscitate with blood
	Fetal distress present	Deliver by caesarean section
	Fetal distress absent	>37 weeks, induce labour
	Fetus dead	Induce labour. Coagulopathy likely
	Minor preterm abruption	Wait. Serial ultrasound scans

CHAPTER 25

Fetal growth, health and surveillance

Between 24 weeks and term, about 0.5% of babies will die. A further 1 in 500 will develop cerebral palsy. More than 1 in 20 will require admission to a neonatal unit. Furthermore, there is growing evidence that *in utero* health and growth influence health, particularly cardiac disease, in later life. Care of the fetus in pregnancy must be directed towards the causes of these: the principal causes of death and cerebral palsy are outlined in the boxes below. Prominent among these is intrauterine growth restriction. Identification and management of the sick fetus are difficult, not least because of the difficulty in identifying the pregnancy at risk, limited resources and the potential for overmedicalization of pregnancy.

Principal causes of perinatal mortality
Unexplained
Preterm delivery
Intrauterine growth restriction (IUGR)
Congenital abnormalities
Intrapartum, including hypoxia
Placental abruption

Fetal health and growth: terminology

Because there are so many associations of adverse neonatal outcomes, and because their mechanisms of action are poorly understood, our use of terms such as compromise and fetal distress is simplistic.

Small for gestational age (SGA)

Also called small for dates (SFD), this means that the weight of the fetus is less than the tenth centile for its gestation (if at term: 2.7 kg). Other cut-off points (e.g. third centile) can also be used. Traditionally, small size was felt to reflect chronic illness due to placental dysfunction. These babies are at increased risk of complications because they are more likely than normal birthweight babies to be growth restricted, but many are simply constitutionally small, have grown consistently (Fig. 25.1) and are not compromised. Assessment of fetal weight is better at identifying IUGR if customized according to what would be expected for the individual rather than the overall population.

Intrauterine/fetal growth restriction (IUGR or FGR)

This describes fetuses that have failed to reach their own 'growth potential'. Their growth *in utero* is slowed and many end up 'small' (SGA), but some do not: many stillbirths or fetuses distressed in labour are of apparently 'normal' weight. If a fetus was genetically determined to be 4 kg at term and delivers at term weighing 3 kg, its growth has been restricted, and it may have placental dysfunction (Fig. 25.2) (www.gestation.net). Similarly, an ill, malnourished, tall adult may weigh more than a healthy shorter one. This means that whilst most IUGR babies are SGA, a proportion do not appear to be.

Fetal distress

This refers to an acute situation, such as hypoxia, that may result in fetal damage or death if it is not reversed, or if the fetus is delivered urgently. As such, it is usually

Obstetrics & Gynaecology, Fifth Edition. Lawrence Impey, Tim Child.
© 2017 John Wiley & Sons, Ltd. Published 2017 by John Wiley & Sons, Ltd.

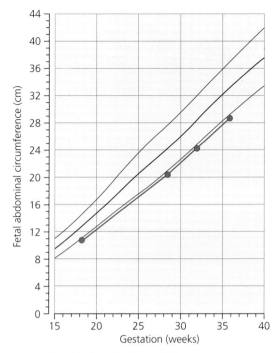

Fig. 25.1 Consistent growth of a small fetus.

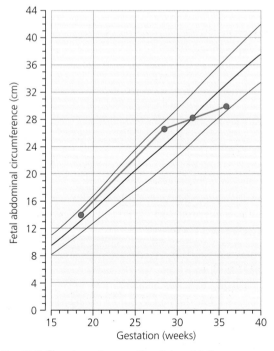

Fig. 25.2 Slowed growth suggestive of placental disease.

used in labour (see Chapter 29). Nevertheless, most babies that subsequently develop cerebral palsy were not born hypoxic.

Fetal compromise

This describes a chronic situation and should be defined as when conditions for the normal growth and neurological development are not optimal. Most identifiable causes involve poor nutrient transfer through the placenta, often called 'placental dysfunction'. Commonly, there is IUGR, but this may also be absent (e.g. maternal diabetes or prolonged pregnancy).

Fetal surveillance

Aims of fetal surveillance

1 Identify the 'high-risk' pregnancy using history or events during pregnancy, or using specific investigations.
2 Monitor the fetus for growth and well-being. The methods used will vary according to pregnancy risk and events during the pregnancy.
3 Intervene (usually expedite delivery) at an appropriate time, balancing the risks of *in utero* compromise against those of intervention and prematurity. The latter is itself a major cause of mortality and morbidity.

Problems with fetal surveillance

All methods of surveillance have a false-positive rate (i.e. they can be overinterpreted). Whilst they may identify problems, they do not necessarily solve them and prevent adverse outcomes. In addition, they 'medicalize' pregnancy by concentrating on the abnormal, and they are expensive. For these reasons, identification of pregnancy risk is important.

Identification of pregnancy risk

Pre-pregnancy risks

History: The traditional methods have centred on history: the mother's age, her previous medical history and obstetric history. Unfortunately, most women who develop pregnancy complications such as IUGR do not have any such risk factors, i.e. the use of

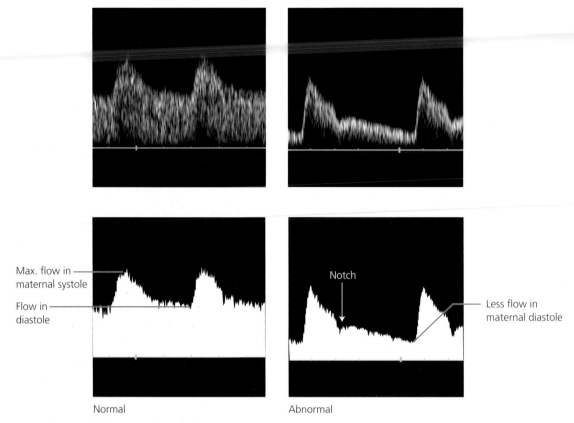

Max. flow in maternal systole

Flow in diastole

Notch

Less flow in maternal diastole

Normal

Abnormal

Fig. 25.3 Normal and abnormal uterine artery Doppler.

history as a screening test is not sensitive. Further, taking all minor risk factors such as age >35 years into account will mean that many women who would have had normal pregnancy outcomes are considered high risk, i.e. the use of history as a screening test is not specific.

Early pregnancy

Blood tests: Pregnancy-associated plasma protein A (PAPPA) is a placental hormone, the maternal level of which is reduced in the first trimester with chromosomal abnormalities. It is therefore used in screening for Down's syndrome. It is now known that a low level constitutes a high risk for IUGR, placental abruption and consequent stillbirth (*JAMA* 2004; **292**: 2249).

Maternal uterine artery Doppler (Fig. 25.3): The uterine circulation normally develops a very low

resistance in normal pregnancy. Abnormal waveforms, suggesting failure of development of a low resistance circulation, identify 75% of pregnancies at risk of adverse neonatal outcomes in the early third trimester, particularly early pre-eclampsia, IUGR or placental abruption. This test is less predictive of later problems. Uterine artery Doppler can be performed from 12 weeks to term but is most sensitive at 20–23 weeks.

Integrated screening for pregnancy risk: Using integration of (the above) different independent risk factors as in screening for chromosomal abnormalities will increase the accuracy of screening. In this way, factors in the history and investigations can be used to identify more high-risk women (with a lower false-positive rate). This is currently under evaluation but is likely to enable more appropriate targeting of hospital-based and high-risk antenatal care.

Later pregnancy

Pregnancy events: With the occurrence of pre-eclampsia or vaginal bleeding, or if routine abdominal palpation suggests an SFD fetus, more close examination is required and the risk level will change.

Methods of fetal surveillance

Routine pregnancy care

The tests outlined below are not routine in low-risk pregnancy. Here, the cornerstone of the identification of the small or compromised fetus is serial measurement of the symphysis fundal height and other aspects of antenatal visits.

Ultrasound assessment of fetal growth

What it is: Ultrasound scan is used to measure fetal size after the first trimester, particularly the abdominal and head circumferences. These changes are recorded on centile charts (Fig. 25.4). Three factors help to differentiate between the healthy small fetus and the 'growth-restricted' fetus.
1 The rate of growth can be determined by previous scans, or a later examination, at least 2 weeks apart.
2 The pattern of 'smallness' may help: the fetal abdomen will often stop enlarging before the head, which is 'spared'. The result is a 'thin' fetus or 'asymmetrical' growth restriction. A reduction in the rate of growth of the abdominal circumference by >30% is suggestive of IUGR.
3 Allowance for constitutional non-pathological determinants of fetal growth enables 'customization' of individual fetal growth, assessing actual growth according to expected growth.
Benefits: Serial ultrasound is safe and useful in confirming consistent growth in high-risk and multiple pregnancies, and is essential to the management of such pregnancies. The use of ultrasound in dating and identification of abnormalities is discussed elsewhere.
Limitations: 'One-off' ultrasound scans in later pregnancy are of limited benefit in 'low-risk' pregnancies (*Cochrane* 2008; CD001451). Inaccurate measurements are common, misleading and potentially harmful. Mothers with diabetes often have large babies, particularly with a large abdominal circumference, although these babies are still more vulnerable.

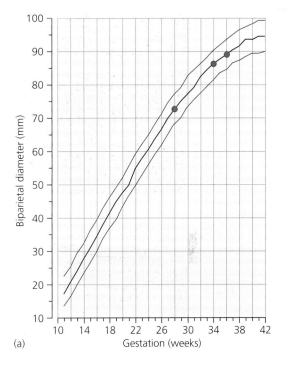

(a)

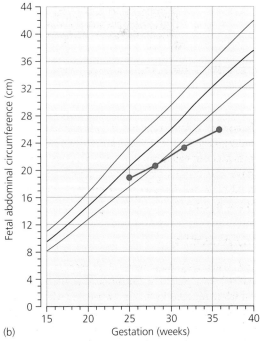

(b)

Fig. 25.4 (a) Normal growth of the head; (b) slowed growth of the abdomen.

Doppler waveforms of the umbilical artery

What it is: Doppler is used to measure velocity wave-forms in the umbilical arteries (Fig. 25.5). Evidence of a high-resistance circulation, i.e. reduced/absent flow in fetal diastole compared to systole, suggests placental dysfunction. Resistance is described according to end-diastolic flow (i.e. high or >95th centile), absent (AEDF) or reversed (REDF). The latter two findings indicate severe placental dysfunction.

Benefits: Umbilical artery waveforms help identify which small fetuses are actually growth restricted and therefore compromised and is best performed before 34 weeks. Its usage improves perinatal outcome in high-risk pregnancy whilst reducing intervention in those not compromised. The absence or reversal of flow in diastole usually predates cardiotocograph (CTG) abnormalities and correlates well with severe compromise.

Limitations: Doppler is not a useful screening tool in low-risk pregnancies and is less effective at identifying the normal-weight but compromised fetus. It is also not sensitive alone after 34 weeks gestation when it is used in conjunction with the middle cerebral artery (MCA) as the cerebroplacental ratio (CPR) is better.

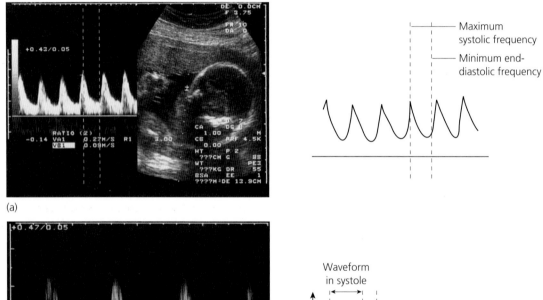

(a)

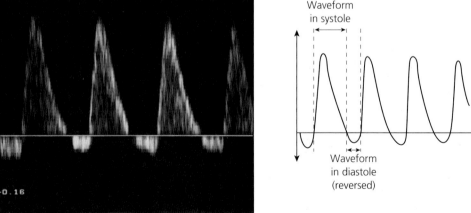

(b)

Fig. 25.5 (a) Normal umbilical artery end-diastolic flow; (b) reversed end-diastolic flow.

Doppler waveforms of the fetal cerebral circulation

What it is: Doppler is used to assess the resistance or velocity of the middle cerebral artery (Fig. 25.6). With fetal compromise, the MCA often develops a low-resistance pattern in comparison to the thoracic aorta or renal vessels. This reflects a head-sparing effect. The velocity of MCA flow also increases with fetal anaemia.

Benefits: The ratio of the pulsatility index (PI) of this vessel to that of the umbilical artery PI (MCA PI/umbA PI) is currently the best method of assessing chronic placental dysfunction after 34 weeks (*Am J Obstet Gynecol* 2015; **213**(1): 54.e1–10). The velocity of the MCA is routinely used to assess pregnancies at risk of fetal anaemia.

Limitations: The use of these is currently restricted to high-risk pregnancy, specific situations (e.g. suspected anaemia and SGA). Even with SGA babies beyond 34 weeks, they are not widely used. Their routine use has not yet been shown to reduce perinatal mortality or morbidity.

Doppler waveforms of the fetal venous circulation

What it is: All major fetal vessels can be seen, but the most commonly measured is the ductus venosus (Fig. 25.7).

Benefits: The ductus venosus waveform is a measure of a cardiac function, and is used to assess extremely preterm fetuses (<28 weeks) as an alternative to CTG monitoring, and is better <26 weeks. It is also useful for assessing disease severity in babies with heart failure and twin–twin transfusion syndrome.

Limitations: It requires expertise and is seldom used outside fetal medicine centres.

Cardiotocography or non-stress test

What it is: The fetal heart is recorded electronically for up to an hour. Accelerations and variability >5 beats/minute should be present, decelerations absent and the rate in the range of 110–160 (Fig. 25.8). Antenatal abnormalities represent a late stage in fetal compromise.

Benefits: CTGs give immediate information about fetal status at ≥26 weeks gestation. Computerized interpretation of short-term variability (STV) is of benefit in 'buying time': delaying delivery of chronically compromised preterm (usually <34 weeks) fetuses.

Limitations: CTGs alone are of no use as an antenatal screening test. Indeed, reliance on occasional CTGs as tests of well-being leads to increased perinatal mortality. The best a normal antenatal CTG means is that, barring an acute event, the fetus will not die in the next 24 hour. Therefore, to be useful in high-risk pregnancy, it needs to be performed daily. CTG analysis is discussed in Chapter 29.

Kick chart

What it is: The mother records the number of individual movements that she experiences every day.

Benefits: Most compromised fetuses have reduced movements in the hours before demise. A reduction in fetal movements is an indication for more sophisticated testing. Kick charts are simple and cheap.

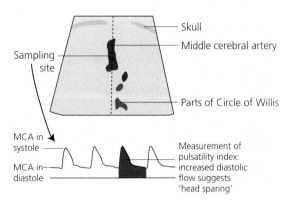

Fig. 25.6 Ultrasound of middle cerebral artery.

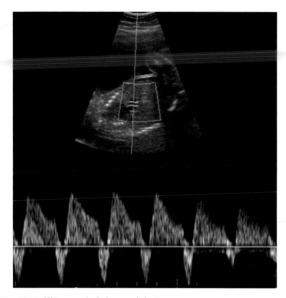

Oblique view of fetus

Sampling site in fetus

Reversal of flow (away from heart) in atrial systole

Fig. 25.7 Ultrasound of abnormal ductus venosus.

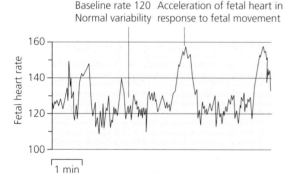

Baseline rate 120   Acceleration of fetal heart in
Normal variability   response to fetal movement

Fetal heart rate

1 min

Fig. 25.8 Normal antenatal CTG.

Limitations: Compromised fetuses stop moving only shortly before death. Routine counting is of very limited benefit in reducing perinatal mortality, may lead to unnecessary intervention and increases maternal anxiety. Kick charts should not be used routinely.

The small for gestational age fetus and the IUGR fetus

Epidemiology

Small for gestational age (SGA) means small for the gestation, usually <10th centile. By definition, 10% of babies are below the 10th centile, 3% below the third, for that gestation. Because of the difficulties in quantifying IUGR, its frequency is uncertain. IUGR is a major cause of stillbirth.

Aetiology

Fetal size and health are determined by a combination of genetic and acquired factors.

Constitutional determinants affect growth and birth weight without causing IUGR. Low maternal height and weight, nulliparity, Asian (as opposed to Caucasian or Afro-Caribbean) ethnic group and female fetal gender are all associated with smaller babies.

Pathological determinants of fetal growth, causing IUGR, include pre-existing maternal disease (e.g. renal disease and autoimmune disease), maternal pregnancy complications (e.g. pre-eclampsia), multiple pregnancy, smoking, drug usage, infection such as cytomegalovirus (CMV), extreme exercise and malnutrition and congenital (including chromosomal) abnormalities. In addition, maternal obesity and diabetes are associated with an increased risk of adverse outcomes.

'Customization' of fetal growth: Whilst adjustment for constitutional factors such as gender is clearly appropriate, there is debate as to whether adjustment, particularly for ethnicity, is also correct. Fetal

growth charts in healthy women of whatever race show similar trajectories (*Lancet* 2014; **384**(9946): 869–879). However, adjusting estimated fetal weight for constitutional factors appears to improve prediction of the at-risk fetus.

Complications

Stillbirth, fetal distress in labour, neonatal unit admission and *long-term handicap* are increased. Up to a half of all so-called 'unclassified' stillbirths are SGA or have IUGR. *Preterm delivery*, both iatrogenic and spontaneous, is more common. *Maternal risks* are greater because pre-eclampsia may coexist and because caesarean delivery is often used.

Diagnosis

In the absence of routine third-trimester ultrasound, most babies with SGA and IUGR are missed.

History: Reduced fetal movements is not a consistent feature of IUGR because a compromised fetus stops moving only when very unwell, and because most events of reduced movements are transient, insignificant and in well babies.

Examination: Serial measurement of the symphysis fundal height may be reduced or slow down. The blood pressure and urine must be checked as pre-eclampsia commonly coexists with IUGR, particularly <34 weeks.

Investigations: The diagnosis of SGA is made using *ultrasound*. Investigations are to determine both the cause (e.g. placental or fetal abnormality of infection) and the severity of compromise. The anomaly scan is repeated to look for malformations; testing for infection (CMV) or for chromosomal abnormalities with non-invasive prenatal testing (NIPT) or *amniocentesis* should be considered. To tell which SGA fetuses are actually IUGR and how severely, ultrasound and *umbilical artery Doppler*, which, after 34 weeks, are combined with the *middle cerebral artery* as the CPR, are used. A reduction in growth velocity by >30% of the abdominal circumference also suggests IUGR *The amniotic fluid volume is often reduced* (oligohydramnios). *Cardiotocography* is also used but will become abnormal usually only when severe compromise or 'fetal distress' is present.

'At booking' major risk factors for SGA
Previous history of SGA or stillbirth
Heavy smoking
Cocaine usage
Heavy daily exercise
Maternal illness, e.g. diabetes
Parental SGA

Management of IUGR

SGA only

Preterm: Growth is rechecked with ultrasound at 2–3-weekly intervals.

Gestation >37 weeks: Current UK recommendations are that delivery should be arranged. However, in some fetuses that are not very small (e.g. >3rd centile), with normal umbA and CPR Dopplers, it may be more appropriate to wait until 40–41 weeks to allow labour to be spontaneous.

IUGR

Gestation <34 weeks (Fig. 25.9): The aim is to prevent *in utero* demise or neurological damage associated with ongoing placental dysfunction, whilst maximizing the gestation to avoid complications of prematurity. The threshold for intervention therefore varies with gestation. In general, an estimated fetal weight needs to be >500 g and the gestation >25–26 weeks for a fetus to be potentially viable once delivered. The IUGR fetus with abnormal umbA Doppler values is reviewed at least twice a week; if AEDF is seen the mother is admitted and given steroids. If the gestation is >32 weeks, delivery by caesarean is usual; if the gestation is <32 weeks, a daily computerized CTG is performed and delivery arranged if this is abnormal. Bedrest does not increase fetal growth, but admission or even delivery may be needed for other indications, particularly severe pre-eclampsia. The severely preterm IUGR fetus is usually delivered by caesarean; delivery before 34 weeks should be immediately preceded by maternal administration of magnesium sulphate.

Gestation 34–37 weeks: At this gestation, delivery can sometimes be deferred in the absence of severely abnormal Doppler indices. Delivery can be by induction, or caesarean if the CTG is abnormal.

Gestation >37 weeks: Delivery is indicated, by induction or caesarean if the CTG is abnormal.

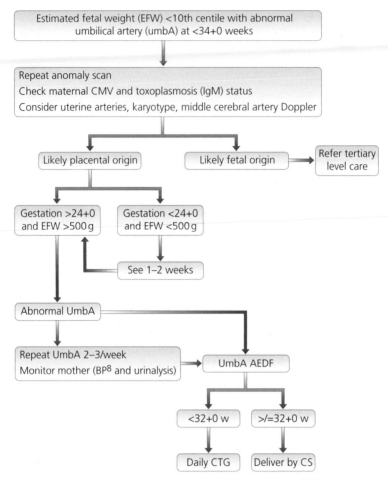

Fig. 25.9 Management of preterm IUGR. AEDF, absent end-diastolic flow; BP, blood pressure; CMV, cytomegalovirus; CS, caesarean section; CTG, cardiotocography.

Stillbirth

Definition and epidemiology

Stillbirth occurs when a fetus is delivered after 24 completed weeks' gestation showing no signs of life. In the UK, the rate is 1 in 200 pregnancies; it is slightly lower in most developed countries; only about 10% occur intrapartum. In developing countries, the rate is much higher, and most are at term or intrapartum. Women who have had one stillbirth are 3–5 times more likely to experience another. Fetal disease of whatever aetiology is a major cause of early neonatal mortality: the rates of the two are often combined as 'perinatal mortality'.

Aetiology

- *Intrauterine growth restriction*, whether SGA, is the most common. Smoking and multiple pregnancy are important risk factors.
- *Unexplained* cases are often due to the pathology behind IUGR.
- *Fetal and chromosomal congenital abnormalities* vary in incidence according to the level of prenatal diagnosis.
- *Pre-existing maternal disease*, e.g. diabetes, autoimmune disease, sickle cell disease, renal disease.
- *Pregnancy-related maternal disease*, e.g. pre-eclampsia, gestational diabetes. Much of the risk is via placental disease, i.e. IUGR.

- *Infection* (bacterial, e.g. group B streptococcus (GBS), or viral, e.g. parvovirus and CMV). In developing countries syphilis and malaria are important causes.
- *Placental abruption.*
- *Intrapartum*, usually hypoxia.
- *Rare*: fetal exsanguination, as feto-maternal haemorrhage or vasa praevia, fatty liver and cholestasis.

Diagnosis

The majority of antepartum stillbirths present as reduced or absent fetal movements. The diagnosis is made using ultrasound.

Prevention of stillbirth

Risk identification allows targeted surveillance or even intervention. Examples are women at increased risk of IUGR, e.g. smokers, multiple pregnancy or those with a previous history. Risk identification on history alone performs poorly; most stillbirths occur in women considered at low risk. Integrated screening using multiple risk factors including uterine artery Doppler is better.

Those at risk of IUGR undergo serial ultrasound for fetal growth scanning. Screening for women with other disease, e.g. gestational diabetes, is also performed. Those at low risk undergo routine antenatal care; accurate serial measurement of the symphysis fundal height is the cornerstone of identification of the SGA fetus. Fetuses with SGA are monitored as described.

Potentially beneficial routine interventions

Glucose tolerance testing is currently only used in the UK when women are considered at high risk (e.g. obese). Testing is frequently omitted by accident.

Ultrasound in the third trimester: This has the capacity to detect SGA and some cases of IUGR, but is currently not recommended in the UK due to fears abut cost, overintervention and a lack of clear evidence regarding management.

Early induction of labour will prevent stillbirth beyond the gestation at which it is performed (Fig. 25.10). Several hundred inductions, however, will be needed to prevent one stillbirth; further, induction can be unpleasant, and may increase intrapartum risk and that of caesarean section. Induction before 38 weeks is associated with increased infant mortality and short-term complications.

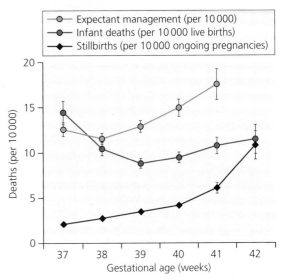

Fig. 25.10 Risk of stillbirth and infant mortality according to gestational age.

Management of stillbirth

Investigations re cause: Placental histology and culture, and postmortem (PM) and microarray (comparative genomic hybridization) are advised. If a PM is declined, MRI may provide information. The neonate is weighed. The mother's blood should be checked for previously undiagnosed autoimmune, liver, renal and thyroid disease, and for diabetes.

Investigations re maternal health: Severe maternal illness, for example pre-eclampsia and infection, can cause stillbirth. Assessment of maternal health is essential.

Induction of labour is usually arranged. Caesarean section should be avoided if possible.

Postnatal management: A meeting or frank 'debrief' is required when all results are available and a prognosis and plan made for a future pregnancy. The mother is at high risk of mental illness.

The prolonged pregnancy

Epidemiology and aetiology

A pregnancy is prolonged if ≥42 weeks' gestation are completed. However, the risk of perinatal mortality and morbidity rises rapidly, albeit still at a low absolute risk, between 41 and 42 weeks (see Fig. 25.10). Approximately 10% of pregnancies apparently reach 42 weeks, although with accurate early pregnancy dating with ultrasound, the figure is nearer 6%. The aetiology of prolonged pregnancy is not understood, but it is more common if previous pregnancies have been prolonged and in nulliparous women, and is rarer in South Asian and black women.

Risks

The rate of stillbirth per 1000 continuing pregnancies rises from 0.35 at 37 weeks to 2.12 at 43 weeks. Neonatal illness and encephalopathy, meconium passage and a clinical diagnosis of fetal distress are more common. The risks are greater in women of South Asian origin (*BMJ* 2007; **334**: 833). The absolute risk of a problem nevertheless remains small.

Management

The problem is that induction of labour medicalizes it and may fail to establish labour and lead to caesarean section. However, prolonged pregnancy increases the chances of fetal distress when labour does start: this also leads to an increased chance of a caesarean section. The aim is to balance the risks of obstetric intervention against those of prolonged pregnancy.

By 41–42 weeks, this balance is clearly in favour of induction of labour. This prevents one fetal death for every 500 women induced, and is associated with a *lower* caesarean rate than waiting (*Cochrane* 2006; CD004945). It is therefore usual to induce labour between 41 and 42 weeks, but in appropriately counselled women who prefer not to be induced, surveillance with daily CTG is an alternative. 'Sweeping' the cervix (usually at 40–41 weeks) helps spontaneous labour start earlier.

Management of the prolonged pregnancy	
Check the gestation carefully; counsel patient appropriately	
If correct, induction before 41 weeks is inappropriate unless complications are present	
From 41 weeks	Examine the patient vaginally and offer induction *unless* she prefers to wait
If no induction	Sweep cervix and arrange daily cardiotocography (CTG)
If CTG abnormal	Deliver whatever the condition of the cervix, by caesarean

Further reading

Hussain AA, Yakoob MY, Imdad A, Bhutta ZA. Elective induction for pregnancies at or beyond 41 weeks of gestation and its impact on stillbirths: a systematic review with meta-analysis. *BMC Public Health* 2011; **11**(Suppl. 3): S5.

Papageorghiou AT, Ohuma E, Altman D, et al. International standards for fetal growth based on serial ultrasound measurements: the Fetal Growth Longitudinal Study of the INTERGROWTH-21st Project. *Lancet* 2014; **384**(9946): 869–879. Available at: www.thelancet.com/pdfs/journals/lancet/PIIS0140-6736(14)61490-2.pdf (accessed 19 July 2016).

Royal College of Obstetricians and Gynaecologists. *The Investigation and Management of the Small-for-Gestational-Age Fetus*. Green-top Guideline No. 31. Available at: www.rcog.org.uk/globalassets/documents/guidelines/gtg_31.pdf (accesssed 19 July 2016).

Smith GCS. Prevention of stillbirth. *Obstetrician & Gynaecologist* 2015; **17**(3): 183–187.

Fetal growth surveillance at a glance

Screening for the high-risk pregnancy	Maternal, past obstetric and pregnancy history for risk factors
	Uterine artery Doppler at, e.g., 12 or 23 weeks to identify some high-risk pregnancies
	Maternal blood tests abnormal (e.g. pregnancy-associated plasma protein A (PAPPA)): high risk if in absence of an anomaly
	Integration of above likely to prove best in future

(Continued)

Fetal growth surveillance at a glance (Continued)

	Antenatal care including symphysis–fundal height measurements: refer for ultrasound if less than expected, and repeat at 2–3-weekly intervals if fetus small for gestational age (SGA) 'One-off' ultrasound, umbilical artery Doppler or cardiotocography (CTG) little use
Methods of surveillance in the high-risk pregnancy or if proven SGA	Ultrasound (2–4 weekly) to establish consistent growth If SGA <34 weeks: umbilical artery Doppler If SGA >34 weeks: umbilical artery and middle cerebral artery (cerebroplacental ratio) CTG on a daily basis in preterm fetus with severely abnormal Dopplers, or to establish that fetus healthy at time of test Methods specific to disorder, e.g. blood pressure in pre-eclampsia

Small for gestational age (SGA) and intrauterine growth restriction (IUGR) at a glance

Definition	SGA	Smaller than the 10th centile for the gestation
	IUGR	Small compared to genetic determination, and compromised
Aetiology		Predominantly physiological determinants of size: race, parity, fetal gender, maternal size
		Pathological determinants of fetal growth: maternal illness, e.g. renal disease, pre-eclampsia; also multiple pregnancy, chromosomal abnormalities, infections, smoking
Clinical features		Low symphysis–fundal height. Features of pre-eclampsia
Investigations		Ultrasound to determine size Check for fetal abnormalities and cytomegalovirus status ± chromosomes Umbilical artery Doppler (umbA) if <34 weeks Umbilical artery and middle cerebral artery (MCA) Doppler (cerebroplacental ratio: CPR) if >34 weeks Cardiotocography (CTG) if Dopplers severely abnormal, e.g. umbA absent end-diastolic flow (AEDF)
Management	SGA	<37 weeks: Monitor growth with ultrasound every 2–3 weeks <37 weeks: No intervention if growth consistent and umbA normal Consider delivery
	IUGR	<34 weeks: Twice-weekly umbA Doppler if abnormal but not AEDF Give steroids Daily CTG if umbA shows AEDF <32 weeks Deliver if umbA shows AEDF >32 weeks or CTG abnormal Give magnesium just prior to delivery
		>34 weeks: Monitor CPR Consider delivery anyway
		>34 weeks: Deliver

CHAPTER 26

Abnormal lie and breech presentation

Abnormal (transverse and oblique) lie

Definitions and epidemiology

The lie of the fetus describes the relationship of the fetus to the long axis of the uterus. If it is lying longitudinally within the uterus, the lie is longitudinal (Fig. 26.1a) and the *presentation* will be cephalic (head) or breech: either will be palpable at the pelvic inlet. If neither is present, the fetus must be lying across the uterus, with the head in one iliac fossa (oblique lie) or in the flank (transverse lie; Fig. 26.1b). Abnormal lie occurs at 1 in 200 births, but is more common earlier in the pregnancy: before term, it is normal.

Aetiology

Preterm labour is more commonly complicated by an abnormal lie than labour at full term. *Circumstances that allow more room to turn*, e.g. polyhydramnios or high parity (more lax uterus), are the most common causes, frequently resulting in an 'unstable' or continually changing lie. *Conditions that prevent turning*, e.g. fetal and uterine abnormalities and twin pregnancies, may also cause persistent transverse lie, as may *conditions that prevent engagement*, e.g. placenta praevia and pelvic tumours or uterine deformities (Fig. 26.2). Unstable lie in nulliparous women is rare and usually signifies obstruction.

Complications

If the head or breech cannot enter the pelvis, labour cannot deliver the fetus. An arm or the umbilical cord (Fig. 26.3) may prolapse when the membranes rupture, and if neglected, the obstruction eventually causes uterine rupture. Both fetus and mother are at risk.

Management

No action is required for transverse or unstable lie before 37 weeks unless the woman is in labour. After 37 weeks, the woman is often admitted to hospital in case the membranes rupture and an ultrasound scan is performed to exclude particular identifiable causes, notably polyhydramnios and placenta praevia. External cephalic version (ECV) is unjustified because the fetus usually turns back. If spontaneous version occurs and persists for more than 48 hours, the mother is discharged. In the absence of pelvic obstruction, an abnormal lie will usually stabilize before 41 weeks. At this stage, or if the woman is in labour, the persistently abnormal lie is delivered by caesarean, but in expert hands ECV and then amniotomy (stabilizing induction) is an alternative.

Breech presentation

Definitions and epidemiology

The presentation refers to the part of the fetus that occupies the lower segment of the uterus or the pelvis. Presentation of the buttocks is breech presentation (Fig. 26.4). It occurs in 3–4% of term pregnancies but, like the abnormal lie, is common earlier in the pregnancy and is therefore more common (25%) if labour occurs preterm. The extended breech (70%) has both

Obstetrics & Gynaecology, Fifth Edition. Lawrence Impey, Tim Child.
© 2017 John Wiley & Sons, Ltd. Published 2017 by John Wiley & Sons, Ltd.

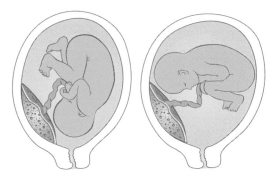

Fig. 26.1 (a) Longitudinal lie. (b) Transverse lie.

legs extended at the knee. The flexed breech (15%) has both legs flexed at the knee. In the footling breech (15%, more common if preterm), one or both feet present below the buttocks.

Aetiology

No cause is found with most. A previous breech presentation has occurred in 8%. *Prematurity* is commonly associated with breech presentation. Conditions that prevent movement, such as *fetal* and *uterine abnormalities* or *twin pregnancies*, or that prevent engagement of

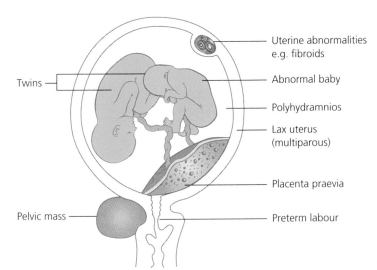

Twins

Pelvic mass

Uterine abnormalities
e.g. fibroids

Abnormal baby

Polyhydramnios

Lax uterus
(multiparous)

Placenta praevia

Preterm labour

Fig. 26.2 Causes of transverse lie and breech presentation.

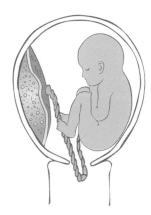

Fig. 26.3 Cord prolapse.

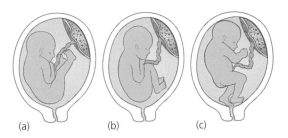

(a)   (b)   (c)

Fig. 26.4 Types of breech presentation. (a) Extended. (b) Flexed. (c) Footling.

the head, such as *placenta praevia, pelvic tumours* and *pelvic deformities* are more common (see Fig. 26.2).

Diagnosis

Breech presentation is commonly missed (30%), but diagnosis is only important from 37 weeks or if the woman is in labour. Upper abdominal discomfort is common: the hard head is normally palpable and ballottable at the fundus. Ultrasound confirms the diagnosis, helps detection of a fetal abnormality, pelvic tumour or placenta praevia and ensures the prerequisites for ECV are met.

Complications

Perinatal and long-term morbidity and mortality are increased. Fetal abnormalities are more common, but even 'normal' breech babies have slightly higher rates of long-term neurological handicap which is mostly independent of the mode of delivery. In addition, labour has additional hazards of hypoxia and birth trauma, although these are commonly overestimated.

Management

External cephalic version

From 37 weeks, an attempt is made to turn the baby to a cephalic presentation (Fig. 26.5). This reduces breech presentation at term and therefore caesarean section (*Cochrane* 2015; CD000083). The success rate is about 50%; approximately 3% of successfully turned breeches will turn back. Where ECV fails, only about 3% will turn spontaneously before delivery.

Technique: ECV is done without anaesthetic, but is made easier and more successful by administering a uterine relaxant (tocolytic) to the mother. With both hands on the abdomen, the breech is disengaged from the pelvis, pushed upwards and to the side, and rotation in the form of a forward somersault is attempted. This is performed under ultrasound guidance and in hospital to allow immediate delivery if complications occur. Cardiotocography (CTG) is performed straight after and anti-D is given to Rhesus-negative women.

Safety of ECV: In expert hands, the risk of fetal damage is extremely low, although placental abruption and

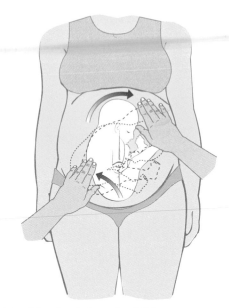

Fig. 26.5 External cephalic version (ECV).

uterine rupture have been reported. Immediate emergency caesarean section is required in 0.5%.

Factors affecting success of ECV: Lower success rates are seen in nulliparous women, in Caucasians, where the breech is engaged, where the head is not easily palpable or uterine tone is high, with obese women and if the liquor volume is reduced. Fetal size makes little difference.

Contraindications to ECV: ECV is not performed if the fetus is compromised, if vaginal delivery is contraindicated (e.g. placenta praevia), if there are twins, if the membranes are ruptured or if there has been recent antepartum haemorrhage. One previous caesarean section is not a contraindication.

Labour after a successful ECV is slightly more likely to end in caesarean section than if the fetus has always been cephalic.

Mode of birth

If ECV has failed or is contraindicated, or the breech presentation was missed, the alternatives are planned caesarean section at 39 weeks or planned vaginal breech birth. Caesarean section probably very slightly reduces perinatal mortality which is 1 in 3–500 with planned breech birth with expert care (*Acta Obstet Gynecol Scand*

2014; **93**(9): 888–896). The difference in risk is very small, and probably largely due to the earlier gestation of elective caesarean section (39 weeks) than spontaneous labour (40 weeks). Caesarean section also reduces the incidence of neonatal morbidity including birth trauma, low Apgar scores and neonatal unit admission. However, this morbidity is short term, and caesarean section is not clearly protective against long-term handicap (*AJOG* 2004; **191**: 864). Short-term maternal morbidity is not increased by caesarean section. Complications of subsequent pregnancies, particularly placenta accreta are, however, more common. Parents should be counselled as to these findings: most in the West undergo caesarean section.

Some women wish to deliver vaginally; further, breech presentation is often diagnosed only in late labour and second twins often present as breech. Under such circumstances, vaginal breech delivery is usually appropriate, as it is with a second twin, yet skills are being lost due to lack of experience. This renders such births more risky and knowledge of the management of vaginal breech birth remains essential.

Vaginal breech birth

Patient selection: Vaginal breech birth is probably more risky with a fetus >3.8 kg, with evidence of fetal compromise, an extended head or footling legs.

Intrapartum care: Pushing is discouraged until the buttocks are visible. Cardiotocography is advised. In about 30%, there is slow cervical dilatation in the first stage or, particularly, poor descent in the second. Under these circumstances augmentation with oxytocin is unwise and caesarean section is advised.

Breech birth: Most breech babies deliver (Fig. 26.6) easily: it is perhaps in 10% where real skill is required. A difficult delivery is often the result of injudicious traction causing extension of the head, or operator panic. Once the buttocks distend the perineum, an episiotomy can be made but is not essential. The fetus delivers with maternal effort as far as the umbilicus, and should not be touched. The legs can be flexed out of the vagina, whilst the back is kept anterior. Once the scapula is visible, the anterior and then the posterior arms are 'hooked' down by a finger over the shoulder sweeping across the chest. If the arms cannot be reached because they are extended above the neck, then *Lovset's procedure* is required: placing the hands around the body with the thumbs on the sacrum and rotating the baby

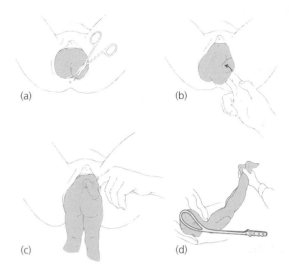

Fig. 26.6 Breech delivery. (a) As the buttocks distend the perineum, perform the episiotomy. (b) A finger behind the knee delivers the legs. (c) A finger hooks each arm down. (d) Forceps delivering the head once the arms are delivered.

180° clockwise and then counter-clockwise with gentle downward traction. This allows the anterior shoulder and then the posterior shoulder to enter the pelvis. Once the back of the neck is visible, the operator supports the entire weight of the fetus on one palm and forearm, with their finger in its mouth to guide the head over the perineum and maintain flexion. With the same intent, the other hand presses against the occiput. This is the *Mauriceau–Smellie–Veit manoeuvre*. If this fails to deliver the head, an assistant holds the legs up whilst forceps are applied, and with the next contraction the head is lifted slowly out of the vagina.

It is often maintained that an all-fours position for birth is most effective. There is reason to believe this is correct: the pelvic dimensions enlarge, aortocaval compression is less and the baby is much more visible when emerging, This has not been subjected to scientific scrutiny.

Further reading

Royal College of Obstetricians and Gynaecologists. *External Cephalic Version and Reducing the Incidence of Breech Presentation*. Green-top Guideline No. 20a. Available at: www.rcog.org.uk/globalassets/documents/guidelines/gt20aexternalcephalicversion (accessed 21 July 2016).

Royal College of Obstetricians and Gynaecologists. *The Management of Breech Presentation.* Green-top Guideline No. 20b. Available at: www.rcog.org.uk/globalassets/documents/guidelines/gtg-no-20b-breech-presentation.pdf (accessed 21 July 2016).

Vlemmix F, Bergenhenegouwen L, Schaaf J, *et al.* Term breech deliveries in the Netherlands: did the increased cesarean rate affect neonatal outcome? A population-based cohort study. *Acta Obstetricia et Gynecologica Scandinavica* 2014; **93**(9): 888–896.

Transverse/oblique lie at a glance

Definition	Lie of fetus not parallel to long axis of uterus
Epidemiology	1 in 200 births
Aetiology	Preterm labour, polyhydramnios, multiparity, placenta praevia, pelvic mass, fetal or uterine abnormality, twins
Management	Admit if >37 weeks. Ultrasound to find cause
	If not stabilized by 41 weeks, or if pelvis obstructed, elective caesarean

Breech presentation at a glance

Types	Extended (70%), flexed (15%), footling (15%)
Epidemiology	3% at term, more if preterm labour or previous breech presentation
Aetiology	Idiopathic, uterine/fetal anomalies, placenta praevia, pelvic mass, twins
	More common preterm
Complications	Increased perinatal mortality and morbidity due to:
	Unknown but unrelated to vaginal delivery
	Congenital anomalies
	Intrapartum problems (1% excess mortality)
Management	External cephalic version (ECV) from 37 weeks, 50% success. Not if antepartum haemorrhage, ruptured membranes, fetal compromise, twins
	Elective caesarean section very slightly safer than vaginal birth. Vaginal breech birth remains appropriate with careful selection, counselling and management

CHAPTER 27
Multiple pregnancy

Epidemiology

Twins occur in 1 in 80 pregnancies, triplets in 1 in 1000. There is considerable geographic variation. The incidence of twins is increasing because of subfertility treatment and the increasing number of older mothers, although in the UK triplets and higher order multiples have become fewer again with better fertility treatment regulation.

Types of multiple pregnancy

Dizygotic (DZ) twins (two-thirds of all multiple pregnancies) or triplets result from fertilization of different oocytes by different sperm (Fig. 27.1). Such fetuses may be of different sex and are no more genetically similar than siblings from different pregnancies.

Monozygotic (MZ) twins result from mitotic division of a single zygote into 'identical' twins. Whether they share the same amnion or placenta depends on the time at which division into separate zygotes occurred (see Fig. 27.1). Division before day 3 (approximately 30%) leads to twins with separate placentas and amnions (dichorionic diamniotic: DCDA). Division between days 4 and 8 (approximately 70%) leads to twins with a shared placenta but separate amnions (monochorionic diamniotic: MCDA). Later division (9–13 days) is very rare and causes twins with a shared placenta and a single amniotic sac (monochorionic monoamniotic: MCMA). Incomplete division leads to conjoined twins. Monochorionic (MC) twins have a higher fetal loss rate, particularly before 24 weeks.

Aetiology

Assisted conception, genetic factors and increasing maternal age and parity are the most important factors, largely affecting DZ twinning. About 20% of all *in vitro* fertilization (IVF) conceptions and 5–10% of clomiphene-assisted conceptions are multiple. Embryo transfer of more than two fertilized ova at IVF is now performed in the UK only under exceptional circumstances, but is common elsewhere.

Diagnosis

Vomiting may be more marked in early pregnancy. The uterus is larger than expected from the dates and palpable before 12 weeks. Later in pregnancy, three or more fetal poles may be felt. Most are diagnosed only at ultrasound; as this is now performed in most pregnancies, the diagnosis is seldom missed.

Maternal complications

Virtually all obstetric risks are exaggerated in multiple pregnancies (Fig. 27.2). *Gestational diabetes* and *pre-eclampsia* particularly are more frequent. *Anaemia* is common, partly because of a greater increase in blood volume causing a dilutional effect and partly because more iron and folic acid are needed.

Fetal antenatal complications

All multiples

Twins have greater mortality (sixfold increase) and long-term handicap (fivefold increase). Triplets fare even worse with an 18-fold increase in handicap. The major risk factors are preterm delivery, intrauterine growth restriction (IUGR) and monochorionicity (see below).

Obstetrics & Gynaecology, Fifth Edition. Lawrence Impey, Tim Child.
© 2017 John Wiley & Sons, Ltd. Published 2017 by John Wiley & Sons, Ltd.

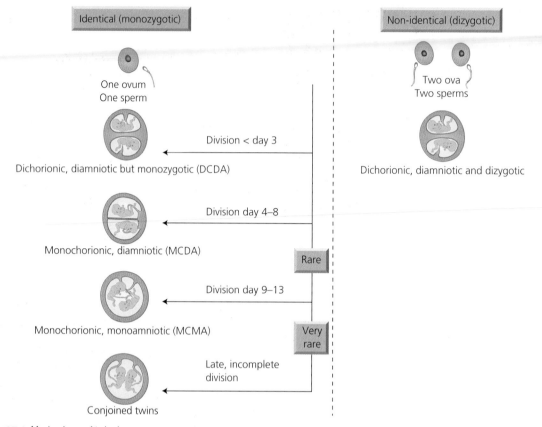

Fig. 27.1 Mechanisms of twinning.

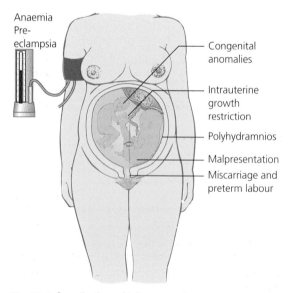

Fig. 27.2 Complications of twin pregnancies.

Miscarriage: One of a twin or more of a higher multiple pregnancy can 'vanish', where there is first-trimester death. Late miscarriage is also more common, particularly in MC twins as a complication of twin–twin transfusion syndrome (see below).

Preterm labour is the main cause of perinatal mortality: 40% of twin and 80% of triplet pregnancies deliver before 36 weeks; 10% of twins deliver before 32 weeks.

Intrauterine growth restriction (IUGR) (Fig. 27.3) is much more common.

Congenital abnormalities are not more common per baby in dichorionic, but they are in monochorionic pregnancies.

Complications of monochorionicity

These largely result from the shared blood supply in the single placenta (Fig. 27.4).

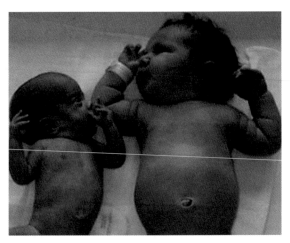

Fig. 27.3 Twins with growth discordancy.

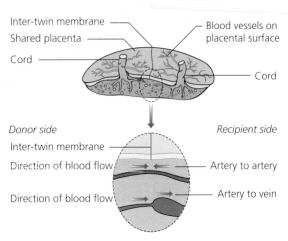

Fig. 27.4 Monochorionic twin placenta with shared blood vessels.

Twin–twin transfusion syndrome (TTTS): This occurs only in MCDA twins, the most common form of identical twins, and in about 15%. It results from unequal blood distribution through vascular anastomoses of the shared placenta (see Fig. 27.4). One twin, the 'donor', is volume depleted and develops anaemia, IUGR and oligohydramnios. The other or 'recipient' twin becomes volume overloaded and may develop polycythaemia, cardiac failure and massive polyhydramnios, causing, *in extremis*, massive distension of the uterus. Disease is staged according to Quintero in stages 1–5. Both twins are at very high risk of *in utero* death or severely preterm delivery.

Twin anaemia polycythaemia sequence (TAPS) occurs where there are marked haemoglobin differences between MC twins but in the absence of the liquor volume changes characteristic of TTTS. Occurring as a consequence of small placental anastomoses, it can follow incomplete laser ablation for TTTS.

Twin reversed arterial perfusion (TRAP) is a rare abnormality of MC twins. An abnormal, often acardiac fetus is perfused by a normal 'pump' twin, which is therefore at risk of cardiac failure.

Intrauterine growth restriction is more common in MC twins, in the absence of clear blood volume discordancy. A particular problem is where the umbilical artery waveform of the smaller twin is very erratic (selective IUGR with intermittent absent or reversed end-diastolic flow, abbreviated to sIUGR with iAREDF). This may be the result of the superficial artery–artery anastomoses,

shown in Fig. 27.4; an ultrasound of these is shown in Fig. 27.5. Sudden *in utero* death occurs in up to 20%, handicap in 8%.

Co-twin death: If one of an MC twin pair dies, due to TTTS or any other cause, the drop in its blood pressure allows acute transfusion of blood from the other twin. This rapidly leads to hypovolaemia and, in about 30% of cases, death or neurological damage. The survivor of a dichorionic twin pregnancy is not at risk, except of preterm delivery, because the circulation is not shared.

Monoamniotic twins: In this rare situation, not only the placenta but also the amniotic sac is shared. The cords are always entangled (Fig. 27.6). *In utero* demise is common, probably because of this and/or sudden acute shunting of blood between the two babies in anastomoses between the close cord insertions.

Intrapartum complications

Malpresentation of the first twin occurs in 20% (Fig. 27.7): this is an indication for caesarean section.

Fetal distress in labour is more common. The second twin delivered has an increased risk of death (fivefold), after the first has been delivered because of hypoxia, cord prolapse, tetanic uterine contraction or placental abruption, and may present as a breech. However, routine caesarean section does not improve neonatal outcome.

Postpartum haemorrhage is more common (10%).

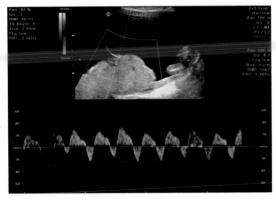
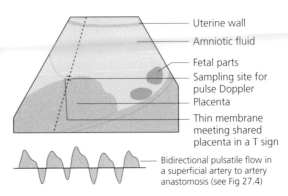

Uterine wall
Amniotic fluid
Fetal parts
Sampling site for
pulse Doppler
Placenta
Thin membrane
meeting shared
placenta in a T sign
Bidirectional pulsatile flow in
a superficial artery to artery
anastomosis (see Fig 27.4)

Fig. 27.5 Ultrasound of monochorionic diamniotic twin placenta.

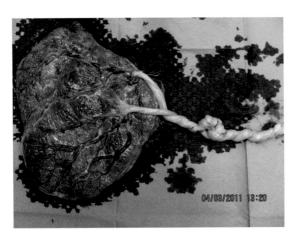

Fig. 27.6 Monochorionic monoamniotic twin placenta.

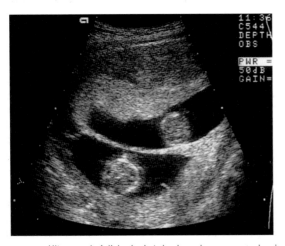
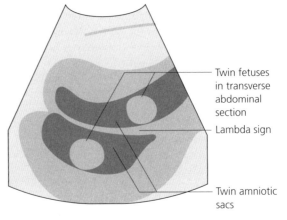

Twin fetuses
in transverse
abdominal
section
Lambda sign
Twin amniotic
sacs

Fig. 27.7 Ultrasound of dichorionic twins in early pregnancy showing the lambda sign.

Complications of twin pregnancies

Perinatal mortality increased fourfold
Preterm labour and miscarriage
Congenital abnormalities
Placental insufficiency/intrauterine growth restriction (IUGR)
Twin–twin transfusion syndrome (monochorionic twins only)
Antepartum and postpartum haemorrhage
Pre-eclampsia, diabetes, anaemia
Malpresentation

Outcomes of multiple pregnancies

Type	8–24-week loss 1+ baby*	Perinatal mortality (per baby)*	Cerebral palsy (per baby)*
DC twins	2.5%	3–5%	1%
MCDA twins	15%	5–12%	2–5%
Triplets	5–15%	10%	2–3%

DC, dichorionic; MCDA, monochorionic diamniotic.
* Approximate figures.

Antepartum management

All multiples

General: The pregnancy should be considered 'high risk'. Care should be consultant led, although not every visit need be in the hospital. Iron and folic acid supplements are prescribed; low-dose aspirin is advised if there are other risk factors to prevent pre-eclamspia. Multiple pregnancies increase maternal tiredness and anxiety, and may result in financial problems. Postnatal home help should be discussed. In the UK, NICE recommends that a specialist, multidisciplinary team supervises pregnancy care.

Early ultrasound: Screening for chromosomal abnormalities is offered as usual. Chorionicity is most accurately ascertained in the first trimester: in dichorionic twins, the dividing membrane is thicker as it meets the placentas (lambda sign) (see Fig. 27.7); in monochorionic twins it is thin (T sign) (see Fig. 27.5) and perpendicular to the shared placenta. Twins of opposite gender are always DZ.

Identification of risk of preterm delivery: Transvaginal ultrasound of cervical length is not advised in the UK but may identify those at most risk. In contrast to singletons, neither progesterone nor cervical cerclage prevents preterm birth in multiple pregnancies.

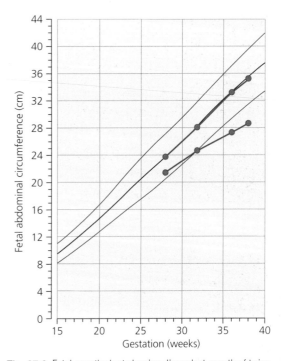

Fig. 27.8 Fetal growth chart showing discordant growth of twins.

Identification of IUGR: As this is both more common and more difficult to detect in multiple pregnancies compared with singleton pregnancies, serial ultrasound examinations for growth are usually routinely performed at 28, 32 and 36 weeks (Fig. 27.8) and more often with monochorionic twins.

Timing of delivery: Delivery at 37 weeks is advised in the UK for dichorionic twins, and at 36 weeks for uncomplicated monochorionic twins.

Monochorionic twins

Ultrasound surveillance of MC twin pregnancies starts by 12 weeks. Ultrasound is advised every 2 weeks until 24 weeks and every 2–3 weeks thereafter.

TTTS is most commonly diagnosed between 16 and 24 weeks. Growth and liquor volume discordancies with polyhydramnios are evident, with evidence of fluid overload in the recipient, e.g. tricuspid regurgitation (Fig. 27.9). Except where disease is very mild, laser ablation of the entire placental interface in a fetal medicine centre, using ultrasound and fetoscopy, is the preferred treatment. Even with optimal treatment, survival of both twins occurs in only 50%, with one twin in 80%;

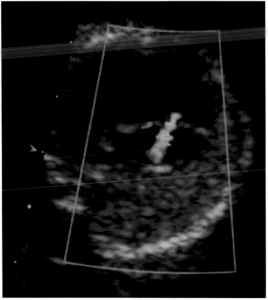

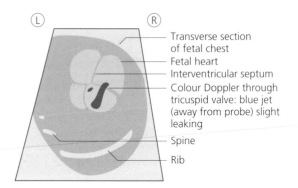

Transverse section of fetal chest

Fetal heart

Interventricular septum

Colour Doppler through tricuspid valve: blue jet (away from probe) slight leaking

Spine

Rib

Fig. 27.9 Ultrasound of fetal heart showing tricuspid regurgitation.

about 10% of survivors have neurological disability. Pregnancies complicated by TTTS after 26 weeks are usually delivered.

IUGR is managed by careful surveillance and iatrogenic preterm delivery. Occasionally laser ablation or umbilical cord occlusion are appropriate if at 'previable' gestations.

High order multiple pregnancy

Selective reduction to a twin pregnancy at 12 weeks should be discussed with women with triplets or higher order pregnancies. This is highly emotive (Fig. 27.10). Whilst this slightly increases early miscarriage rates, it reduces the chances of preterm birth and therefore cerebral palsy, including where there is a monochorionic twin pair (*BJOG* 2015; **122**: 1053–1060). This is safest before 14 weeks.

Surveillance is according to the chorionicity; delivery by 36 weeks is usually advised.

Fetal abnormality

Where one twin has an abnormality, selective termination should be discussed. In DC twins this can be by intracardiac injection of KCl; this is best before 14 weeks as miscarriage is less common. Where late (>24

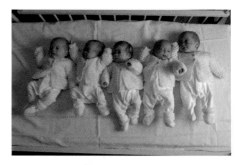

Fig. 27.10 Quintuplet girls delivered in Oxford in 2007. By kind permission of the parents.

weeks' gestation) termination of pregnancy is legal, as in the UK, it can be offered from 32 weeks so that if delivery ensues, the remaining twin will survive. In monochorionic twins, the cord must be occluded using bipolar diathermy, or its insertion ablated, because the circulation is shared.

Intrapartum management

Mode of delivery

Caesarean section, provided the presenting twin is cephalic, does not improve perinatal outcome. It is indicated if the first fetus is a breech or a transverse lie

(20%), with high order multiples, if there have been antepartum complications and, in some hospitals, with all monochorionic twins. Vaginal delivery when the first fetus is cephalic, whatever the lie or presentation of the second, remains commonplace (Fig. 27.11).

Method of delivery

Induction (or caesarean) is usual at 37 weeks (DC twins) or 36 weeks (MC twins), after which time perinatal mortality is increased. Cardiotocography (CTG) is advised as the risk of intrapartum hypoxia is increased, particularly for the second twin. Epidural analgesia is not mandatory but is helpful if difficulty is encountered with the second twin. The first twin is delivered in the normal manner.

At this stage particularly, good communication with, and a comfortable position for, the mother are essential. Continuous fetal monitoring is essential. Contractions often diminish after the first twin. Usually these return within a few minutes; oxytocin can be started if not. The lie of the second twin is checked and external cephalic version (ECV) is performed if it is not longitudinal. Once the head or breech enters the pelvis, the membranes are ruptured and pushing again begins. Delivery is usually easy whether cephalic or breech. Excessive delay is associated with increased morbidity for the second twin, but excessive haste is equally dangerous. If the head does not descend, a malpresentation (particularly a brow) is likely and caesarean section is very occasionally required. If fetal distress or cord prolapse occurs, vaginal delivery can be expedited with a ventouse or breech extraction. The latter must be performed under general, epidural or spinal anaesthesia, and only by experienced personnel. It involves inserting a hand into the uterus, grasping the feet and guiding them down. After delivery, a prophylactic oxytocin infusion is used to prevent postpartum haemorrhage.

Pitfalls in delivering twins
Scaring the mother, too many people present Failure to monitor the second twin properly Overstimulation of the uterus with oxytocin Rupture of the membranes too early Postpartum haemorrhage

Further reading

Benoit RM, Baschat AA. Twin-to-twin transfusion syndrome: prenatal diagnosis and treatment. *American Journal of Perinatology* 2014; **31**(7): 583–594.

Dodd JM, Deussen AR, Grivell RM, Crowther CA. Elective birth at 37 weeks' gestation for women with an uncomplicated twin pregnancy. *Cochrane Database of Systematic Reviews* 2014; **2**: CD003582.

Royal College of Obstetricians and Gynaecologists. *Management of Monochorionic Twin Pregnancy.* Green-top Guideline No. 51. Available at: www.rcog.org.uk/globalassets/documents/guidelines/t51management monochorionictwinpregnancy2008a.pdf (accessed 21 July 2016).

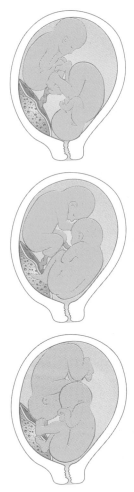

Fig. 27.11 Different presentations of twins.

Multiple pregnancy at a glance

Incidence	Twins 1.3%, triplets 0.1%; incidence of twins increasing because of fertility treatment and older mothers	
Terms	Dizygotic (DZ)	Different oocytes fertilized by different sperm
	Monozygotic (MZ)	Division of zygote after fertilization by one sperm
	Dichorionic: (DC)	Two placentas (DZ or MZ)
	Monochorionic (MC)	Shared placenta (always MZ)
Twin types	DC (approx. 70%)	Can be identical (MZ) or not (DZ); do not share placenta or sac
	MCDA (approx. 30%)	Identical (MZ), share placenta (MC) but not amniotic sac (DA)
	MCMA (approx. 1%)	Identical (MZ), share placenta (MC) and amniotic sac (MA)
Aetiology	Ovulation induction and *in vitro* fertilization (IVF), genetic factors, increasing age and parity	
Diagnosis	Usually at ultrasound scan. Vomiting, 'large for dates', 3+ fetal poles	
Complications	Maternal	Pre-eclampsia, anaemia, gestational diabetes, operative delivery
	All twins	Increased morbidity and mortality due to most obstetric complications, particularly miscarriage, preterm labour, placental insufficiency/intrauterine growth restriction (IUGR), antepartum and postpartum haemorrhage and malpresentations
	MC twins	Congenital abnormalities, twin–twin transfusion (TTTS), IUGR
Management	All twins	Early diagnosis, identification of chorionicity. Consultant care. Iron and folic acid supplements. Anomaly scan
		Increased surveillance for pre-eclampsia, diabetes, anaemia
		Serial ultrasound at 28, 32 and 36 weeks
	MC twins	Ultrasound fortnightly from 12 weeks for TTTS and IUGR. Laser treatment if TTTS
	Delivery	37 if DC; 36 weeks if MC
	Labour	Caesarean section if first twin not cephalic and usual indications as for singletons. Cardiotocography. After first twin, lie of second twin checked: external cephalic version (ECV) to longitudinal lie if necessary. Amniotomy when presenting part engaged, then maternal pushing. Ventouse or breech extraction if fetal distress

Twin–twin transfusion syndrome (TTTS) at a glance

Incidence	15% of all MC twins
Pathology	Unequal blood distribution in shared placenta leading to discordant blood volumes, liquor and often growth
Diagnosis	Discordant liquor volumes. Recipient twin larger, polyhydramnios, fluid overload, heart failure Donor twin smaller, 'stuck' with oligohydramnios
Complications	Late miscarriage and severe preterm delivery, *in utero* death, neurological damage
Management	Ultrasound surveillance from 12 weeks. Laser ablation if TTTS diagnosed
Prognosis	Very poor untreated. With laser, approx. 50% both twins survive; 80% one twin survives

CHAPTER 28

Labour 1: Mechanism – anatomy and physiology

Labour is the process whereby the fetus and placenta are expelled from the uterus, which normally occurs between 37 and 42 weeks' gestation. The diagnosis is made *when painful uterine contractions accompany dilatation and effacement of the cervix*. It is divided into stages. In the *first stage*, the cervix opens to 'full dilatation' to allow the head to pass through. The *second stage* is from full dilatation to delivery of the fetus. The *third stage* lasts from delivery of the fetus to delivery of the placenta.

Labour	
Diagnosis	Painful contractions lead to dilatation of the cervix
First stage	Initiation to full cervical dilatation
Second stage	Full cervical dilatation to delivery of fetus
Third stage	Delivery of fetus to delivery of placenta

Mechanical factors of labour

Three mechanical factors determine progress during labour.
1 The degree of force expelling the fetus (the powers).
2 The dimensions of the pelvis and the resistance of soft tissues (the passage).
3 The diameters of the fetal head (the passenger).

The powers (Fig. 28.1)

Once labour is established, the uterus contracts for 45–60 seconds about every 2–4 minutes. This pulls the cervix up (effacement) and causes dilatation, aided by the pressure of the head as the uterus pushes the head down into the pelvis. Poor uterine activity is a common feature of the nulliparous woman and in induced labour, but is rare in multiparous women.

The passage

The bony pelvis

This has three principal planes. At its *inlet*, the transverse diameter is about 13 cm, wider than the 11 cm antero-posterior (AP) diameter (Fig. 28.2). The *mid-cavity* is almost round as the transverse and AP diameters are similar. At the *outlet*, the AP diameter (12.5 cm) is greater than the transverse diameter (11 cm). In the lateral wall of the round mid-pelvis, bony prominences called *ischial spines* are palpable vaginally. These are used as landmarks by which to assess the descent of the head on vaginal examination. The level of descent is called 'station' and is crudely measured in centimetres in relation to these 'spines'. Station 0 means the head is at the level of these spines; station +2 means it is 2 cm below and station −2 means it is 2 cm above (Fig. 28.3). A variety of pelvic shapes have been described, but diagnosis and therefore description of these are seldom useful in clinical practice.

The soft tissues

Cervical dilatation is a prerequisite for delivery and is dependent on contractions, the pressure of the fetal head on the cervix and the ability of the cervix to soften

---

Obstetrics & Gynaecology, Fifth Edition. Lawrence Impey, Tim Child.
© 2017 John Wiley & Sons, Ltd. Published 2017 by John Wiley & Sons, Ltd.

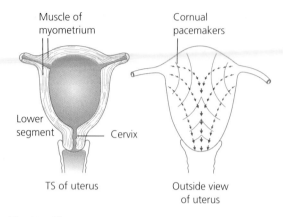

Fig. 28.1 The powers.

and allow distension. The soft tissues of the vagina and perineum need to be overcome in the second stage: the perineum often tears or is cut (episiotomy) to allow the head to deliver.

The passenger

The head is oblong in transverse section. Its bones are not yet fused and, on vaginal examination, spaces between them are palpable as sutures and fontanelles. The anterior fontanelle (bregma) lies above the forehead. The posterior fontanelle (occiput) lies on the back of the top of the head. Between these two is the area called the vertex. In front of the bregma is the brow (Fig. 28.4). Because the head is not round, several factors determine how easily it fits through the pelvic diameters.

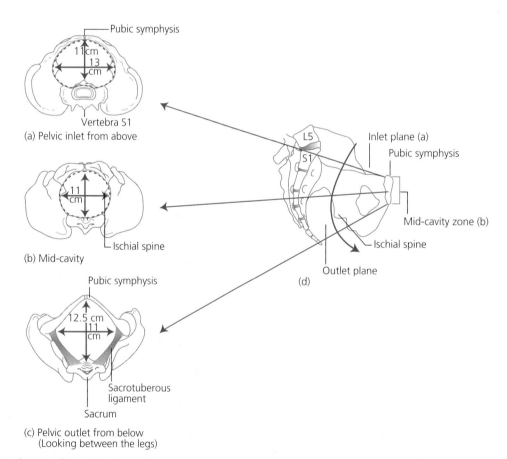

Fig. 28.2 Anatomy of the pelvis showing the three planes (a, b and c), and where they are on a lateral view of the pelvis (d).

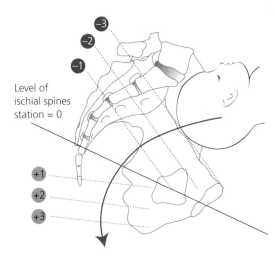

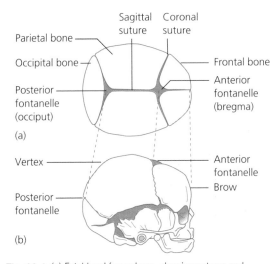

Fig. 28.3 Descent of the head in labour in relation to the ischial spines.

Fig. 28.4 (a) Fetal head from above, showing sutures and fontanelles. (b) Fetal head from the side.

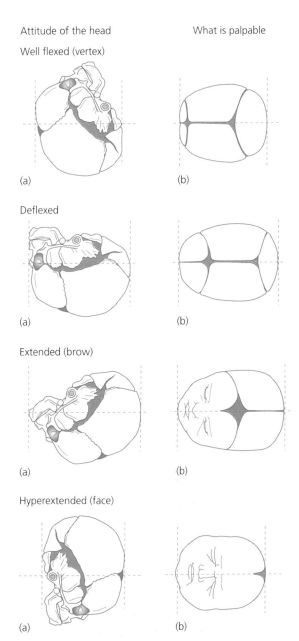

Fig. 28.5 Attitude of the fetal head showing how extension of the head changes the presenting diameter and what is palpable on vaginal examination.

Attitude: extension/flexion

The attitude is the degree of flexion of the head on the neck (Fig. 28.5). The ideal attitude is maximal flexion, keeping the head bowed. This is called *vertex presentation*, and the presenting diameter is 9.5 cm, running from the anterior fontanelle to below the occiput at the back of the head. A small degree of extension results in a larger diameter. Extension of 90° causes a *brow presentation*, and a much larger diameter of 13 cm. A further 30° of extension (with the face looking parallel and away from the body) is a *face presentation*. Extension of the head can mean that the fetal diameters are too large to deliver vaginally.

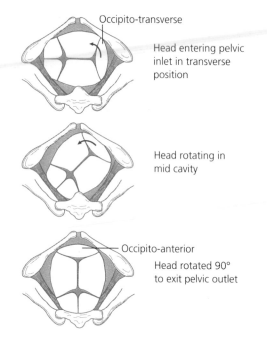

Occipito-transverse

Head entering pelvic inlet in transverse position

Head rotating in mid cavity

Occipito-anterior

Head rotated 90° to exit pelvic outlet

Fig. 28.6 View from below showing rotation of the head (position) according to the three planes of the pelvis.

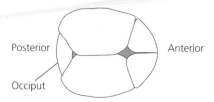

Posterior · · · · Anterior

Occiput

Fig. 28.7 Diagram of moulding showing compression and overlap of sutures.

Position: rotation

The position is the degree of rotation of the head on the neck (Fig. 28.6). If the sagittal suture is transverse, the oblong head will fit the pelvic inlet best. But at the outlet the sagittal suture must be vertical for the head to fit. The head must therefore normally rotate 90° during labour. It is usually delivered with the *occiput anterior* (occipito-anterior: OA). In 5% of deliveries it is occipito-posterior (OP) and more difficulty may be encountered. Persistence of the occipito-transverse (OT) position implies non-rotation and delivery without assistance is impossible.

Size of the head

The head can be compressed in the pelvis because the sutures allow the bones to come together and even overlap slightly. This slightly reduces the diameters of the head and is called *moulding* (Fig. 28.7). Pressure of the scalp on the cervix or pelvic inlet can cause localized swelling or *caput*. It is relatively unusual for a normally formed head to be simply too big to pass through a normal bony pelvis (cephalopelvic disproportion),

although a larger head may cause a longer and more difficult labour.

Terms describing the fetal head
Presentation is the part of the fetus that occupies the lower segment or pelvis, i.e. head (cephalic) or buttocks (breech)
Presenting part is the lowest part of the fetus palpable on vaginal examination: the lowest part of the head or breech. For a cephalic presentation, this can be the vertex, the brow or the face, depending on the attitude. For simplicity, these are often described as separate 'presentations'
Position of the head describes its rotation: occipito-transverse (OT), occipito-posterior (OP) or occipito-anterior (OA)
Attitude of the head describes the degree of flexion: vertex, brow or face

Movements of the head (Fig. 28.8)
Engagement in occipito-transverse (OT)
Descent and flexion
Rotation 90° to occipito-anterior (OA)
Descent
Extension to deliver
Restitution and delivery of shoulders

Cervical dilatation: the 'stages' of labour

Initiation and diagnosis of labour

Involuntary contractions of uterine smooth muscle occur throughout the third trimester and are often felt as Braxton Hicks contractions. How this leads to labour is not fully understood, but the fetus has a role, and prostaglandin production is important both in reducing cervical resistance and increasing release of the

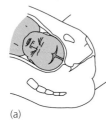

(a)

Engagement: The oblong-shaped head normally enters the pelvis in the occipito-transverse (OT) position, because the transverse diameter of the inlet is greater than the antero-posterior diameter.

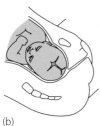

(b)

Descent and flexion: The head descends into the round mid-cavity and flexes as the cervix dilates. Descent is measured by comparison with the level of the ischial spines (see Fig. 28.3) and is called station.

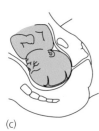

(c)

Rotation: In the mid-cavity, the head rotates 90° (internal rotation) so that the face is facing the sacrum and the occiput is anterior, below the symphysis pubis (occipito-anterior, OA). This enables it to pass through the pelvic outlet which has a wider antero-posterior than transverse diameter. In 5% of cases, the head rotates to occipito-posterior (OP).

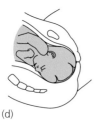

(d)

Rotation completed, further descent: The perineum distends.

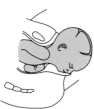

(e)

Extension and delivery.

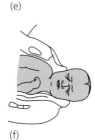

(f)

Restitution: The head then rotates 90° (external rotation) to the same position in which it entered the inlet, facing either right or left, to enable delivery of the shoulders.

hormone oxytocin from the posterior pituitary gland. This aids stimulation of contractions, which arise in one of the pacemakers situated at each cornu of the uterus.

Labour is diagnosed when painful regular contractions lead to effacement and dilatation of the cervix. Effacement is when the normally tubular cervix is drawn up into the lower segment until it is flat (Fig. 28.9). This is commonly accompanied by a 'show' or pink/white mucus plug from the cervix and/or rupture of the membranes, causing release of liquor. Labour in multiparous women is often much faster than in nulliparous ones.

The first stage

This lasts from the diagnosis of labour until the cervix is dilated by 10 cm (fully dilated). The descent, flexion and internal rotation described occur to varying degrees. If the membranes have not already ruptured, they normally do so now.

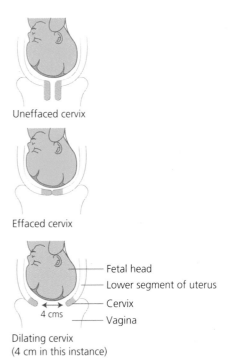

Uneffaced cervix

Effaced cervix

Fetal head
Lower segment of uterus
Cervix
4 cms
Vagina

Dilating cervix
(4 cm in this instance)

Fig. 28.9 Effacement and dilatation of the cervix.

Fig. 28.8 (a–f) Movement of the head in labour.

The latent phase is where the cervix usually dilates slowly for the first 4 cm and may take several hours.

The active phase follows. Average cervical dilatation is at the rate of 1 cm/h in nulliparous women and about 2 cm/hour in multiparous women. The active first stage should not normally last longer than 16 hours.

The second stage

This lasts from full dilatation of the cervix to delivery. Descent, flexion and rotation are completed and followed by extension as the head delivers.

The passive stage lasts from full dilatation until the head reaches the pelvic floor and the woman experiences the desire to push. Rotation and flexion are commonly completed. This stage may last a few minutes, but can be much longer.

The active stage is when the mother is pushing. The pressure of the head on the pelvic floor produces an irresistible desire to bear down, although epidural analgesia may prevent this. The woman gets in the most comfortable position for her, but not supine, and pushes with contractions. The fetus is delivered, on average, after 40 minutes (nulliparous) or 20 minutes (multiparous). This stage can be much quicker but if it takes >1 hour, spontaneous delivery becomes increasingly unlikely.

Delivery

As the head reaches the perineum, it extends to come up out of the pelvis (Fig. 28.10). The perineum begins to stretch and often tears, but can be cut (episiotomy), usually only if progress is slow or fetal distress is present. The head then restitutes, rotating 90° to adopt the transverse position in which it entered the pelvis. With the next contraction, the shoulders deliver. The anterior shoulder comes under the symphysis pubis first, usually aided by lateral body flexion in a posterior direction; the posterior

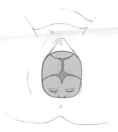

Fig. 28.10 Head delivery over the perineum by extension.

shoulder is aided by lateral body flexion in an anterior direction. The rest of the body follows.

The third stage

This is the time from delivery of the fetus to delivery of the placenta. It normally lasts about 15 minutes and normal blood loss is up to 500 mL. Uterine muscle fibres contract to compress the blood vessels formerly supplying the placenta, which shears away from the uterine wall.

Perineal trauma

The perineum is intact in about one-third of nulliparous women and in half of multiparous women. A *first-degree tear* involves minor damage to the fourchette. *Second-degree tears* and *episiotomies* involve perineal muscle. *Third-degree tears* involve the anal sphincter also and occur in 1% of deliveries. They are subclassified according to the degree of damage. *Fourth-degree tears* also involve the anal mucosa.

Further reading

Smith R. Parturition. *New England Journal of Medicine* 2007; **356**: 271–283.

Mechanism of normal labour at a glance

When	37–42 weeks
Diagnosis	Contractions with effacement and dilatation of the cervix
First stage	Average duration: 8 h, nulliparous; 5 h, multiparous
	Uterus contracts every 2–3 min
	Latent (<4 cm) and active (4–10 cm) phases
	Cervix dilates until the widest diameter of head passes through
	Head descends, remaining flexed to maintain the smallest diameter
	(Variable descent occurs before labour: 'engagement')
	90° rotation from occipito-transverse (OT) to occipito-anterior (OA) (or occipito-posterior (OP)) begins
	Amniotic membranes usually rupture or are ruptured artificially
Second stage	Contractions continue
	Head descends and flexes further, rotation usually completed
	Pushing starts when head reaches pelvic floor (active second stage)
Delivery	Head now extends as it is delivered over perineum
	Head restitutes, rotating back to transverse before the shoulders deliver
Third stage	Placenta is delivered. Average duration 15 min

CHAPTER 29
Labour 2: Management

Labour is a normal physiological process and most women will deliver safely without any management. Nevertheless, advances in obstetric care have contributed to its safety. The principal difficulty is that, in attempting to prevent rare but serious bad outcomes whilst not knowing who is at most risk, we cannot target intervention accurately enough. An example of this is induction of labour for post dates: this will prevent approximately one stillbirth for every 300 women induced at 41–42 weeks, and is usually advised, because we cannot predict the stillbirth. But such 'medicalization' of a natural process can initiate a cascade of intervention. For instance, induction of labour means epidural analgesia is more likely to be used. Epidural analgesia increases the chances of an instrumental delivery. Obstetricians therefore spend much of their time sorting out problems that they have themselves created.

Many women also fear labour, for its pain, for interventions such as instrumental deliveries and because it is a time of risk to the fetus. Such fear can be reduced by information, reassurance, accommodating reasonable wishes and, most importantly, by not treating labour as a disease. Such support, particularly in labour, improves outcomes and reduces the need for intervention (Fig. 29.1). This is not surprising because, albeit simplistically, fear leads to adrenaline secretion, and adrenaline is a potent inhibitor of uterine contractions.

General care of the woman in labour

Physical health in labour

Observations: The temperature and blood pressure should be monitored every 4 hours, the pulse every hour (first stage) and then every 15 minutes (second stage).

If abnormal, measurements should be more frequent. Contraction frequency is recorded every 30 minutes.

Mobility and delivery positions: Freedom of movement is encouraged. Most women deliver semi-recumbent: squatting, kneeling or the left-lateral position all probably increase the dimensions of the pelvis. The supine position is avoided: the gravid uterus compresses the main blood vessels, reducing cardiac output and causing hypotension, and often fetal distress. This is called aortocaval compression (Fig. 29.2). In the supine position this is prevented by maintaining at least 15° of left lateral tilt.

Hydration: Women should be encouraged to drink isotonic drinks or water. Intravenous fluid may be necessary if labour is prolonged.

Stomach and food: Eating is appropriate during labour, although only small amounts are usually eaten. In the unlikely event of a general anaesthetic being required, the stomach contents can be aspirated (Mendelson's syndrome), so eating is often discouraged if the labour is high risk, and ranitidine is often given to reduce the stomach acidity.

Pyrexia in labour: This is best defined as >37.5 °C. This is associated with an increased risk of neonatal illness and is not always a result of chorioamnionitis. It is more common with epidural analgesia and prolonged labour. Cultures of the vagina, urine and blood are taken. Paracetamol is administered; intravenous antibiotics and cardiotocography (CTG) monitoring are warranted if the fever reaches 38 °C.

The urinary tract: Neglected retention of urine can irreversibly damage the detrusor muscle. An epidural usually removes bladder sensation. The woman must be encouraged to micturate frequently in labour; if she has an epidural, catheterization may be needed, but routine catheterization is unnecessary.

Obstetrics & Gynaecology, Fifth Edition. Lawrence Impey, Tim Child.
© 2017 John Wiley & Sons, Ltd. Published 2017 by John Wiley & Sons, Ltd.

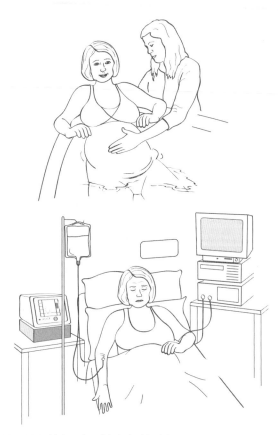

Fig. 29.1 Maternal anxiety is bad for labour.

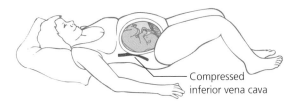

Fig. 29.2 Aortocaval compression. If the patient is allowed to lie flat on her back, the inferior vena cava is compressed.

Mental health in labour

The importance of psychological well-being in labour is crucial. The impact of this is seldom remembered but fear and anxiety cause adrenaline secretion and adrenaline slows labour.

Environment: This need not be too clinical. Resuscitation equipment can be hidden. Music and privacy may help. More women now choose to deliver at home, or in less clinical atmospheres such as birthing centres.

The birth attendant: The continuous presence of a 'caregiver' is reassuring (1:1 care). This reduces the length of labour, the use of analgesia and the need for augmentation and obstetric intervention. Continuous support, explanation and encouragement are needed.

The partner or accompanying person is an important potential source of support for the woman. He/she may need support too.

Control: Women have differing expectations of labour. Some want labour to be safe, quick and reasonably painless. Others have definite views, possibly because they view labour as a positive experience rather than a means to an end. They should be encouraged to write their views on a 'birth plan', which can be discussed so that expectations are realistic and the woman does not regard deviation from the plan as failure. Most requests in uncomplicated labour can then be safely accommodated, as most labours need little or no intervention.

Progress in labour: problems and their treatment

Monitoring progress: the partogram

Progress in labour is dependent on the powers, the passage and the passenger. A partogram (Fig. 29.3) is used to record progress in dilatation of the cervix and descent of the head. This is assessed on vaginal examination and plotted against time. After the latent phase (i.e. at about 4 cm dilated), the usual minimum rate of dilatation is 1 cm/hour: 'alert' and 'action' lines on the partogram indicate slow progress. Debate remains as to exactly where they should be placed; NICE recommends that slow progress is diagnosed if there is <2 cm dilatation in 4 hours. This visual record therefore aids identification of abnormal progress and also forms a record of maternal vital signs, fetal heart rate (FHR), contraction frequency and liquor colour.

The powers

'Inefficient uterine action' is the most common cause of slow progress in labour. Classifications are meaningless. It is common in nulliparous women and in induced labour, but is rare in multiparous women. Continuous support during labour is associated with a

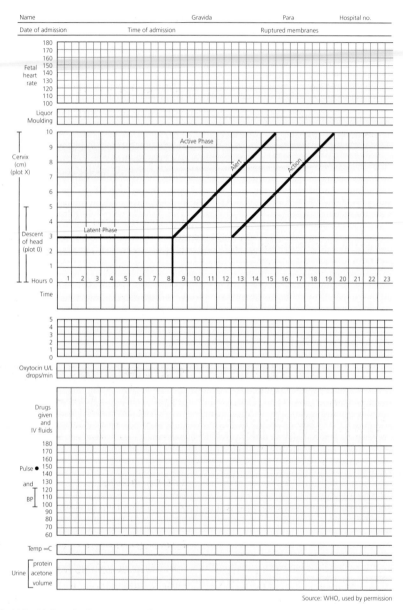

Fig. 29.3 Former World Health Organization partogram. Reproduced with permission of WHO.

reduction in the length of labour probably because it reduces anxiety. Mobility should also be encouraged. Persistently slow progress is treated by augmentation, initially with amniotomy (Fig. 29.4) and then oxytocin (Fig. 29.5). Although oxytocin reduces the duration of labour, it has not been shown to reduce the rate of caesarean section.

Hyperactive uterine action occurs with excessively strong or frequent or prolonged contractions. Fetal distress occurs as placental blood flow is diminished and labour may be very rapid. It is associated with placental abruption, with too much oxytocin, or as a side effect of prostaglandin administration to induce labour. Treatment depends on the cause: if there is no evidence of an

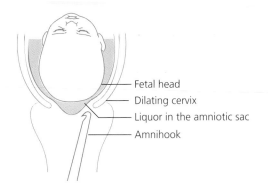

- Fetal head
- Dilating cervix
- Liquor in the amniotic sac
- Amnihook

Fig. 29.4 Amniotomy.

abruption, a tocolytic such as salbutamol can be given intravenously or subcutaneously, but caesarean section is often indicated because of fetal distress.

Nulliparous labour

The first stage: Slow progress in the nulliparous woman is usually due to inefficient uterine action, even if contractions are frequent or feel strong. Strengthening the powers artificially is called augmentation, and this can even sometimes correct passenger problems of attitude or position. This is performed by artificially rupturing the membranes (ARM or amniotomy); if this fails to further cervical dilatation in 2 hours, artificial oxytocin is administered intravenously as a dilute solution and the dose is gradually increased. Provided electronic fetal monitoring is used, this approach is safe because of the relative immunity of the nulliparous uterus to rupture.

Oxytocin will usually increase cervical dilatation within 4 hours if it is going to be effective. If full dilatation is not imminent within 12–16 hours, the diagnosis is reconsidered and caesarean section is performed: problems with the passage or passenger are more likely and the immunity of the uterus to rupture is diminished. *The passive second stage*: If descent is poor, an oxytocin infusion should be started; pushing is not encourage until the mother feels the urge. If an epidural has been used, the urge to push that is characteristic of the active second stage is diminished. *The active second stage*: Pushing need not be directed unless ineffective or an epidural is present. If the stage lasts longer than 1–2 hours, spontaneous delivery becomes less likely because of maternal exhaustion;

fetal hypoxia and maternal trauma are also more common. Traction is often applied to the fetal head with a ventouse or forceps.

Multiparous labour

The first stage: Slow progress in the multiparous woman is unusual. The multiparous uterus is seldom 'inefficient' and the pelvic capacity has been 'proven' in the previous labour unless delivery has previously been by caesarean section. The cause is therefore more likely to be the fetal head: its attitude or position, or because it is much bigger than before. Further, the multiparous uterus is more prone to rupture than the nulliparous uterus. Augmentation of labour with oxytocin must therefore be preceded by careful exclusion of a malpresentation.

The second stage: For the reasons described above, oxytocin should not be started for the first time, and instrumental delivery, although rarely needed, requires similar caution.

Augmentation and induction

Augmentation is the artificial strengthening of contractions in established labour
Induction is the artificial initiation of labour

The passenger

The fetus can contribute to poor progress in labour.

Occipito-posterior (OP) position

This common disorder of rotation is often combined with varying degrees of extension, and causes a larger diameter to negotiate the pelvic outlet. Labour is often longer and more painful, with backache and an early desire to push. The occiput is palpated posteriorly near the sacrum on vaginal examination (Fig. 29.6). If progress in labour is normal, no action is needed: many fetuses rotate to occipito-anterior (OA) spontaneously or deliver OP. If labour is slow, augmentation is used. If the position is persistent (5% of deliveries), delivery will be 'face to pubis' and completed by flexion rather than extension over the perineum. A few do not progress to full dilatation and caesarean section

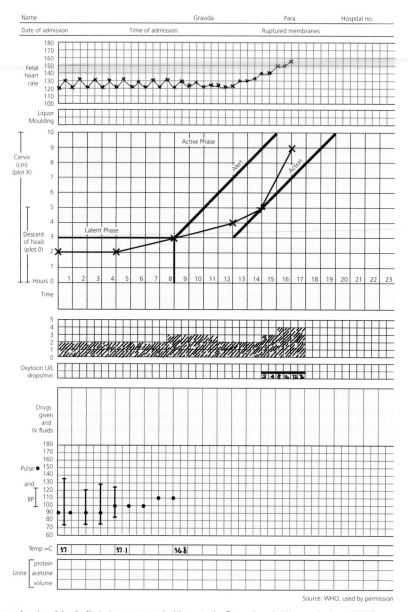

Fig. 29.5 A partogram showing delay in first stage managed with oxytocin. Reproduced with permission of WHO.

is required. If associated with a prolonged active second stage, instrumental delivery is usually achievable with rotation to OA position using a ventouse or with manual rotation. Kielland's forceps, requiring particular expertise, are associated with most success in these circumstances.

Occipito-transverse (OT) position

This occurs when normal rotation has been incomplete. The occiput lies on the left or the right, and this is palpated on vaginal examination (Fig. 29.7). This is the position in which the head normally enters the pelvis and is a normal finding in the first stage. Only if vaginal

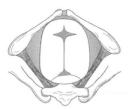

Fig. 29.6 The occipito-posterior (OP) position associated with extension of the head.

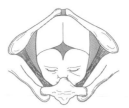

Fig. 29.8 Brow presentation.

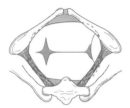

Fig. 29.7 The occipito-transverse (OT) position: delivery is impossible without rotation.

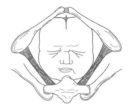

Fig. 29.9 Face presentation (chin is posterior).

delivery has not been achieved after 1 hour of pushing in second stage is the position significant. This is common and usually associated with poor 'powers', so rotation with traction is required for delivery to occur: this is usually achieved with the ventouse.

Brow presentation

This is rare, occurring in 1 in 1000 labours. Extension of the fetal head on the neck (see Fig. 28.5) results in a large (13 cm) presenting diameter that will not normally deliver vaginally (Fig. 29.8). The anterior fontanelle, supraorbital ridges and the nose are palpable vaginally. Caesarean section is required.

Face presentation

This is also rare, occurring in 1 in 400 labours. Complete extension of the head results in the face being the presenting part. Fetal compromise in labour is more common. The mouth, nose and eyes are palpable vaginally. The presenting diameter is 9.5 cm, allowing vaginal delivery in most cases so long as the chin is anterior (mento-anterior position): delivery is completed by flexion over the perineum. If the chin is posterior (mento-posterior position; Fig. 29.9), extension of the head over the perineum is impossible, as it is already maximally extended, and caesarean section is indicated.

Fetal abnormality

Rarely, abnormalities such as fetal hydrocephalus may obstruct delivery. Breech presentation and transverse or oblique lie in labour are discussed in Chapter 26.

Common causes of failure to progress in labour	
Powers	Inefficient uterine action
Passenger	Fetal size Disorder of rotation, e.g. occipito-transverse (OT), occipito-posterior (OP) Disorder of flexion, e.g. brow
Passage	Cephalo-pelvic disproportion Possible role of cervix

The passage

Cephalo-pelvic disproportion

This implies that the pelvis is simply too small to allow the head to pass through, but it can almost never be diagnosed with certainty. It depends on fetal as well as pelvic size: therefore, although commonly used to describe a person, it is applicable to a pregnancy. In the absence of a gross pelvic deformity, which is extremely rare in healthy women, it is a *retrospective* diagnosis best defined as the inability to deliver a particular fetus despite: (i) the presence of adequate uterine activity and (ii) the absence of a malposition or presentation. The word 'retrospective' means that it can normally only be diagnosed after labour has failed to progress and not with any accuracy before labour. Measuring the pelvis clinically or with X-rays or computed tomography (CT) scanning is unhelpful as the pelvis is not completely rigid and the scalp bones can overlap (see Fig. 28.7). Cephalo-pelvic disproportion is more likely with large babies, with very short women or where the head in a nulliparous woman remains high at term. Elective caesarean section is usually inappropriate in such women, but the term 'trial of labour' is sometimes thoughtlessly used.

Pelvic variants and deformities

Normal variants in pelvic shape have been extensively classified but this is virtually never useful in modern practice. The 'gynaecoid' or ideal pelvis is found in 50–80% of Caucasian women. The 'anthropoid' pelvis (20%) has a narrower inlet, with a transverse diameter often less than the antero-posterior (AP) diameter. The android pelvis (5%) has a heart-shaped inlet and a funnelling shape to the mid-pelvis. In the platypelloid pelvis (10%) the oval shape of the inlet persists within the mid-pelvis.
Abnormal pelvic architecture is usually confined to developing countries where health and nutrition are poor. Rickets and osteomalacia, poorly healed pelvic fractures, spinal abnormalities (such as major degrees of kyphosis or scoliosis), poliomyelitis and congenital malformations are very rare in the developed world.

Other pelvic abnormalities

Rarely, a pelvic mass such as an ovarian tumour or uterine fibroid blocks engagement and descent of the head. This will be palpable vaginally and caesarean section is indicated.

The cervix

The role of the cervix is to prevent the fetus from literally dropping out before term. During normal labour, it is not simply the strength of contractions that removes this natural obstruction but a complex mechanism involving hydration of the cervical collagen. The cervix itself, in addition to the contractions, may determine the course of labour, but the clinical relevance of this is poorly understood.

Care of the fetus

Permanent fetal damage attributable to labour is uncommon: only about 10% of cases of cerebral palsy are attributed solely to intrapartum problems. Nevertheless, fetal death or damage, usually neurological, has devastating effects. There are several causes of damage/

1 Fetal hypoxia, commonly described as 'distress', is the best known.
2 Infection/inflammation in labour, e.g. group B streptococcus.
3 Meconium aspiration leading to chemical pneumonitis.
4 Trauma is rarely spontaneous and more commonly due to obstetric intervention, e.g. forceps.
5 Fetal blood loss.

Fetal distress and hypoxia

Definition

The term 'fetal distress' is a clinical diagnosis made by indirect methods and is widely abused. It should be defined as *hypoxia that might result in fetal damage or death if not reversed or the fetus delivered urgently*. Delivery allows *ex utero* resuscitation. In reality, hypoxia is simply the best known cause of intrapartum fetal damage and its effects are unpredictable and vary considerably.

The convention is that a pH of <7.20 in the fetal scalp (capillary) blood (see below) indicates significant hypoxia. In reality, the mean cord arterial pH at birth is about 7.22, so a capillary pH of <7.20 will not be uncommon in labour, and conventional practice over-diagnoses fetal distress. Indeed, it is only below 7.00 that neurological damage is considerably more common. Even at this level, most babies have no sequelae; further, most babies with neurological damage actually had a normal pH at birth. This reflects the influences of other factors, antepartum, e.g. intrauterine growth restriction (IUGR) or intrapartum (e.g. maternal fever), on neonatal outcome.

Aetiology

Why hypoxia occurs is poorly understood. Contractions temporarily reduce placental perfusion and may compress the umbilical cord, so longer labours and those with excessive time (>1 hour) spent pushing are more likely to produce hypoxia. Acute hypoxia in labour can be due to placental abruption, hypertonic uterine states and the use of oxytocin, prolapse of the umbilical cord and maternal hypotension.

Epidemiology

Prediction of the 'at-risk' fetus is imprecise. Intrapartum risk factors include long labour, meconium, the use of epidurals and oxytocin; antepartum factors include pre-eclampsia and IUGR. Fetuses with these risk factors are usually monitored in labour with CTG.

Diagnosing fetal distress

As hypoxia is a relatively rare cause of handicap, the effects of attempts to prevent it will be limited. The diagnosis of fetal distress is usually made from the finding of significant fetal acidosis (scalp pH <7.20) or ominous FHR abnormalities. The following are methods employed in the detection of fetal distress.

Colour of the liquor: meconium
Meconium is the bowel contents of the fetus that stains the amniotic fluid. It is rare in preterm fetuses but common after 41 weeks. Meconium very diluted in amniotic fluid is seldom significant, but with undiluted meconium ('pea soup'), perinatal mortality is increased fourfold. Nevertheless, the presence or absence of meconium is not a reliable indicator of fetal well-being (*Obstet Gynecol* 2003; **102**: 89). It is an indication for caution (and hence closer surveillance with a CTG) because (i) the fetus may aspirate it, causing meconium aspiration syndrome, and (ii) hypoxia is more likely.

Fetal heart rate auscultation
The heart is auscultated every 15 minutes during the first stage, and every 5 minutes in the second, with a Pinard's stethoscope (Fig. 29.10) or a hand-held Doppler for 60 seconds after a contraction. The distressed or potentially distressed fetus normally exhibits abnormal heart rate patterns, which can be heard. This method of intrapartum fetal surveillance is considered appropriate for low-risk pregnancies, and if abnormalities are detected or risk factors develop, a CTG is indicated.

Cardiotocography
This records the FHR on paper and electronically, either from a transducer placed on the abdomen or from a

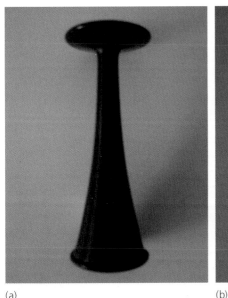

(a)

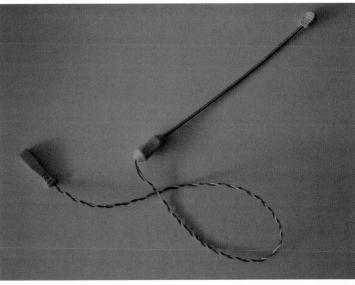

(b)

Fig. 29.10 (a) Pinard's stethoscope for intermittent auscultation in labour. (b) Fetal scalp electrode for electronic fetal monitoring in labour.

clip or probe in the vagina attached to the fetal scalp. Another transducer synchronously records the uterine contractions. Wireless technology allows maternal mobility. Interpretation is complex and difficult, requiring experience (see below) (Fig. 29.11).

Fetal electrocardiogram monitoring
Limited evidence suggests that if used in conjunction with a CTG, this improves neonatal outcomes whilst preventing some of the associated increase in operative delivery.

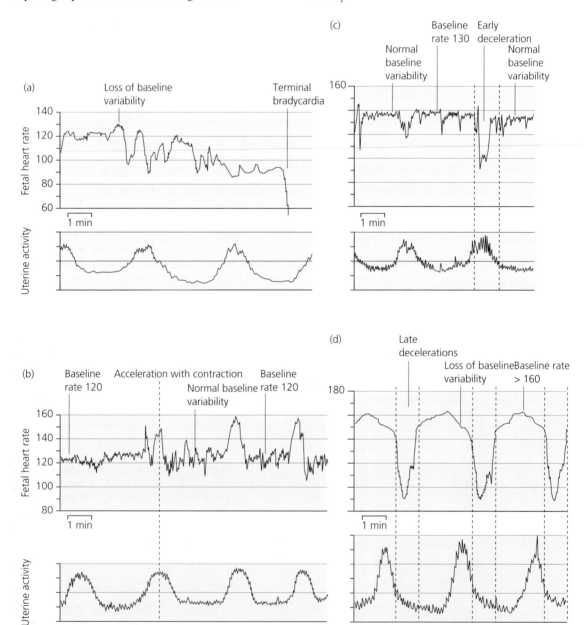

Fig. 29.11 (a) Acute fetal distress; the fetus is dying. (b) Normal cardiotocography (CTG); acceleration of the fetal heart with contractions. (c) Early decelerations are synchronous with a contraction. (d) Late decelerations, tachycardia, reduced variability suggestive of fetal distress.

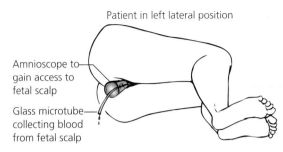

Fig. 29.12 Fetal blood sampling from scalp in labour.

Fetal blood (scalp) sampling (FBS)

A metal tube called an amnioscope is inserted vaginally through the cervix. The scalp is cleaned and a small cut is made, from which blood is collected in a microtube (Fig. 29.12). The pH ± lactate are immediately analysed. If the pH is <7.20, delivery, unless imminent, is expedited by the fastest route possible. As discussed above, because most acidotic babies have no problems, this conventional threshold for intervention leads to an overdiagnosis of fetal distress but less so than if CTG monitoring is used without it.

CTG monitoring for fetal distress

The CTG should be assessed in conjunction with the clinical situation, the contraction frequency, the level of risk (e.g. meconium, maternal fever or IUGR fetus) and the progress of the labour. A combination of abnormal patterns increases the likelihood of fetal distress. Risk management tools such as 'fresh eyes stickers', prompting regular assessments of the pattern by two people, may reduce errors. CTGs are classified as normal, non-reassuring or abnormal, according to four key features.

1 *Baseline rate*: this should be 110–160 beats/minute. *Tachycardias* are associated with fever, fetal infection and, if in conjunction with other abnormalities, fetal hypoxia. *A steep, sustained deterioration in rate* suggests acute fetal distress (see Fig. 29.11a).

2 *Baseline variability*: the short-term variation in FHR should be >5 beats/minute (see Fig. 29.11b), except during episodes of fetal sleep, which usually last less than 45 minutes. Prolonged reduced variability, particularly with other abnormal features, *suggests hypoxia* (see Fig. 29.11d).

3 *Accelerations* of the fetal heart with movements or contractions are reassuring (see Fig. 29.11b).

4 *Decelerations*:

- *Early decelerations* are synchronous with a contraction as a normal response to head compression and therefore are usually benign (see Fig. 29.11c).
- *Variable decelerations'* vary in timing and classically reflect cord compression, which can ultimately cause hypoxia.
- *Late decelerations* persist after the contraction is completed and are *suggestive* of fetal hypoxia (see Fig. 29.11d). The depth of the deceleration is usually unimportant.

A classification using these features has been developed by NICE (2015), although the 2015 FIGO classification (www.jsog.or.jp/international/pdf/CTG.pdf) is easier to use.

A normal CTG is reassuring, but the false-positive rate of abnormal patterns is high; confirmation of hypoxia should be made by fetal scalp pH sampling to avoid unnecessary intervention, except in acute situations (e.g. prolonged fetal bradycardia) or if access to the fetal scalp is not possible. The use of CTG is widespread; in high-risk situations, its use is logical but is poorly evaluated. In 'low-risk' labour, it does reduce the incidence of neonatal seizures but does not improve long-term neonatal outcome, whilst increasing the rates of caesarean section and other obstetric interventions. Despite these disadvantages, many of the problems with CTGs are associated with poor interpretation, inappropriate timing or a failure to use fetal blood sampling in conjunction. Regular training in CTG interpretation is necessary and now mandatory. However, computer-based interpretation systems have so far failed to help significantly and are not currently recommended by NICE.

Fetal distress: simplified scheme for screening and diagnosis
Level 1 — Intermittent auscultation of fetal heart. If abnormal, or meconium, or long, or high-risk labour, *proceed to*
Level 2 — Continuous cardiotocography (CTG). If sustained bradycardia >5 min, deliver. If abnormal on other criteria, simple measures to correct. If these fail, *proceed to*
Level 3 — Fetal blood sampling (FBS). If abnormal, *proceed to*
Level 4 — Delivery by quickest route

Indications for using a CTG

Prelabour risk factors include pre-eclampsia, IUGR, previous caesarean section, induction.

In labour risk factors include the presence of meconium, the use of oxytocin, the presence of a temperature >38 °C, during the administration of epidural analgesia. *IA abnormalities,* if detected, should prompt the use of a CTG.

The pros and cons of cardiotocography	
Advantages	Visual record that includes variability High sensitivity for fetal distress/hypoxia Reduction in short-term neurological morbidity
Disadvantages	Cumbersome; reduces maternal mobility Increased rate of obstetric intervention No proven reduction in mortality or long-term handicap More puerperal sepsis

Management of fetal distress

In utero resuscitation: Fetal distress is not always progressive and resuscitative measures are taken before FBS or delivery. The woman is placed in the left lateral position to avoid aortocaval compression; oxygen and intravenous fluid are administered. Any oxytocin infusion is stopped; contractions can also be stopped with beta-2 agonists such as terbutaline. A vaginal examination is also made to exclude cord prolapse or very rapid progress.

Confirmation of distress and delivery: If simple measures fail, FBS (see Fig. 29.12) is performed: delivery is expedited if the pH is <7.20. If the pH is >7.20 but the abnormal FHR pattern continues or deteriorates, a second sample will be needed in about 30 minutes. If scalp sampling is impossible or the fetal heart shows a sustained bradycardia, delivery is undertaken anyway.

Other causes of fetal damage and their treatment

Fetal infection and the inflammatory response

Severe fetal infection due to group B streptococcus affects about 1.7 per 1000 live births where strategies to prevent it are not used. Treatment encompasses screening for the organism and treatment of high-risk groups, which in labour comprise women with a maternal fever or prolonged rupture of the membranes.

There is increasing evidence that even a low-grade maternal fever is a strong risk factor for seizures, fetal death and cerebral palsy, even in the *absence* of evidence of infection. The combination of this with fetal hypoxia is particularly dangerous (*AJOG* 2008; **49**: e1–6). It is still unknown whether this is due to causes of the fever (in addition to infection) or to the fever itself (i.e. overheating), so that the therapeutic role for antibiotics or antipyretics is unknown. Nevertheless, this appears to be independent of fetal hypoxia and is probably much more important than is currently thought.

Meconium aspiration

Meconium is aspirated by the fetus into its lungs, where it causes a severe pneumonitis. This is more common in the presence of fetal hypoxia, but it can occur without it. Where the meconium is thick, amniofusion of saline into the uterus to dilute the meconium reduces the incidence of meconium aspiration (*Cochrane* 2000; CD00014). Maternal safety, however, remains unproven and this is seldom performed.

Fetal trauma

Fetal trauma may be iatrogenic, principally from instrumental vaginal delivery or breech delivery. Shoulder dystocia often results in trauma, but prediction and therefore prevention are imprecise.

Fetal blood loss

This is very rare and is due to vasa praevia (Fig. 29.13), feto-maternal haemorrhage or, on occasion, placental abruption.

Care of the mother

The need for continuous support in labour, usually from 'one-to-one' midwifery, cannot be overemphasized.

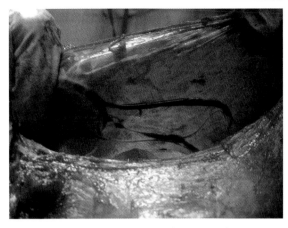

Fig 29.13 Fetal vessels in membranes in vasa praevia.

Pain relief in labour

Labour is normally extremely painful, but analgesia is a mother's choice: tolerance of pain and attitudes to childbirth differ widely. At opposite ends of a spectrum, some women prefer maximal analgesia while others prefer a more natural approach. There are also instances where analgesia, particularly epidural anaesthesia, is medically advisable. The methods employed can modify either pain or the emotional response to pain.

Non-medical

Preparation at antenatal classes, the presence of a birth attendant and the maintenance of mobility all help women cope with labour pain. Immersion in water at body temperature is effective and should be distinguished from water birth, where the baby is actually delivered under water. Other methods that have not been adequately scientifically validated but are helpful to some include transcutaneous electrical nerve stimulation (TENS), hypnotherapy, acupuncture, localized pressure on the back, the application of superficial heat or cold, massage and aromatherapy.

Inhalational agents

Entonox is an equal mix of nitrous oxide and oxygen. It has a rapid onset and is a mild analgesic. However, it is insufficient for all but the most 'motivated' mothers and can cause light-headedness, nausea and hyperventilation as women attempt to obtain the maximum effect.

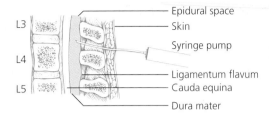

Fig. 29.14 Epidural analgesia; transverse section of the spinal column of L3–4.

Systemic opiates

Pethidine and Meptid (occasionally diamorphine) are widely used as intramuscular injections. However, the analgesic effect is small and many patients become sedated, confused or feel out of control. Antiemetics are usually needed. Opiates also cause respiratory depression in the newborn, which requires reversal with naloxone, and may reduce breastfeeding rates.

Epidural anaesthesia

This is the injection of a combination of an opiate (e.g. fentanyl) and local anaesthetic (e.g. bupivacaine or ropivacaine), delivered via an indwelling 'epidural catheter' into the epidural space, between the vertebrae L3–4 or L4–5. A loading dose is best followed by intermittent 'low-dose' top-ups which can be patient controlled (Fig. 29.14). The effect is variable, but in ideal circumstances pain sensation is abolished but motor blockade does not occur. It is suitable for the entire labour; in addition, a top-up of a higher dosage achieves enough anaesthesia for obstetric procedures.

Advantages

This is the only method in labour that can make women pain free, and is very popular. It can also be advised on purely medical grounds, if labour is long, to help reduce blood pressure in hypertensive women and to abolish a premature urge to push.

Disadvantages

The anaesthesia is occasionally ineffective or incomplete. Intravenous access is required. Transient hypotension is common after the loading dose. Mobility is usually reduced; indeed, pressure sores may occur without careful nursing. Reduced bladder sensation causes urinary retention. Maternal fever is more common. The caesarean section rate is not increased, although instrumental delivery is more common. Pushing may need to be 'directed' as sensation is reduced and the active second stage is usually delayed by an hour after full dilatation is diagnosed. Transient fetal bradycardias are also common, but seldom precipitate fetal distress.

Contraindications to epidural analgesia
Severe sepsis
Coagulopathy or anticoagulant therapy (unless low-dose heparin)
Active neurological disease
Some spinal abnormalities
Hypovolaemia

Major complications of technique

'Spinal tap' (0.5%) is inadvertent puncture of the dura mater causing leakage of cerebrospinal fluid (CSF) and often a severe headache. Characteristically, the pain is worse when sitting up and alleviated by lying down. It is treated with analgesics and, if persistent for >48 hours, with the administration of a 'blood patch' to seal the leak. *Very rarely*, inadvertent intravenous injection produces convulsions and cardiac arrest. Or inadvertent injection of local anaesthetic into the CSF combined with progression up the spinal cord causes 'total spinal analgesia' and respiratory paralysis.

Epidural analgesia is very safe in expert hands but needs increased midwifery care and modification of the second stage of labour.

Problems with epidurals
Spinal tap
Total spinal analgesia
Hypotension
Local anaesthetic toxicity
Higher instrumental delivery rate
Poor mobility
Urinary retention
Maternal fever

Anaesthesia for obstetric procedures

Spinal anaesthesia

Local anaethetic is injected as a 'single shot' through the dura mater into the CSF (Fig. 29.15). This rapidly

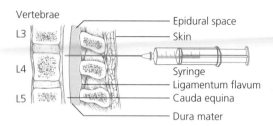

Fig. 29.15 Spinal analgesia, transverse section of the spinal column.

produces a short-lasting but effective total analgesia (and motor blockade) that is suitable for caesarean section or mid-cavity instrumental vaginal delivery. The principal complications are hypotension and, rarely, 'total spinal' analgesia causing respiratory paralysis.

Epidural anaesthesia

Higher dose epidural analgesia can be used for both instrumental delivery and caesarean section. For the latter, a combination of spinal and epidural anaesthesia (CSE) is best, allowing a rapid onset due to the spinal and longer lasting anaesthesia with the opportunity for top-ups, due to the epidural.

Pudendal nerve block

Local anaesthetic is injected bilaterally around the pudendal nerve where it passes by the ischial spine. This is suitable for low-cavity instrumental vaginal deliveries.

Conduct of labour

Initiation and diagnosis of labour

The woman is advised to contact her maternity services if contractions are regular, painful, lasting at least 30 seconds and occurring every 3–4 minutes, or if the membranes have ruptured. A brief history of the pregnancy and past obstetric history is taken, and temperature, blood pressure, pulse and urinalysis are recorded. The presentation is checked and a vaginal examination is performed to check for cervical effacement and dilatation to confirm the diagnosis of labour. The degree of descent is also assessed. The colour of any leaking liquor is noted. Every 15 minutes, the fetal heart is listened to for 1 minute following a contraction; if the pregnancy is high risk or meconium is seen or there is maternal fever, a CTG is started.

At this stage, account must be taken of the woman's wishes for labour, and the birth plan should be read. These wishes should be respected as far as possible and the care that she is given should be adjusted accordingly (see Different approaches to delivery). Described below is the basic care that should be given to all labouring women.

First stage of labour (Fig. 29.16)

The mother

The mother is made comfortable and encouraged to remain mobile. The supine position is avoided. Continuous support, attention and explanation are needed. Pain is better tolerated when progress is made. If analgesia is requested, nitrous oxide provides short-term relief but commonly an epidural is used. The vital signs and fluid balance are monitored; catheterization is often needed if an epidural is used, but should not be routine.

The fetus

The colour of the liquor is observed. The fetal heart is auscultated as above every 15 minutes or it is monitored with CTG if the pregnancy is 'high risk' or a heart rate abnormality is detected. If the heart rate pattern is abnormal, the fetus may be hypoxic. Intravenous fluid and the left lateral position (to avoid aortocaval compression) are used. Any oxytocin is usually stopped. If the abnormal heart rate pattern persists, a fetal scalp blood sample is taken. If there is fetal distress (i.e. scalp blood pH <7.20), expedition of delivery in the first stage can only be accomplished by caesarean section.

Progress

Progress is assessed, usually 4 hourly, by vaginal examination. Dilatation is estimated digitally in centimetres and descent of the head is measured by its relationship to the ischial spines; these measurements are recorded on the partogram (see Fig. 29.5). Slow dilatation after the latent phase can be treated with ARM (or amniotomy). If progress continues to be slow, oxytocin is used in a nulliparous woman; in a multiparous woman a malpresentation or malposition must be carefully excluded first. If the cervix is not fully dilated by 12–16 hours, caesarean delivery is usually appropriate unless delivery can be anticipated in the next hour or two.

Observations in labour		
	Mother	*Fetus*
First stage	Every 30 min: contraction frequency Every hour: pulse (+ check apparent FHR is not maternal HR) Every 4 hours: BP, temperature, vaginal examination	Every 15 min: FHR
Second stage	Every 15 min: pulse (+ check apparent FHR is not maternal HR)	Every contraction: FHR

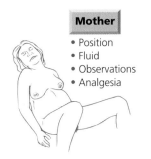
Mother
• Position
• Fluid
• Observations
• Analgesia

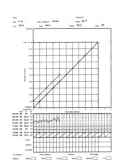
Fetus
• Intermittent auscultation or
• Cardiotocography
• Resuscitation +/– fetal blood sample if heart rate abnormal
• LSCS if fetal distress

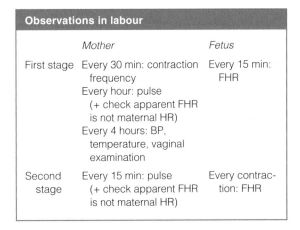

Progression
• Vaginal examination
• Augmentation with ARM +/– oxytocin if nulliparous and progress is slow
• LSCS if full dilation not imminent by 12 hours

Fig. 29.16 Management of first stage. ARM, artificial rupture of membranes; LSCS, lower segment caesarean section.

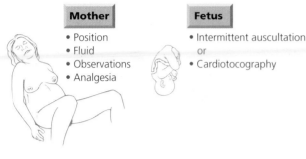

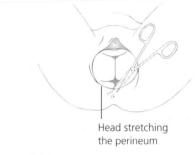

Fig. 29.17 Management of second stage.

Second stage of labour (Fig. 29.17)

If there is no epidural, 'non-directed' pushing is encouraged only when the mother has the desire to push or the head is visible. If an epidural is *in situ*, it is normal to wait at least an hour before pushing, and oxytocin is administered if the woman is nulliparous and descent is poor. If numb from an epidural, she is encouraged to push about three times for about 10 seconds during each contraction (directed pushing). During this time, considerable support and encouragement are required. Fetal distress is normally diagnosed in the same manner as for the first stage.

If delivery is not imminent after 2 hours of pushing (1 hour if multiparous), or there is fetal distress, expedition of delivery is usually recommended, with the ventouse or forceps. Careful assessment is required to ensure that all the prerequisites for these are met.

Normal delivery

As the head approaches the perineum, the attendant's hands are scrubbed and gloved. The mother should be positioned however she feels most comfortable, but *not* flat on her back. The routine use of an episiotomy has no benefit: episiotomy should be reserved for where there is fetal distress, where the head is not passing over the perineum despite maternal effort, or a large tear is likely. If it is performed, the perineum is infiltrated with local anaesthetic and a 3–5 cm cut is made with scissors from the centre of the fourchette at a 45° angle to the (mother's) right side of the perineum (Fig. 29.18).

Whilst the head progressively distends the perineum, the attendant waits with 'hands poised'. The mother is asked to stop pushing as the head starts to deliver and to

Head stretching
the perineum

Fig. 29.18 Episiotomy.

pant slowly; the attendant may press on the perineum and head ('hands on') to prevent a rapid delivery and perineal damage. The head then restitutes. With the next contraction, maternal pushing and gentle downward traction on the head lead to delivery of the anterior shoulder; traction is then directed upwards to deliver the posterior shoulder. Unless requiring resuscitation, the baby is delivered onto the mother's (preferably bare) chest and wrapped to keep warm; the umbilical cord should not be clamped for at least a minute unless resuscitation is urgently required (Fig. 29.19).

Third stage of labour (Fig. 29.20)

Oxytocin is administered intramuscularly to help the uterus contract once the shoulders are delivered (not until after the last fetus if it is a multiple pregnancy). A combination of ergometrine and oxytocin (Syntometrine) is often used but frequently leads to maternal vomiting. This 'active management' of the third stage can be unpopular, but reduces the incidence of postpartum haemorrhage and need for blood transfusion.

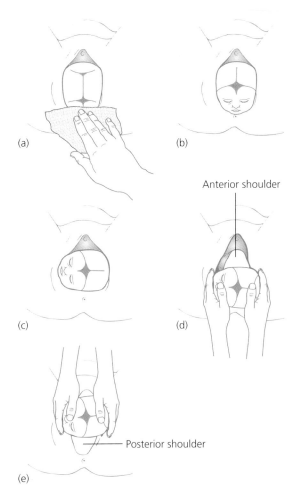

Fig. 29.19 Normal delivery. (a) 'Guarding' the perineum as the head distends it. (b) The head delivers. (c) The head restitutes. (d) The anterior shoulder is delivered by gentle downward traction until the next contraction. (e) The posterior shoulder is delivered by gentle upward traction.

Once placental separation is evident from lengthening of the cord and the passage of blood, continuous gentle traction on the cord allows delivery of the placenta (controlled cord traction). At the same time, the left hand pushes down suprapubically to prevent uterine inversion.

The placenta is checked for missing cotyledons and the vagina and perineum for tears. Once these are sutured, a swab and needle count is performed, blood loss is recorded, the mother is cleaned, made comfortable and encouraged to breastfeed. Maternal observation should continue for at least 2 hours.

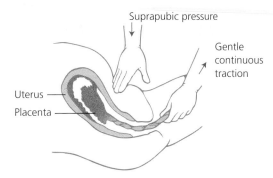

Fig. 29.20 Management of third stage. Delivery of the placenta.

Retained placenta

This is defined as a third stage longer than 30 minutes, and occurs after 2.5% of deliveries. Partial separation may provoke considerable blood loss into the uterus, causing it to enlarge and leading to hypovolaemia. In the absence of bleeding, an hour is usually left for natural separation, after which the placenta is 'manually removed'. A hand in the uterus, under general or spinal anaesthesia, gently separates the placenta from the uterus, with the second hand on the abdomen preventing the uterus from being pushed up. Blood is usually cross-matched and intravenous antibiotics are given.

Classification of perineal trauma	
First degree	Injury to skin only
Second degree	Involving perineal muscles but not anal sphincter
Episiotomy	Equivalent to second degree but may extend to third/fourth
Third degree	Involving anal sphincter complex 3a: <50% of external anal sphincter torn 3b: >50% of external anal sphincter torn 3c: internal anal sphincter also involved
Fourth degree	Involving anal sphincter and anal epithelium

Perineal repair (Fig. 29.21)

First- and second-degree tears and uncomplicated episiotomies without anal sphincter damage are sutured under local anaesthetic. Failure to suture reduces healing and may cause more pain. Absorbable synthetic material is used (e.g. Dexon or Vicryl): continuous

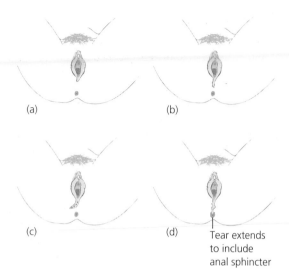

Fig. 29.21 Perineal trauma. (a) First-degree tear. (b) Second-degree tear. (c) Mediolateral episiotomy. (d) Third-degree tear.

Tear extends
to include
anal sphincter

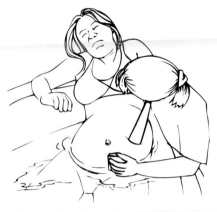

Fig. 29.22 Water birth.

rather than separate sutures for the muscle, and a sub-cuticular layer for the skin. A rectal and vaginal examination excludes sutures that are too deep and retained swabs, respectively.

Third- and fourth-degree tears occur in 1–3% of deliveries. Risk factors include forceps delivery, large babies, nulliparity and the (now obsolete) use of mid-line episiotomy. The sphincter is repaired under epidural or spinal anaesthetic with the visualization and asepsis afforded by an operating theatre. The torn ends of the external sphincter are mobilized and sutured, usually overlapping, with the internal sphincter sutured separately if damaged. Adequate repair requires experience. Antibiotics and laxatives are given, as well as analgesia. Physiotherapy assessment, sometimes with anal manometry, is usual. Long term, up to 30% of women have sequelae, usually incontinence of flatus or urgency, but occasionally frank incontinence.

Different approaches to delivery

Natural approaches to labour

Childbirth is a major life event. Whilst safety is the most important factor, it is usually taken for granted. The experience can be 'negative' for other reasons, particularly if the woman is immobile and attached to monitors or 'drips'. Whilst the safety of childbirth has increased, this cannot all be attributed to the increased

'medicalization' that has occurred in the last few years, much of which has been without scientific basis. There is increasing pressure among women to have more choice and participation in decisions about their labours: now that labour is safer, we should try to make it more rewarding.

Both *home birth* and birth in a *midwifery-led unit*, whether stand-alone or alongside an obstetric unit, are actively encouraged for appropriate low-risk women. The 'Birthplace study' (*BMJ* 2011; **343**: d740) demonstrated that in 'low-risk' multiparous women these options were as safe for the baby, that transfer to an obstetric unit was approximately 10% and that intervention including caesarean section was less. In low-risk nulliparous women, intervention was also considerably less, although fetal outcomes were slightly worse and transfer rates were 35–45%.

Water birth (Fig. 29.22): The labour and delivery are conducted in a large bath of water maintained at 37 °C. Water is relaxing and analgesic. The baby is delivered under water and does not breathe until brought rapidly to the surface. It is used for motivated low-risk women, provided that trained personnel are available. Despite its widespread usage, there is still incomplete evidence regarding the safety of this method.

Fast labour: 'active management'

Some women prefer labour to be quick and painless. For these, the early use of an epidural and 'active management of labour' (*BJOG* 1999; **106**: 183–187) may help. The principles apply to nulliparous women and are: (i) early diagnosis of labour; (ii) 2-hourly vaginal examinations; (iii) early correction of slow progress with amniotomy and oxytocin (augmentation); and (iv) caesarean section by 12 hours if delivery is not imminent. In addition, there is one-to-one midwifery care, a comprehensive antenatal education programme and continuous audit. This policy shortens labour and the 'latent phase' so long as it is only used once the cervix is fully effaced, but it does not reduce the rate of caesarean section. This policy has been widely vilified but with informed consent should remain open to women.

Avoiding labour: caesarean section for maternal request

For discussion see Chapter 31.

Criteria for home birth
Woman's request
'Low risk' on basis of antenatal or past obstetric and medical complications
37–41 weeks
Cephalic presentation
Clear liquor
Normal fetal heart rate
All maternal observations normal

Further reading

Birthplace in England Collaborative Group. Perinatal and maternal outcomes by planned place of birth for healthy women with low risk pregnancies: the Birthplace in England national prospective cohort study. *BMJ* 2011; **343**: d7400. Available at: www.bmj.com/content/343/bmj.d7400 (accessed 22 July 2016).

Hodnett ED, Gates S, Hofmeyr GJ, Sakala C, Weston J. Continuous support for women in childbirth. *Cochrane Database of Systematic Reviews* 2011; 2: CD003766.

National Institute for Health and Care Excellence. *Intrapartum Care. Care of Healthy Women and Their Babies During Childbirth.* Clinical Guideline No. 190. Available at: www.nice.org.uk/guidance/cg190/evidence/full-guideline-248734765 (accessed 22 July 2016).

Reuwer P, Bruinse H, Franx A. *Proactive Support of Labor: The Challenge of Normal Childbirth*, 2nd edn. Cambridge: Cambridge University Press, 2015.

Silva M, Halpern S. Epidural analgesia for labor: current techniques. *Local and Regional Anesthesia* 2010; **3**: 143–153.

Slow progress in labour at a glance

Definitions	'Slow labour' is progress slower than 0.5 cm/h after 4 cm (latent phase) 'Prolonged labour' is >12 h duration after latent phase	
Epidemiology	Common in nulliparous women; rare in multiparous	
Aetiology	Powers	Inefficient uterine action
	Passenger	Fetal size, disorder of rotation, e.g. occipito-transverse (OT), occipito-posterior (OP) Disorder of flexion, e.g. brow
	Passage	Cephalo-pelvic disproportion, rarely cervical resistance (if induction)
Management	General	Wait if natural labour wanted, mobilize, improve support
	Nulliparou	Amniotomy; oxytocin
	Multiparous	Amniotomy; oxytocin if malpresentation/malposition excluded
	If this fails	Caesarean section if first stage Instrumental delivery if second stage (if prerequisites met)

Occipito-posterior (OP) position at a glance

Definition	Abnormality of rotation, with face upwards. Some extension common
Epidemiology	5% of deliveries, more common in early labour
Aetiology	Idiopathic, inefficient uterine action, pelvic variants
Features	Slow labour. Back pain, early desire to push. Occiput posterior on vaginal examination
Management	Nil required if progress normal If slow progress, amniotomy and oxytocin (caution if multiparous) If these fail in first stage, caesarean section If second stage, >1–2 h of pushing, rotational instrumental delivery if criteria met

Fetal monitoring in labour at a glance

Modes of fetal injury	Hypoxia, meconium aspiration, trauma, infection/inflammation, blood loss
Fetal distress	Hypoxia that may result in fetal damage or death if not reversed or the fetus delivered urgently
High-risk situations	Fetal conditions, e.g. intrauterine growth restriction (IUGR), prolonged pregnancy Medical complications, e.g. diabetes and pre-eclampsia Intrapartum factors: long labours, presence of meconium, maternal fever
Monitoring methods	Intermittent auscultation (IA), inspection for meconium: If IA abnormal or high-risk situation: cardiotocography (CTG) 　Normal features: rate 110–160, accelerations, variability >5 beats/minute 　Abnormal features: tachy- or bradycardias, decelerations, reduced variability If CTG shows bradycardia: resuscitate, deliver if not improved If CTG shows other abnormality: resuscitate; fetal blood sample
Intervention	If fetal blood sample abnormal, delivery by quickest route: 　Caesarean section if first stage 　Instrumental vaginal delivery if second stage and criteria met

Pain relief in labour at a glance

Types	Non-medical	Support, water
	Medical	Entonox, opiates, epidural
Epidural	Injection of local anaesthetic into epidural space via indwelling catheter	
	Advantages	Best pain relief
	Disadvantages	Increased supervision, maternal fever, reduced mobility, increased instrumental delivery rate, hypotension, urinary retention
	Complications	Spinal tap, 'total spinal analgesia', local anaesthetic toxicity
	Contraindications	Severe sepsis, coagulopathy, active neurological disease, hypovolaemia, severe spinal abnormalities, severe cardiac outflow obstruction

CHAPTER 30

Labour 3: Special circumstances

Induction of labour

Labour that is started artificially is induced. It is different from augmentation, when the contractions of established labour are strengthened. Theoretically, induction is performed in situations where allowing the pregnancy to continue would expose the fetus and/or mother to risk greater than that of induction. In practice, there are many instances when labour is induced and quantification of risk is virtually impossible.

Methods of induction

Whether induction is successful partly depends on the state, or 'favourability', of the cervix. This is related to 'consistency', the degree of effacement or early dilatation, how low in the pelvis the head is (station) and the cervical position (anterior or posterior within the vagina). These are often scored out of 10, as the 'Bishop's score': the lower the score, the more unfavourable the cervix (Fig. 30.1). Transvaginal ultrasound assessment may also be used.

Induction with prostaglandins

Prostaglandin E_2 (PGE$_2$) as gel or a slow-release preparation is inserted into the posterior vaginal fornix. This is the best method in nulliparous women, and in most multiparous women unless the cervix is very favourable. It either starts labour or the 'ripeness' of the cervix is improved to allow amniotomy.

Induction with amniotomy ± oxytocin

The forewaters are ruptured with an instrument called an amnihook (artificial rupture of the membranes (ARM)). An oxytocin infusion is then usually started within 2 hours if labour has not ensued. Oxytocin is often used alone if spontaneous rupture of the membranes has already occurred, although prostaglandins are as effective.

Methods of induction		
Medical	Prostaglandins	
	Oxytocin (after amniotomy/membrane rupture)	
Surgical	Amniotomy	

Natural induction

Cervical sweeping involves passing a finger through the cervix and 'stripping' between the membranes and the lower segment of the uterus (Fig. 30.2). At 40 weeks, this reduces the chance of induction and postdates pregnancy. However, it can be uncomfortable.

Indications for induction

Fetal indications include high-risk situations such as prolonged pregnancy, suspected intrauterine growth restriction (IUGR) or compromise, antepartum haemorrhage, poor obstetric history and prelabour term rupture of the membranes.

Obstetrics & Gynaecology, Fifth Edition. Lawrence Impey, Tim Child.
© 2017 John Wiley & Sons, Ltd. Published 2017 by John Wiley & Sons, Ltd.

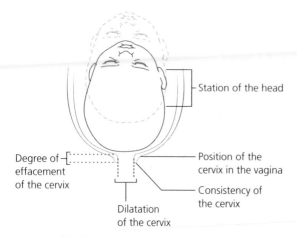

Fig. 30.1 The Bishop's score.

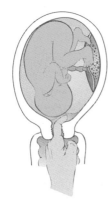

Fig. 30.2 Sweeping the membranes. A finger is inserted through the cervix and rotated: the membranes are peeled off the lower segment.

Materno-fetal indications, where both mother and fetus should benefit, include pre-eclampsia and maternal disease such as diabetes.

Maternal indications are social reasons and *in utero* death. In practice, the decision to induce, and the choice of method and timing, are dependent on each individual case.

Routine induction: There is a trend towards increased induction of labour, because of the probable reduction in rare, late-pregnancy complications, such as stillbirth, achieved by earlier delivery. Epidemiological data suggest that the lowest perinatal and infant mortality rate is achieved by delivery at 38 weeks. Such a policy should, however, be weighed against the large numbers of women needing to be induced to prevent one adverse outcome, the increased medicalization of labour and the possibly increased risk of adverse fetal outcome as a result of the induction process.

Common indications for induction
Prolonged pregnancy
Suspected growth restriction
Prelabour term rupture of the membranes
Pre-eclampsia
Medical disease: hypertension and diabetes

Contraindications

Absolute contraindications include acute fetal compromise (including an abnormal cardiotocograph (CTG)), abnormal lie, placenta praevia or pelvic obstruction such as a pelvic mass or pelvic deformity causing cephalopelvic disproportion. It is usually considered inappropriate after more than one caesarean section.

Relative contraindications include one previous caesarean section (increased scar rupture rate) and prematurity.

Management of induced labour

Because of both the indication for induction and the use of drugs, the fetus is at increased risk in labour. Cardiotocography should be used for an hour, 1 hour after the use of prostaglandins or when they stimulate uterine activity. Oxytocin is commonly required in labour, and also warrants CTG monitoring. Induction commonly increases the time spent in 'early labour', and the woman should be warned of this.

Complications

Labour may fail to start or be slow due to *inefficient uterine activity*. Paradoxically, overactivity of the uterus can occur. This *hyperstimulation* is rare but causes fetal distress and even uterine rupture. *Postpartum haemorrhage* (PPH) is more likely, as is *intrapartum and postpartum infection*. *Prematurity* can follow, by accident (incorrect gestation) or design. Although induced labour has a higher risk of *instrumental delivery* or *caesarean section* than does spontaneous labour, this does not mean that induction at a given term gestation necessarily increases an individual's risk when compared with expectant management (*BMJ* 2012; **344**: e2838).

Labour/vaginal birth after a previous caesarean section

Repeat, elective caesarean sections account for more than one-quarter of all caesarean sections performed, yet vaginal birth after caesarean (VBAC) can often be safely achieved.

Contraindications

These include the usual absolute indications for caesarean section, a vertical uterine scar, previous uterine rupture and multiple previous caesareans. After two caesareans, vaginal delivery is in practice very seldom attempted in the UK.

Factors influencing vaginal delivery after one caesarean section

Prediction of success: If a vaginal delivery is attempted, 72–75% of women will deliver vaginally; the others will require an emergency caesarean section in labour. Prediction of success is not reliable but factors associated with increased success include spontaneous labour, interpregnancy interval less than 2 years, low age and body mass index, Caucasian race, a previous vaginal delivery (chance of vaginal delivery 90%) and when the previous caesarean section had been performed electively (e.g. for breech presentation) or for fetal distress, as opposed to dystocia. Further, a smaller subsequent fetus and engagement of the head are good prognostic features.

Safety of vaginal delivery after caesarean section

No randomized controlled trials have been performed to compare VBAC with elective caesarean. Women should be fully apprised of the risk and benefits. Both maternal (placenta praevia, accreta, difficult surgery) and fetal risks (perinatal death) increase with increasing number of caesarean sections, and very few women with two or more previous caesareans attempt a vaginal birth. Therefore, planned family size should be an important factor to consider.

Maternal

This is related to the chance of vaginal delivery: vaginal delivery is safest, emergency caesarean least safe, with elective caesarean between. Therefore, when attempting

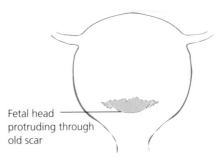

Fig. 30.3 Rupture of scar from previous caesarean section.

Fetal head protruding through old scar

a VBAC, maternal safety depends on the chance of such an emergency delivery. Overall, the risk of infection and blood transfusion is similar between a planned VBAC and planned caesarean, although the risk of maternal death is approximately doubled at 13/100 000. Planned caesarean increases risk in subsequent pregnancies.

Fetal

A small overall increased fetal risk with VBAC is mainly because caesarean section, performed at 39 weeks, eliminates the 0.1% risk of antepartum stillbirth beyond that time. The risk of labour itself is small: the usual, rare risks of labour, and rupture of the old uterine scar (Fig. 30.3). This occurs in 0.5% of VBAC attempts after one caesarean, and about 1.3% after two, but has at least a 10% perinatal mortality. These amount to a 0.04% risk of delivery-related death with planned VBAC. The risk is higher with an unsuccessful VBAC (i.e. emergency caesarean) and if prostaglandins or oxytocin are used, because of an up to 2% risk of uterine rupture. Nevertheless, the overall risk of mortality with VBAC is approximately the same risk as found in a first labour. In contrast, transient tachypnoea of the newborn (TTN) is more common (5%) where elective caesarean has been performed.

Risks of planned vaginal birth versus elective repeat lower segment caesarean section (LSCS)		
	VBAC	Repeat LSCS
Fetal		
Antepartum stillbirth >39 weeks	0.1%	0
Delivery-related death	0.04%	~0
Serious morbidity	0.1%	~0
Respiratory morbidity	2%	5%
Maternal		
Maternal death	4/100 000	13/100 000
Uterine rupture	0.5%	<0.1%
Blood transfusion	2%	1–2%

Management of labour after a caesarean section

Delivery in hospital and CTG monitoring are advised because of the risk of scar rupture. Induction is usually avoided as it is associated with a higher risk of rupture: caesarean is preferable unless the cervix is ripe or the fetal head is engaged. Augmentation also increases the risk of scar rupture and is performed with extreme caution. Epidural analgesia is safe, but labour should not be prolonged. Scar rupture usually presents as fetal distress, sometimes accompanied by scar pain, cessation of contractions, vaginal bleeding and even maternal collapse. Immediate laparotomy and caesarean are indicated if rupture is suspected.

Prelabour, term rupture of the membranes

In 10% of women after 37 weeks, the membranes rupture before the onset of labour; 60% will start to labour within 24 hours.

Diagnosis of prelabour term rupture of the membranes

Typically, there is a gush of clear fluid, which is followed by an uncontrollable intermittent trickle. This is occasionally initially confused with urinary incontinence. 'Point of care tests' such as Actim PROM, may help where the diagnosis is not clear. A few have only a 'hindwater' rupture: that is, liquor is definitely leaking but membranes remain present in front of the fetal head.

Risks of prelabour term rupture of the membranes

Cord prolapse is rare and usually a complication of transverse lie or breech presentation. There is a small but definite risk of neonatal infection; this is increased by vaginal examination (Fig. 30.4), the presence of group B streptococcus (GBS) and increased duration of membrane rupture.

Management

Confirmation is made by identification of liquor. The lie and presentation are checked. Digital vaginal

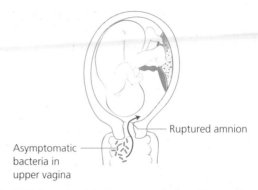

Fig. 30.4 Ascending infection can complicate prelabour rupture of the membranes.

examination is usually avoided, but may be performed in a sterile manner if there is a risk of cord prolapse (abnormal lie or fetal distress). Fetal auscultation or CTG is performed. Management options are to await the spontaneous onset of labour, or to induce labour. *Induction of labour* does not increase the risk of caesarean section, and is associated with a lower chance of maternal infection. It is also associated with a lower risk of the baby being admitted to the neonatal unit. This policy is therefore slightly safer, particularly if the mother is a GBS carrier.

Waiting for spontaneous labour up to 24 hours is common practice. Ideally, the maternal pulse, temperature and fetal heart rate are measured every 4 hours, although many women are not admitted. The presence of meconium or evidence of infection warrants immediate induction. After 18–24 hours, it is usual to prescribe antibiotics as a prophylaxis against GBS, and to induce labour.

Further reading

Dare MR, Middleton P, Crowther CA, Flenady VJ, Varatharaju B. Planned early birth versus expectant management (waiting) for prelabour rupture of membranes at term (37 weeks or more). *Cochrane Database of Systematic Reviews* 2006; **2**: CD005302. Available at: http://onlinelibrary.wiley.com/doi/10.1002/14651858. CD005302/pdf (accessed 22 July 2016).

National Institute for Health and Care Excellence. *Inducing Labour*. Clinical Guideline No. 70. Available at: www.nice.org.uk/guidance/cg70 (accessed 22 July 2016).

Royal College of Obstetricians and Gynaecologists. Birth after Previous Caesarean Birth. Green-top Guideline No. 45. Available at: www.rcog.org.uk/globalassets/documents/guidelines/gtg_45.pdf (accessed 22 July 2016).

Delivery after caesarean section at a glance

Incidence	Many (~50%) still undergo elective caesarean; usual practice if >1 prev lower segment caesarean section (LSCS)
Success	72–75% vaginal delivery rate if labour attempted
Contraindications	Vertical uterine scar; usual indications for caesarean
Safety	Maternal: related to chance of success Similar morbidity for vaginal delivery after caesarean (VBAC) or elective LSCS Mortality slightly higher with elective LSCS Fetal: threefold increase in risk with VBAC, but absolute risk of antepartum stillbirth 0.1% and delivery-related death 0.04%. Scar rupture rate 0.5%, higher if prostaglandins or oxytocin used Elective caesarean makes subsequent pregnancies higher risk for both
Management	Cardiotocography, careful monitoring of progress, rapid recognition and delivery if scar rupture

Induction of labour at a glance

Definition	Labour is started artificially	
Methods	Vaginal prostaglandin E_2, or amniotomy and oxytocin, or both	
Main indications	Fetal	Prolonged pregnancy, prelabour term spontaneous rupture of membranes, intrauterine growth restriction
	Materno-fetal	Pre-eclampsia, diabetes
Contraindications	Absolute	Acute fetal distress; where elective caesarean indicated
	Relative	Previous lower segment caesarean section
Complications	LSCS, other interventions in labour, longer labour, hyperstimulation, postpartum haemorrhage	

Prelabour term rupture of the membranes at a glance

Definition	Membranes rupture after 37 weeks before the onset of labour
Incidence	10%: 60% start labour in <24 h
Features	Gush of fluid
Investigations	Cardiotocography, point of care test
Management	Check for infection, lie/presentation. Avoid vaginal examination Consider immediate induction as risks lower, or wait Advise induction and antibiotics if >18–24 h duration

CHAPTER 31
Instrumental and operative delivery

Forceps or ventouse delivery

These allow the use of traction if delivery needs to be expedited in the second stage of labour. The shape of the pelvis will only allow delivery if the occiput is anterior, or occasionally posterior. Rotation is therefore sometimes also needed. In the absence of rotation, instrumental delivery simply adds power. No instrument can drag a fetus that is too large through the pelvis, and technique and judgement are required. The aim is to prevent fetal and maternal morbidity associated with a prolonged second stage or expedite delivery where the fetus is compromised.

A 'normal' vaginal delivery usually produces less blood loss, requires less analgesia and is safer and more pleasant for mother and baby unless a valid indication for intervention is present. In the UK, approximately 20% of nulliparous and 2% of multiparous women are delivered by forceps or ventouse.

Ventouse

Also known as the vacuum, this consists of a plastic, rubber or metal cap, connected to a handle; the cap is fixed near the fetal occiput by suction (Fig. 31.1). Traction during maternal pushing will deliver the occipito-anterior (OA) positioned head, but also often allows the shape of the pelvis to simultaneously rotate a malpositioned head to the OA position. The ventouse can be used for most instrumental deliveries.

Obstetric forceps

These come in pairs that fit together for use. Each has a 'blade', shank, lock and handle. When assembled, the blades fit around the fetal head and the handles fit together (Fig. 31.2). The lock prevents them from slipping apart. *Non-rotational forceps* (e.g. Simpson's, Neville–Barnes) grip the head in whatever position it is and allow traction. They are therefore only suitable when the occiput is anterior. These forceps have a 'cephalic' curve for the head and a 'pelvic curve' which follows the sacral curve. *Rotational forceps* (e.g. Kielland's) have no pelvic curve and enable a malpositioned head to be rotated by the operator to the OA position, before traction is applied.

Safety of ventouse and forceps

Failure: Both methods of delivery can fail: this is more common with the ventouse, particularly if the cup is placed inaccurately.

Maternal complications and the need for analgesia are greater with forceps, but use of either instrument can cause vaginal lacerations or third-degree tears and postpartum haemorrhage. Cervical and uterine tears are very rare.

Fetal complications are slightly worse with the ventouse. An unsightly 'chignon', a swelling of the area of scalp that was drawn into the cup by suction, is usual. It diminishes over a period of hours, but a mark may be visible for days. Scalp lacerations, cephalhaematomata

Obstetrics & Gynaecology, Fifth Edition. Lawrence Impey, Tim Child.
© 2017 John Wiley & Sons, Ltd. Published 2017 by John Wiley & Sons, Ltd.

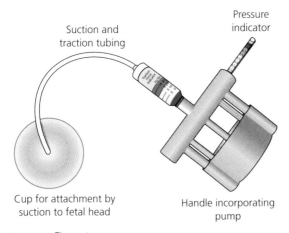

Fig. 31.1 The ventouse.

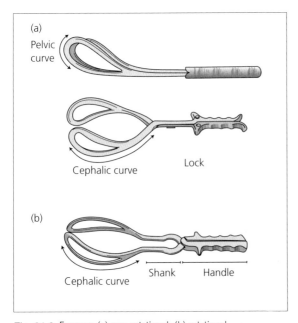

Fig. 31.2 Forceps: (a) non-rotational; (b) rotational.

and neonatal jaundice are more common with the ventouse. Facial bruising, facial nerve damage and even skull fractures occasionally occur with injudicious use of forceps, and prolonged traction by either instrument is dangerous.

Changing instrument: This is associated with increased fetal trauma, and is usually only appropriate, and only once, if a ventouse has achieved descent to the pelvic outlet, but then comes off the head and is replaced by a low-cavity forceps delivery (see below).

Indications for instrumental vaginal delivery

Prolonged second stage is the most common indication. Instrumental vaginal delivery is usual if 1–2 hours of pushing (active second stage) has failed to deliver the baby. If the mother is exhausted it may be performed earlier. The length of passive second stage is less important.

Fetal distress: This is more common in the second stage: delivery can be expedited.

Prophylactic use of instrumental vaginal delivery is indicated to prevent pushing in some women with medical problems such as severe cardiac disease or hypertension.

In a breech delivery, forceps are occasionally applied to the after-coming head.

Prevention of instrumental vaginal delivery

Whilst the ventouse and forceps have clear benefits, e.g. delayed second stage, avoidance of such circumstances is preferable.

All labours: Continuous support is essential (*Cochrane 2011*; CD003766), and delivery should be in the most comfortable maternal position possible. Epidural analgesia and cardiotocography (electronic fetal monitoring (EFM)) predispose to instrumental delivery.

Where epidural analgesia is used: In spite of its excellent analgesia and consequent popularity, epidural analgesia increases the risk of instrumental delivery. If used, maternal pushing should be delayed at least an hour after the diagnosis of second stage unless the head is low or the mother has the urge to push, oxytocin should be considered if descent of the head is poor (only in nulliparous women), and pushing should be directed.

Types of instrumental vaginal delivery

The type of delivery and choice of instrument are determined by the *position* and *descent* of the head. No instrument should be regarded as 'first choice' for all situations, but an overall comparison of forceps and ventouse is given below. With either instrument, if moderate traction does not produce immediate and progressive descent, caesarean section is indicated. 'High' forceps deliveries (the head is not engaged) are dangerous and obsolete. Caesarean section at full cervical dilatation is increasingly used but is often difficult surgically and is associated with increased maternal trauma and neonatal unit admission (*Lancet* 2001; **358**: 1203). Skill at instrumental delivery remains essential.

Low-cavity delivery

The head is well below the level of the ischial spines, bony prominences palpable vaginally on the lateral wall of the mid-pelvis, and is usually occipito-anterior (OA) (Fig. 31.3a). Forceps or a ventouse are appropriate (see box), the former being better if maternal effort is poor. A pudendal block with perineal infiltration is usually sufficient analgesia.

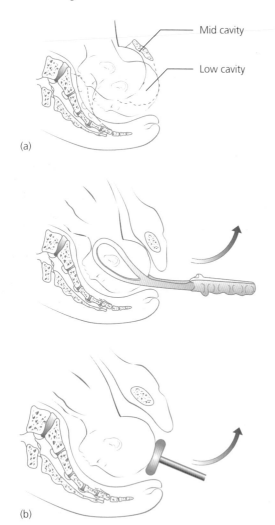

Mid cavity

Low cavity

(a)

(b)

Fig. 31.3 (a) Side view of pelvis showing level of head for mid-cavity and low-cavity forceps delivery. (b) Forceps and ventouse in position on the fetal head showing direction of traction.

Mid-cavity delivery

The head is engaged, but is at or just below the level of the ischial spines (see Fig. 31.3a). Epidural or spinal anaesthesia is usual. If there is any doubt that delivery will be successful, it is attempted in the operating theatre, with full preparations for a caesarean section. This is called a 'trial' of forceps or ventouse. The position may be OA, occipito-transverse (OT) or occipito-posterior (OP).

Occipito-anterior position: Forceps or a ventouse can be used.

Occipito-transverse position: Usually this is a result of insufficient descent of the head to make it rotate. Therefore, descent is achieved with the ventouse, with rotation resulting. Non-rotational forceps are contraindicated. Rotation *in situ* followed by descent can also usually be achieved by manual rotation or with Kielland's rotational forceps (see below).

Occipito-posterior position: This is often accompanied by extension of the fetal head, making the presenting diameter too large for the pelvis. One-fifth of the head may still be palpable abdominally. The need for instrumental delivery is unusual in multiparous women and if required, this position should be suspected. Simply dragging out a baby in this position may fail or cause severe perineal damage. Rotation of 180° can be achieved manually, or with the ventouse, but is most successful with Kielland's forceps. Some regard these forceps as dangerous, but in trained, skilled hands, they are extremely effective.

Common indications for ventouse or forceps delivery
Prolonged active second stage Maternal exhaustion Fetal distress in second stage

Prerequisites for instrumental vaginal delivery

Both forceps and the ventouse are potentially dangerous instruments and their use is subject to stringent conditions. *The head must not be palpable abdominally* (therefore deeply engaged); on vaginal examination the head must be *at or below the level of the ischial spines*. *The cervix must be fully dilated*: the second stage must have been reached (occasional exceptions are made by experts delivering with the ventouse for fetal distress). *The position of the head must be known*: incorrect placement of forceps or ventouse may cause fetal and maternal trauma as well as result in failure. There must be *adequate analgesia*. The *bladder should be empty*: catheterization is normally required. The operator must be skilled and delivering for a *valid reason*.

Failure of instrumental vaginal delivery

If one instrument fails to achieve any descent, the procedure should be abandonned and caesarean section performed. However, if descent has been achieved with the ventouse but the cup has come off, a gentle attempt at forceps is permitted. Prolonged traction and more than one change of instruments increase risks to the fetus and are not more appropriate.

Forceps or ventouse?

Ventouse causes:
Higher failure rate (but lower segment caesarean section [LSCS] not more common if forceps then used)
More fetal trauma
No difference in Apgar scores
Less maternal trauma

Prerequisites for instrumental delivery

Head not palpable abdominally
Head at/below ischial spines on vaginal examination
Cervix fully dilated
Position of head known
Adequate analgesia
Valid indication for delivery
Bladder empty

Caesarean section

Delivery by caesarean section occurs for about 25% of births in the developed world. The usual operation is the lower segment operation (LSCS), in which the abdominal wall is opened with a suprapubic transverse incision and the lower segment of the uterus is also incised transversely to deliver the baby (Fig. 31.4). Occasionally, such as with extreme prematurity, multiple fibroids or where the fetus is transverse, the uterus may be incised vertically: this is called a classical caesarean section. After delivery of the placenta, the uterus and abdomen are sutured.

Indications

Emergency caesarean section

This is usually performed in labour, but may also occur with acute antepartum problems, e.g. placental abruption.

Prolonged first stage of labour is diagnosed when full dilatation is not imminent by 12–16 hours, or earlier if labour was initially rapid. Occasionally, full dilatation is achieved but not all the criteria for instrumental delivery are met. Most commonly, it is due to abnormalities of the 'powers': inefficient uterine action. The 'passenger' (malposition or malpresentation) or 'passage' (pelvic abnormalities and cephalo-pelvic disproportion) can also contribute.

Fetal distress is diagnosed from abnormalities of the fetal heart rate, normally in conjunction with fetal

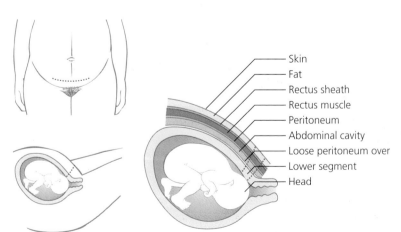

Skin
Fat
Rectus sheath
Rectus muscle
Peritoneum
Abdominal cavity
Loose peritoneum over
Lower segment
Head

Fig. 31.4 Layers of the abdominal wall for delivery of fetus by caesarean section.

blood sampling. A caesarean section is performed if it is the quickest route of delivery for the baby.

Elective caesarean section

This is performed to avoid labour. It is normally performed at 39 weeks' gestation as this reduces the risk of transient tachypnoea of the newborn from 6% at 38 weeks to 4%. If earlier, administration of steroids should be considered (*BMJ* 2005; **331**: 662).

Absolute indications are placenta praevia, severe antenatal fetal compromise, uncorrectable abnormal lie, previous vertical caesarean section and gross pelvic deformity.

Relative indications include breech presentation, severe intrauterine growth restriction (IUGR), twin pregnancy, diabetes mellitus and other medical diseases, previous caesarean section and older nulliparous patients.

When delivery is needed before 34 weeks, it is usual to perform a caesarean section rather than induce labour. The most common indications are severe pre-eclampsia and severe IUGR.

Elective caesarean for maternal request

This is becoming increasingly common. Reasons include fear of labour and a bad previous experience. In most cases, if the obstetrician understands and addresses the reasons for the request, both conflict and a caesarean section can be avoided. Caesarean section is commonly perceived to be the answer to many concerns, but in reality such problems and anxieties can usually be addressed within the context of a normal birth. In the UK, NICE currently advises: 'For women requesting a CS, if after discussion and offer of support (including perinatal mental health support for women with anxiety about childbirth), a vaginal birth is still not an acceptable option, offer a planned CS' (NICE 2011). This remains controversial.

Common indications for caesarean section	
Emergency	Failure to progress in labour
	Fetal distress
Elective	Previous caesarean section(s)
	Breech presentation

Definition of type/urgency of caesarean section	
Emergency	Immediate threat to mother or fetus, e.g. severe fetal distress
Urgent	Maternal/fetal compromise not immediately life-threatening, e.g. dystocia
Scheduled	Needing early delivery but no compromise
Elective	At time to suit mother and team
Peri-/postmortem	For fetus and mother during maternal arrest/for fetus after maternal death

Safety and complications of caesarean section

Maternal

Although serious complications are rare, these are greater than with a normal vaginal delivery. They are more common where the procedure is in labour than when it is elective. Complications may also be related to the indication for the caesarean. Complications include *haemorrhage* and the need for *blood transfusion, infection of the uterus or wound* (up to 20%), rare *visceral causes*, e.g. bladder or bowel damage, postoperative pain and immobility, and *venous thromboembolism*. Preoperative prophylactic antibiotics, which reduce the incidence of infection, and thromboprophylactic measures are routine. Overall, approximately 1 in 5000 women will die after a caesarean.

Fetal

By eliminating the risks of labour, a very small reduction in the risk of perinatal mortality can be anticipated, although this is controversial (*BMJ* 2007; **335**: 1025). An elective procedure increases the risk of *fetal respiratory morbidity* at any given gestation, and in an uncomplicated pregnancy is not recommended before 39 weeks. Although usually minor, this occurs in 2% even at this stage. *Fetal lacerations* are rare and usually minor. *Bonding and breastfeeding* are particularly affected by emergency procedures. Increasing evidence suggests an increase in atopic conditions, obesity and even diabetes in children born by caesarean section.

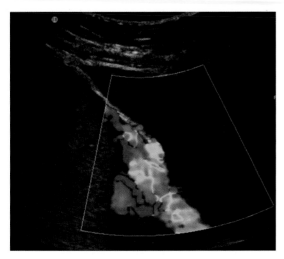

Abdominal wall
Bladder
Bladder and uterine walls
Placenta
Vascular area at placental interface with uterine wall and adjacent bladder wall

Fig. 31.5 Ultrasound of placenta accreta.

Subsequent pregnancies

Caesarean sections become increasingly difficult although in practice, of course, no 'limit' can be set. A small increase (approximately 1.5-fold) in stillbirth in subsequent pregnancies is likely (*BJOG* 2008; **115**: 726). Importantly, the incidence of placenta praevia is more common in pregnancies after a caesarean. Further, the placenta may implant more deeply than normal, in the myometrium (accreta) (Fig. 31.5) or through into surrounding structures (percreta). For a third caesarean section, the overall risk of placenta accreta is 0.57%, and 40% if the placenta is praevia (*Obstet Gynecol* 2006; **107**: 1226). This placental invasion is best diagnosed with 3-D power Doppler (see Fig. 24.3).

Surgery should be performed by an experienced team, with full anaesthetic back-up. Blood must be cross-matched. Facilities for internal iliac or uterine artery embolization are advised. The uterine incision should avoid the placenta, and hysterectomy is performed. Or the uterus and placenta can be left *in situ*, a policy sometimes necessary if there is invasion of the placenta into adjacent structures. In less severe cases, the affected segment of myometrium can be removed. Ultimately, delay in performing hysterectomy can be lethal. This problem is a good argument against the widespread use of caesarean section.

Caesarean section rates

Discussion of caesarean section rates is in Chapter 30.

Further reading

Murphy DJ. Failure to progress in the second stage of labour. *Current Opinions in Obstetrics and Gynecology* 2001; **13**: 557–561.

National Institute for Health and Care Excellence. Intrapartum Care. Care of Healthy Women and Their Babies During Childbirth. Clinical Guideline No. 190. Available at: www.nice.org.uk/guidance/cg190/evidence/full-guideline-248734765 (accessed 22 July 2016).

National Institute for Health and Care Excellence. *Caesarean Section*. Clinical Guideline No. 132. Available at: www.nice.org.uk/guidance/cg132/evidence/full-guideline-184810861 (accessed 22 July 2016).

Royal College of Obstetricians and Gynaecologists. Operative Vaginal Delivery. Green-top Guideline No. 26. Available at: www.rcog.org.uk/globalassets/documents/guidelines/gtg_26.pdf (accessed 22 July 2016).

Forceps and ventouse at a glance

Description	Ventouse attaches by suction, allowing traction with rotation Non-rotational forceps grip and allow traction Rotational forceps grip, allow rotation and then traction	
Rates	20%, nulliparous; 2%, multiparous	
Indications	Prolonged second stage, fetal distress in second stage, when maternal pushing contraindicated	
Prerequisites	Cervix fully dilated, position of head known, head deeply engaged and mid-cavity or below, adequate analgesia, empty bladder, valid indication	
Complications	Maternal trauma	Lacerations, haemorrhage, third-degree tears
	Fetal trauma	Lacerations, bruising, facial nerve injury, hypoxia if prolonged delivery

Caesarean section at a glance

Description	Lower segment (>99%); classical (vertical) rare	
Rates	20–30%	
Common indications	Elective	Breech presentation, previous lower segment caesarean section, placenta praevia
	Emergency	Failure to advance, fetal distress
Complications	Haemorrhage, uterine/wound sepsis, thromboembolism, anaesthetic, subsequent pregnancies	

CHAPTER 32
Obstetric emergencies

Shoulder dystocia

Definition and consequences

This is when additional manoeuvres are required after normal downward traction has failed to deliver the shoulders after the head has delivered. Occurring in approximately 1 in 200 deliveries, it requires urgent and skilled help. Delay in delivery combined with unskilled attempts at delivery may cause brain injury or death; excessive traction on the neck damages the brachial plexus, resulting in Erb's (waiter's tip) palsy, which is permanent in about 10% of cases (Fig. 32.1).

Risk factors and prevention

The principal risks are the large baby, but only about half of all cases occur in babies over 4 kg. Maternal diabetes at least doubles the risk at any given birthweight. Other antenatal risk factors include previous shoulder dystocia and obesity. Intrapartum risk factors are dystocia and instrumental delivery. Antenatal prediction is difficult and further limited by the poor predictive value of even ultrasound at predicting fetal weight. Many cases are therefore considered unpreventable. Nevertheless, in diabetics with a large baby, induction of labour may reduce the incidence, and above 4.5 kg caesarean should be considered.

Management

This requires rapid and skilled intervention: regular mannequin-based teaching and assessment of this is current practice. A calm sequence of actions is recommended. Because the obstruction is at the pelvic inlet, excessive traction is useless, and will cause Erb's palsy: gentle downward traction is used. Initially, senior and neonatal help is requested, and the legs are hyperextended onto the abdomen (McRoberts' manoeuvre); suprapubic pressure is also applied. These methods work in about 90% of cases. If they fail, internal manoeuvres are required, usually necessitating episiotomy to allow the hand to enter the vagina. The shoulders can be rotated, preferably by pressure behind the posterior shoulder to rotate it to the oblique or even 180° degrees (Wood's screw manoeuvre). Alternatively or in addition, the posterior arm is grasped and, by flexion at the elbow, the hand is brought down, narrowing the obstructed diameter by the width of the arm. Last resorts include symphysiotomy, after lateral replacement of the urethra with a metal catheter, and the Zavanelli manoeuvre. This involves replacement of the head and caesarean section, but by this time fetal damage is usually irreversible.

Cord prolapse

Definition and consequences

This occurs when, after the membranes have ruptured, the umbilical cord descends below the presenting part (Fig. 32.2). Untreated, the cord will be compressed or go into spasm and the baby will rapidly become hypoxic. It occurs in 1 in 500 deliveries. The diagnosis is usually made at vaginal examination after the identification of fetal distress.

Risk factors and prevention

Risks include preterm labour, breech presentation, polyhydramnios, abnormal lie and twin pregnancy. More than half occur at artificial amniotomy.

Obstetrics & Gynaecology, Fifth Edition. Lawrence Impey, Tim Child.
© 2017 John Wiley & Sons, Ltd. Published 2017 by John Wiley & Sons, Ltd.

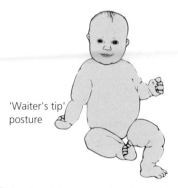

Fig. 32.1 Erb's palsy of right arm in characteristic 'waiter's tip' position.

'Waiter's tip' posture

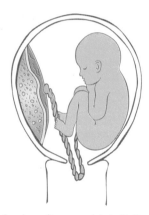

Fig. 32.2 Cord prolapse (here associated with flexed breech presentation).

Management

Initially, the presenting part must be prevented from compressing the cord. It is pushed up by the examining finger, or tocolytics such as terbutaline are given. If the cord is out of the introitus, it should be kept warm and moist but not forced back inside. The patient is asked to go on all fours, whilst preparations for delivery by the safest route are undertaken. Immediate caesarean section is normally used, but instrumental vaginal delivery is appropriate if the cervix is fully dilated and the head is low. With prompt treatment, fetal mortality is rare.

Amniotic fluid embolism

Definition and consequences

This is when liquor enters the maternal circulation, causing anaphylaxis with sudden dyspnoea, hypoxia and hypotension, often accompanied by seizures and cardiac arrest. Acute heart failure is evident. It is extremely rare but is an important cause of maternal mortality because many die: it accounted for 10 of 214 maternal deaths in the UK in the 3 years 2011–13 (MBRRACE-UK). If the woman survives for 30 minutes, she will rapidly develop disseminated intravascular coagulation (DIC), and often pulmonary oedema and adult respiratory distress syndrome (ARDS). In a few, haemorrhage from DIC is the first presentation.

Risk factors

It traditionally occurs when the membranes rupture, but may occur during labour, at caesarean section and even at termination of pregnancy. There are multiple mild predisposing factors and prevention is impossible.

Management

The diagnosis is easily confused with other causes of collapse, and with eclampsia, and is often only made with certainty at postmortem. Resuscitation and supportive treatment as for any cause of collapse are key. Blood for clotting, full blood count, electrolytes and cross-match are undertaken: treatment of massive obstetric haemorrhage (MOH) will be required.

Uterine rupture

Definition and consequences

The uterus can tear *de novo* (Fig. 32.3) or an old scar (e.g. from a caesarean section) can open. The fetus is extruded, the uterus contracts down and bleeds from the rupture site, causing acute fetal hypoxia and massive internal maternal haemorrhage. Rupture of a lower transverse caesarean scar is usually less serious than a primary rupture or one from a classic caesarean; the lower segment is not very vascular and heavy blood loss and extrusion of the fetus into the abdomen are less likely. Nevertheless, the neonatal mortality even from these is about 10%.

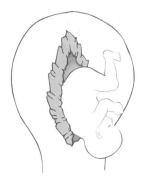

Fig. 32.3 Massive 'primary' rupture of the uterus with extrusion of the fetus.

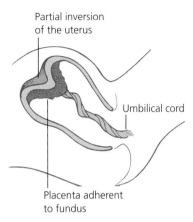

Fig. 32.4 Inverted uterus.

Rupture occurs in 1 in 1500 pregnancies, and in 0.5% of women who attempt a vaginal delivery after a single previous lower segment caesarean section (LSCS). The diagnosis is suspected from fetal heart rate abnormalities or a constant lower abdominal pain; vaginal bleeding, cessation of contractions and maternal collapse may also occur.

Risk factors and prevention

Principal risk factors include *labours with a scarred uterus*: a classic caesarean or deep myomectomy carries higher risks than that of previous LSCS. Rupture of a scarred uterus before labour is rare. *Neglected obstructed labour* is rare in the West but is a common obstetric emergency in developing countries. *Congenital uterine abnormalities* occasionally cause rupture before labour. Preventive measures include avoidance of induction and caution when using oxytocin in women with a previous caesarean section, and elective caesarean section in women with a uterine scar not in the lower segment.

Management

Maternal resuscitation with intravenous fluid and blood is required. Blood is taken for clotting, haemoglobin and cross-match, whilst arranging an immediate laparotomy. The fetus will very rapidly die if extruded from the uterus and blood loss may be faster than can be replaced. The uterus is repaired or removed. Uterine rupture has a high recurrence rate in subsequent pregnancies and early caesarean delivery is required.

Other obstetric emergencies

Uterine inversion

This is when the fundus inverts into the uterine cavity (Fig. 32.4). It usually follows traction on the placenta and occurs in 1 in 20 000 deliveries. Haemorrhage, pain and profound shock are normal. A brief attempt is immediately made to push the fundus up via the vagina. If impossible, a general anaesthetic is given and replacement performed with hydrostatic pressure of several litres of warm saline, which is run past a clenched fist at the introitus into the vagina.

Epileptiform seizures

These are most commonly the result of maternal epilepsy or eclampsia, but can also be due to hypoxia from any cause. The airway is cleared with suction and oxygen administered. Cardiopulmonary resuscitation may be required. The patient is not restrained but is prevented from hurting herself. In the absence of cardiopulmonary collapse, diazepam will normally stop the fit in the first instance. However, it is wise to assume eclampsia is responsible, until this is excluded by the absence of suggestive examination and laboratory findings. Magnesium sulphate is not useful for non-eclamptic seizures and is therefore inappropriate where the diagnosis is uncertain, but it is superior to diazepam in the eclamptic woman.

Local anaesthetic toxicity

Excessive doses or inadvertent intravenous doses of local anaesthetic can cause transient cardiac, respiratory and neurological consequences, occasionally resulting in cardiac arrest. Prevention is most important; treatment involves resuscitation and even intubation until the effects have worn off.

Massive antepartum haemorrhage

This is discussed in the management section. The key is to appreciate that blood loss may be internal, that replacement of normovolaemia and cessation of bleeding are required, and that, provided a coagulopathy (e.g. DIC) is treated, delivery of the fetus may save it and prevent further bleeding.

Massive postpartum haemorrhage

This is discussed on pp. 296–297 (and in the management section). The principles are the same. Surgical management is used only if medical management has failed, but procrastination is lethal.

Pulmonary embolus

This is discussed on p. 197 (and in the management section). Most occur postpartum and can present with cardiac arrest. Thromboprophylaxis is essential to prevent this leading direct cause of maternal death.

Further reading

Kaczmarczyk M, Sparén P, Terry P, Cnattingius S. *Risk factors for uterine rupture and neonatal consequences of uterine rupture: a population-based study of successive pregnancies in Sweden. BJOG* 2007; **114**: 1208–1214.

MBRRACE-UK. *Saving Lives, Improving Mothers' Care. Lessons learned to inform future maternity care from the UK and Ireland Confidential Enquiries into Maternal Deaths and Morbidity 2009–2012.* Available at: www.npeu.ox.ac.uk/downloads/files/mbrrace-uk/reports/Saving%20Lives%20Improving%20 Mothers%20Care%20report%202014%20Full.pdf (accessed 23 July 2016).

Moore L. *Amniotic Fluid Embolism.* Medscape. Available at: http://emedicine.medscape.com/article/ 253068-overview (accessed 23 July 2016).

Nahum G. *Uterine Rupture in Pregnancy.* Medscape. Available at: http://reference.medscape.com/article/275854-overview (accessed 23 July 2016).

Royal College of Obstetricians and Gynaecologists. *Shoulder Dystocia.* Green-top Guideline No. 42. Available at: www.rcog.org.uk/globalassets/ documents/guidelines/gtg42_25112013.pdf (accessed 23 July 2016).

CHAPTER 33
The puerperium

The puerperium is the 6-week period following delivery, when the body returns to its pre-pregnant state. Obstetric involvement is often lacking; midwives conduct most postpartum care. However, maternal morbidity and mortality associated with pregnancy are highest during this period. Many women continue to have problems after discharge, and the lack of medical interest means these problems often go untreated or even unrecognized.

Physiological changes in the puerperium

The genital tract

As soon as the placenta has separated, the uterus contracts and the criss-cross fibres of myometrium occlude the blood vessels that formerly supplied the placenta. Uterine size reduces over 6 weeks: within 10 days the uterus is no longer palpable abdominally (Fig. 33.1). Contractions or 'after-pains' may be felt for 4 days. The internal os of the cervix is closed by 3 days. Lochia, a discharge from the uterus, may be blood-stained for 4 weeks, but thereafter is yellow or white. Menstruation is usually delayed by lactation, but occurs at about 6 weeks if the woman is not lactating.

The cardiovascular system

Cardiac output and plasma volume decrease to pre-pregnant levels within a week. Loss of oedema can take up to 6 weeks. If transiently elevated, blood pressure is usually normal within 6 weeks.

The urinary tract

The physiological dilatation of pregnancy reduces over 3 months and glomerular filtration rate (GFR) decreases.

The blood

Urea and electrolyte levels return to normal because of the reduction in GFR. In the absence of haemorrhage, haemoglobin and haematocrit rise with haemoconcentration. The white blood count falls. Platelets and clotting factors rise, predisposing to thrombosis.

General postnatal care

The mother and baby should not be separated, and privacy is important. Early mobilization is encouraged. Counselling and practical help with breastfeeding are often required. Uterine involution and the lochia, blood pressure, temperature, pulse and any perineal wound are checked daily. Careful fluid balance checks should prevent retention if a woman has had an epidural. Analgesics may be required for perineal pain, which is also helped by pelvic floor exercises. The full blood count may be checked before discharge, and iron is prescribed if appropriate, usually in conjunction with laxatives.

Ideally, the midwife or doctor who attended the delivery should visit the patient after delivery. The circumstances of the delivery should be discussed, particularly if there has been obstetric intervention, and the woman given the opportunity to ask questions about her labour. Discharge should be dependent on the mother's wishes: some like to leave hospital within 6 hours of delivery; others will need a few days in hospital. The GP should be alerted to any complications. Advice regarding contraception is given prior to discharge.

Psychiatric disease and suicide are now recognized as major contributors to maternal death. Most women have a psychiatric history but this is often not recorded. Psychiatric referral is recommended for women with

Obstetrics & Gynaecology, Fifth Edition. Lawrence Impey, Tim Child.
© 2017 John Wiley & Sons, Ltd. Published 2017 by John Wiley & Sons, Ltd.

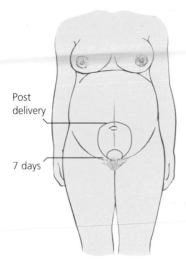

Post delivery

7 days

Fig. 33.1 Diagram of uterine involution.

such a history, and a postnatal plan including the GP is drawn up. Vigilance for evidence of depression is essential.

Lactation

Physiology

Lactation is dependent on prolactin and oxytocin. Prolactin from the anterior pituitary gland stimulates milk secretion. Levels of prolactin are high at birth, but it is the rapid decline in oestrogen and progesterone levels after birth that causes milk to be secreted, because prolactin is antagonized by oestrogen and progesterone. Oxytocin from the posterior pituitary stimulates ejection in response to nipple suckling, which also stimulates prolactin release and therefore more milk secretion. As much as 1000+ mL of milk per day can be produced, dependent on demand. Since oxytocin release is controlled via the hypothalamus, lactation can be inhibited by emotional or physical stress. Colostrum, a yellow fluid containing fat-laden cells, proteins (including immunoglobulin A) and minerals, is passed for the first 3 days, before the milk 'comes in'.

Management

Women should be gently encouraged to breastfeed, when the baby is ready. Early feeding should be on demand. Correct positioning of the baby is vital: the baby's lower lip should be planted below the nipple at the time that the mouth opens in preparation for receiving milk, so that the entire nipple is drawn into the mouth. This could largely prevent the main problems of insufficient milk, engorgement, mastitis and nipple trauma. A restful, comfortable environment is important, not least because oxytocin secretion, and therefore milk ejection, can be reduced by stress. Supplementation is unnecessary, although vitamin K, preferably intramuscularly, should be given to reduce the chances of haemorrhagic disease of the newborn.

Composition of human milk	
Protein	1.0%
Carbohydrate	7.0%
Fat	4.0%
Minerals	0.2%
Immunoglobulins	Mainly immunoglobulin A
Energy	70 kcal/100 mL

Advantages of breastfeeding
Protection against infection in neonate
Bonding
Protection against cancers (mother)
Cannot give too much
Cost saving

Postnatal contraception
Lactation not adequate alone, but important on global scale
Contraception is usually started 4–6 weeks after delivery
Combined contraceptive suppresses lactation and is contraindicated if breastfeeding
Progesterone-only (pill or depot) safe with breastfeeding
Intrauterine device (IUD) safe: screen for infection first. Insert at end of third stage or at 6 weeks

Primary postpartum haemorrhage

Definition and epidemiology

Primary postpartum haemorrhage (PPH) is the loss of >500 mL blood <24 hours of delivery (or >1000 mL after caesarean). It occurs in about 10% of women and remains a major cause of maternal mortality. *Massive*

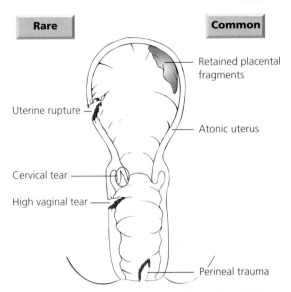

Rare **Common**

Retained placental fragments

Uterine rupture

Atonic uterus

Cervical tear

High vaginal tear

Perineal trauma

Fig. 33.2 Causes and sites of postpartum haemorrhage (PPH).

Risk factors for postpartum haemorrhage (PPH)
Antepartum haemorrhage
Previous history
Previous caesarean delivery
Coagulation defect or anticoagulant therapy
Instrumental or caesarean delivery
Retained placenta
Polyhydramnios and multiple pregnancy
Grand multiparity
Obesity
Prolonged and induced labour

obstetric haemorrhage (MOH) is best defined as blood loss of >1500 mL which is continuing.

Aetiology (Fig. 33.2)

Retained placenta occurs in 2.5% of deliveries. Partial separation can cause blood to accumulate in the uterus, which will rise. Collapse may occur in the absence of external loss.

Uterine causes account for 80%. The uterus fails to contract properly, either because it is 'atonic' or because there is a retained placenta, or part of the placenta. Atony is more common with prolonged labour, with grand multiparity and with overdistension of the uterus (polyhydramnios and multiple pregnancy) and fibroids.

Vaginal causes account for about 20%. Bleeding from a perineal tear or episiotomy is obvious, but a high vaginal tear must be considered, particularly after an instrumental vaginal delivery.

Cervical tears are rare, but associated with precipitate labour and instrumental delivery.

Coagulopathy is rare. Congenital disorders, anticoagulant therapy or disseminated intravascular coagulation (DIC) all cause PPH. If prescribed, antenatal thromboprophylaxis is best stopped at least 12 hours before labour or delivery, although it seldom causes haemorrhage.

Prevention

The routine use of oxytocin in the third stage of labour reduces the incidence of PPH by 60%. Oxytocin is as effective as ergometrine which often causes vomiting and is contraindicated in hypertensive women.

Clinical features

Blood loss should be minimal after delivery of the placenta. An enlarged uterus (above the level of the umbilicus) suggests a uterine cause. The vaginal walls and cervix are inspected for tears. Very occasionally, blood loss may be abdominal: there is collapse without overt bleeding.

Management

The priorities are support, restoration of blood volume, treatment of any developing coagulopathy and cessation of the blood loss. Where blood loss exceeds 1500 mL and is ongoing, a MOH protocol should be activated, with clear algorithms including the use of uncross-matched blood and anaesthetic, haematological and senior obstetric help. The management of massive obstetric haemorrhage is described in the Obstetric management section.

To resuscitate, the patient is nursed flat, oxygen is given, intravenous access is obtained and blood is crossmatched. Fluid ± blood is given.

To prevent/ treat coagulopathy: fresh frozen plasma (FFP) and cryoprecipitate may be required. Tranexamic acid also reduces bleeding.

A retained placenta should be removed manually if there is bleeding, or if it is not expelled by normal methods within 60 minutes of delivery.

To identify and treat the cause of bleeding, vaginal examination is performed to exclude the rare uterine inversion and the uterus is bimanually compressed. Vaginal lacerations are often palpable. Uterine causes are common and oxytocin and/or ergometrine is given intravenously to contract the uterus if trauma is not obvious. If this fails, an examination under anaesthetic (EUA) is performed: the cavity of the uterus is explored manually for retained placental fragments and the cervix and vagina inspected for tears, which should be sutured. If uterine atony persists, prostaglandin F_{2a} (PGF_{2a}) is injected into the myometrium.

Persistent haemorrhage despite medical treatment requires surgery. Bleeding from a placental bed (well-contracted uterus with no trauma) may respond to placement of a Rusch balloon. Other methods to treat haemorrhage include a brace suture (*BJOG* 1997; **104**: 372) and uterine artery embolization. If these fail, hysterectomy should not be delayed.

Other problems of the puerperium

Secondary PPH

Secondary PPH is 'excessive' blood loss occurring between 24 hours and 6 weeks after delivery. It is due to endometritis, with or without retained placental tissue, or, rarely, incidental gynaecological pathology or gestational trophoblastic disease. The uterus is enlarged and tender with an open internal cervical os.

Vaginal swabs and a full blood count are taken, and cross-match in severe cases. Ultrasound may help detect 'retained products' although differentiation between blood clot and retained placental tissue is poor. Antibiotics are given. If bleeding is heavy, evacuation of retained products of conception (ERPC) is used. If the bleeding is more chronic, antibiotics are used initially alone. Characteristically, endometritis due to retained tissue causes bleeding that slows, but does not stop, with antibiotics and gets worse again after the course is finished. Histological examination of the evacuated tissues will exclude gestational trophoblastic disease.

Postpartum pyrexia

This is a maternal fever of ≥38 °C in the first 14 days. *Infection* is the most common cause. Genital tract sepsis is a major cause of maternal mortality. It is most

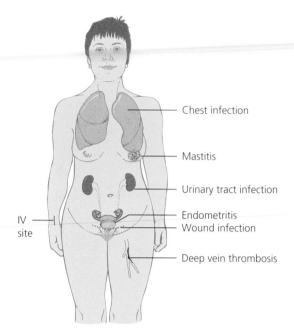

Fig. 33.3 Causes and sites of postpartum pyrexia.

common after caesarean section: prophylactic antibiotics considerably reduce this. Group A streptococcus, staphylococcus and *Escherichia coli* are the most important pathogens in severe cases. The lochia may be offensive and the uterus is enlarged and tender. Urinary infection (10%), chest infection, mastitis, perineal infection and wound infection after caesarean section are also common (Fig. 33.3). *Deep vein thrombosis* (DVT) often causes a low-grade pyrexia.

Postpartum sepsis is initially treated according to the 'Sepsis 6' principles: as soon as possible, blood cultures and venous lactate are taken and regular observations instigated; antibiotics, IV fluid (30 mL/kg), and oxygen area administered. Careful examination of the abdomen, breasts, any intravenous access sites, chest and legs is required. Urine, high vaginal and fetal cultures are also taken. Liaison with microbiology will ensure use of appropriate antibiotics.

Thromboembolic disease

Deep vein thrombosis or pulmonary embolism is a leading cause of maternal mortality, although less than 0.5% of women are affected. Half the deaths are postnatal, usually after discharge from hospital. Early mobility and hydration are important for all women. Risk factors, prevention and treatment are discussed elsewhere.

Psychiatric problems of the puerperium

'Third day blues', consisting of temporary emotional lability, affect 50% of women. Support and reassurance are required.

Postnatal depression affects 10% of women but most do not present and receive no help. Questionnaires such as the Edinburgh Postnatal Depression Scale (EPDS) are helpful in identifying this extremely important problem, but screening is difficult. Depression is more common in women who are socially or emotionally isolated, have a previous history, or after pregnancy complications. Postpartum thyroiditis should be considered. The severity is variable, but symptoms include tiredness, guilt and feelings of worthlessness. Treatment involves social support and psychotherapy. Antidepressants are used in conjunction with these. Postnatal depression frequently recurs in subsequent pregnancies and is associated (70% risk) with depression later in life.

Suicide is a major cause of death postpartum. Most women have a history of depressive or other psychiatric illness. This must be recorded at the booking visit. In general, psychiatric drugs should be continued in pregnancy, but this decision should be made, preferably preconceptually, after assessment of the risks and benefits. For depressive illness, selective serotonin reuptake inhibitors (SSRIs), such as fluoxetine, are preferred. Women with a history of mental illness should see a psychiatrist before delivery, and a multidisciplinary plan for postnatal discharge should be arranged. Urgent referral is indicated if there is a recent significant change in mental state or emergence of new symptoms, or new thoughts or acts of violent self-harm or new and persistent expressions of incompetency as a mother or estrangement from the infant.

Puerperal psychosis affects 0.2% of women and is characterized by abrupt onset of psychotic symptoms, usually around the fourth day. It is more common in primigravid women with a family history. Treatment involves psychiatric admission and major tranquillizers, after exclusion of organic illness. There is usually a full recovery, but some develop mental illness in later life and 10% relapse after a subsequent pregnancy.

Hypertensive complications

Pre-eclampsia and its complications are a major cause of maternal mortality and most deaths occur postpartum. Although delivery is the only cure for pre-eclampsia, it often takes at least 24 hours before the illness improves and the blood pressure, which usually peaks 4–5 days after delivery, may need treatment for weeks. In all pre-eclamptic patients, attention is paid to fluid balance, renal function and urine output, blood pressure and the possibility of hepatic or cardiac failure. Blood pressure measurement continues for 5 days postnatally.

The urinary tract (Fig. 33.4)

Retention of urine is common after delivery, and although it is usually painful it may not be so after epidural analgesia. It may present with frequency, stress incontinence or severe abdominal pain, but the woman or staff may not notice the lack of voiding. Infection, overflow incontinence and permanent voiding difficulties may follow. It can be identified by strict fluid charts and abdominal palpation. Postmicturition ultrasound can be used to assess the residual volume non-invasively. Treatment is with catheterization for at least 24 hours.

Urinary infection occurs in 10% of women. It is usually asymptomatic but, as in pregnancy, often leads to symptomatic infection or pyelonephritis. Routine urine culture is advised.

Incontinence occurs in 20% of women. Overflow and infection should be excluded using postmicturition ultrasound or catheterization and a mid-stream urine (MSU) sample respectively. Obstetric fistulae are very rare in developed countries. Symptoms of stress incontinence

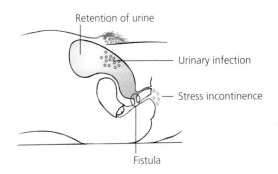

Fig. 33.4 Postpartum urinary problems.

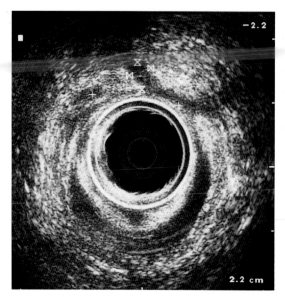
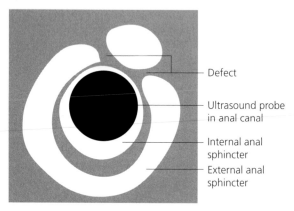

Defect

Ultrasound probe
in anal canal

Internal anal
sphincter

External anal
sphincter

Fig. 33.5 Ultrasound of disrupted anal sphincter.

usually improve, particularly with formal pelvic floor exercises, but these have little preventive role.

Perineal trauma

Perineal trauma is repaired after delivery of the placenta.

Pain persists for more than 8 weeks in 10%. Superficial dyspareunia is common. Pain is less when subcuticular Vicryl sutures have been used. Non-steroidal anti-inflammatory drugs are best; ultrasound, salt baths and Megapulse are of no benefit.

Paravaginal haematoma: Rarely, a woman experiences excruciating pain in the perineum a few hours after delivery. This is almost invariably due to a paravaginal haematoma, which is usually identifiable only on vaginal examination. This is drained under anaesthetic.

Bowel problems

Constipation and haemorrhoids both occur in 20% of women. Laxatives are helpful.

Incontinence of faeces or flatus is a distressing and under-reported symptom affecting 4% of women, mostly transiently. Both pudendal nerve and anal sphincter damage (Fig. 33.5) can be responsible and injury is often unrecognized. Forceps delivery, large babies, shoulder dysto-

cia and persistent occipito-posterior positions are the main risk factors. Affected women are evaluated using anal manometry and ultrasound, and managed according to symptoms. Formal repair may be required, after which deliveries should be by caesarean section.

Further reading

Fraser DM, Cullen L. Postnatal management and breastfeeding. *Current Obstetrics and Gynecology* 2006; **16L**: 65–71.

Jackson E, Curtis KM, Gaffield ME. Risk of venous thromboembolism during the postnatal period: a systematic review. *Obstetrics and Gynecology* 2011; **117**: 691–703.

National Institute for Health and Care Excellence. *Antenatal and Postnatal Mental Health*: *Clinical Management and Service Guidance*. Clinical Guideline No. 45. Available at: www.nice.org.uk/nicemedia/live/11004/30433/30433.pdf (accessed 25 July 2016).

Royal College of Obstetricians and Gynaecologists. *Prevention and Management of Postpartum Haemorrhage*. Green-top Guideline No. 52. Available at: www.rcog.org.uk/globalassets/documents/guidelines/gt52postpartumhaemorrhage0411.pdf (accessed 25 July 2016).

Primary postpartum haemorrhage (PPH) at a glance

Definitions	Primary	Blood loss >500 mL in first 24 h; >1000 mL if after caesarean section
	Secondary	'Excessive' blood loss between 24 h and 6 weeks

Epidemiology   10%; associated with caesarean, forceps, prolonged labour, grand multiparity, antepartum haemorrhage and previous history

Aetiology   Uterine atony, retained placental parts; vaginal, uterine or cervical lacerations

Features   Assess clinical state
Look for poorly contracted uterus, bleeding perineum, vaginal or cervical lacerations

Investigations   Full blood count, clotting, cross-match

Management   Principles are restore blood volume, treat coagulopathy, stop bleeding
Bimanual uterine compression; suture cervical or vaginal tears
Resuscitation with intravenous fluid, blood if necessary
Activate massive obstetric haemorrhage protocol if >1500 mL and continuing
Treat coagulopathy with fresh frozen plasma ± cryoprecipitate
Ergometrine/oxytocin ± prostaglandin F_{2a}; tranexamic acid
Consider Rusch balloon, laparotomy, brace suture, embolization if these fail

Other common serious problems of the puerperium at a glance

Secondary postpartum haemorrhage   Due to endometritis ± retained placental tissue. Give antibiotics, ± evacuation of retained products of conception if no improvement

Pyrexia   Endometritis, wound, perineal, urine, breast, chest infection, thromboembolism
Take: cultures including blood, venous lactate, do ongoing observations
Give: antibiotics, IV fluid, oxygen

Urinary incontinence   20%: exclude fistula and retention. Usually improves with time. Do urine culture and arrange physiotherapy

Urinary retention   Due to epidural or delivery, particularly forceps
CCatheterize for at least 24 h

Faecal incontinence   4%: exclude rectovaginal fistula. Can be due to anal sphincter or pudendal nerve damage; associated with third-degree tears and forceps. Treat with physiotherapy ± sphincter repair

Postnatal depression   10%: identification difficult and poor. Support, psychotherapy, drugs. Risk of suicide most with previous psychiatric illness. Urgent referral if 'red flag signs'

Thrombosis   0.5%: major cause of mortality. Prophylaxis if high risk according to formal risk assessment. Treat with subcutaneous low molecular weight heparin

CHAPTER 34
Birth statistics and audit

Audit

This is the process whereby clinical care is systematically and critically analysed. Comparing what *should be done* with what *is being done* allows changes to be made to what *will be done*. Practice can then be reanalysed, in a completion of the 'audit cycle'. The MBRRACE-UK audits of maternal deaths and perinatal mortality in the UK (www.npeu.ox.ac.uk/mbrrace-uk) is an example of audit in obstetrics. This report, with lay and professional expert input, analyses, criticizes and makes recommendations; reports of later years examine their impact. On a local level, maternal and perinatal mortality are rare, and examination of 'near-miss maternal mortality', perinatal morbidity and intervention in pregnancy and labour is also useful.

Perinatal mortality

Definitions and terms in the UK

- *Stillbirth* occurs when a fetus is delivered after 24 completed weeks' gestation showing no signs of life.
- *Neonatal death* is defined as death occurring within 28 days of delivery.
- *Early neonatal death* occurs within 7 days of delivery.
- *Miscarriage* occurs when a fetus is born with no signs of life before 24 weeks' gestation. However,if a fetus is delivered before 24 weeks, shows clear signs of life but subsequently dies, this is classified as a neonatal death.
- *The perinatal mortality rate* is the sum of stillbirths and early neonatal deaths per 1000 total births.
- *The 'corrected' perinatal mortality rate* excludes those stillbirths and early neonatal deaths that are due to congenital malformations.

Different countries have different definitions concerning gestation and/or birth weight, so comparisons can be misleading. In 1992, in line with improvements in neonatal care, the earliest gestation defined as a stillbirth changed from 28 to the current 24 weeks in the UK and may yet change to 23 weeks. The change of definition is reflected in Fig. 34.1.

Perinatal mortality rate

In developed countries the perinatal mortality rate has been declining since the 1930s. In the UK, it has declined from >50.0 to 7.5 per 1000 births in 2008 (data are collected separately in Scotland) (see Fig. 34.1). The stillbirth rate was 5.1 per 1000 births. The lowest rates are found in Scandinavian countries and the highest in Bangladesh and Central Africa.

Risk factors for perinatal mortality

Perinatal mortality is a reflection of obstetric care to only a limited extent and its decline has been more to do with better general health and nutrition, smaller families and improved neonatal care. The perinatal mortality rate is higher among lower socioeconomic groups, in those below 17 or above 40 years of age, in women who smoke, are obese, abuse drugs or have medical illnesses or poor nutrition. It is higher in highly parous women, in those of Asian or Afro-Caribbean extraction (approximately twofold) and in multiple pregnancies.

Causes of perinatal mortality

Causes of death are classified by the Extended Wigglesworth classification and supplemented by the Obstetric

Obstetrics & Gynaecology, Fifth Edition. Lawrence Impey, Tim Child.
© 2017 John Wiley & Sons, Ltd. Published 2017 by John Wiley & Sons, Ltd.

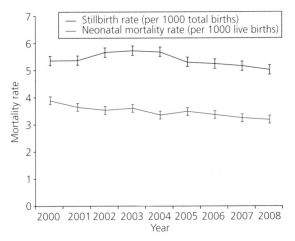

Fig. 34.1 UK stillbirths and neonatal mortality rates (2000–2008). Source: CMACE (2010).

- *Major congenital abnormalities* account for 10% of stillbirths and about 25% of neonatal mortality. Rates vary between regions and are dependent on detection rates and cultural attitudes to termination.
- *Pre-eclampsia* contributes in multiple ways, including preterm delivery and IUGR, but also at term.
- *Infection* contributes to mortality most via preterm birth, but infection may also occur in term labour. Fetal infections in pregnancy (see Chapter 19) are a rare cause of mortality.

Principal causes of perinatal mortality
Unexplained antepartum stillbirth
Intrauterine growth restriction (IUGR) and placental failure Prematurity
Congenital anomalies
Intrapartum hypoxia
Antepartum haemorrhage

Aberdeen classification system, with a new (2010) classification of IUGR defined as <10th centile of birth weight in comparison to what would be expected from constitutional factors such as fetal gender. Many causes overlap; for instance, antepartum haemorrhage is associated with chronic compromise, pre-eclampsia, preterm labour and intrapartum hypoxia. Perinatal mortality recording in the UK has become more sophisticated: rates for individual trusts, adjusted for casemix, are available (www.npeu.ox.ac.uk/mbrrace-uk). Because of separate reporting for stillbirth and neonatal mortality, of overlapping causes and of detailed classification, the list below is a simplification of the results.

- *Unknown*: this represents approximately 20% of perinatal mortality. New data suggest that mothers sleeping not in the left lateral (i.e. allowing aortocaval compression; see Fig. 29.2) may be contributory (*BMJ* 2011: **342**: 3403).
- *Preterm delivery* is the most common cause of neonatal mortality.
- *Intrauterine growth restriction (IUGR) and placental failure*: using current (above) criteria, this accounts for >50% of stillbirths.
- *Antepartum haemorrhage* occurs in at least 10% of deaths.
- *Intrapartum stillbirth* accounts for 9% of stillbirths, but >60% are preterm. Term intrapartum stillbirth is most commonly attributed to hypoxia, but infection and inflammation, trauma and fetal exsanguination can occur.

Maternal mortality

Definitions

A maternal death is the death of a woman during pregnancy, or within 42 days of its cessation, from any cause related to or aggravated by the pregnancy or its management, but not from accidental or incidental causes.

A late maternal death is when a woman dies from similar causes but more than 42 days and less than a year after cessation of the pregnancy.

These are subdivided into 'direct' deaths, which result from obstetric complications of the pregnancy, and 'indirect deaths', which result from previous or new disease, which was not the result of pregnancy but nevertheless aggravated by it.

Recent new classifications are 'coincidental maternal deaths', such as accidents or incidental death, which would have happened irrespective of the pregnancy, and 'pregnancy-related death', including all 'maternal deaths' plus coincidental deaths, and therefore irrespective of the cause of death.

Maternal death rate

In the UK, the maternal death rate (direct and indirect, 2011–13) was 9.02 per 100 000 pregnancies (MBRRACE-UK 2015) (Fig. 34.2). The rate in developed countries has fallen dramatically since the 1930s, when it was similar to that found at present in developing countries. Deaths in less developed countries are far higher: rates of about 500 per 100 000 pregnancies are found in parts of Africa. Improved case ascertainment in the UK makes comparison with other countries difficult.

Maternal mortality has been reported triennially in England and Wales for over 50 years (Fig 34.3). Over

the past 10 years, direct deaths have been consistently falling; indirect deaths have not. Nevertheless, the decline from 13.95/100 000 in 2003–5 has been in spite of immigration and higher numbers of older and obese women.

Factors affecting maternal death rates

Socioeconomic: The persisting high rates in developing countries reflect the contributory factors that have improved in developed countries. These factors include poor general nutrition and health, poverty, poor education and poor access to general and obstetric healthcare. In the UK, new immigrants, those with poor English, those of low socioeconomic class, admitting domestic abuse, from families known to child protection services, and abusing drugs are all over-represented among maternal deaths. The highest risk racial groups are African and Pakistani.

Obstetric: Extremes of maternal age, high parity, multiple pregnancy and multiple previous caesarean deliveries are all associated with increased mortality.

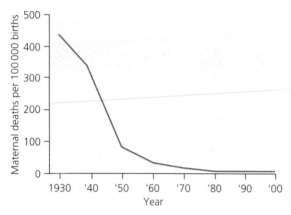

Fig. 34.2 Long-term changes in maternal mortality in the UK.

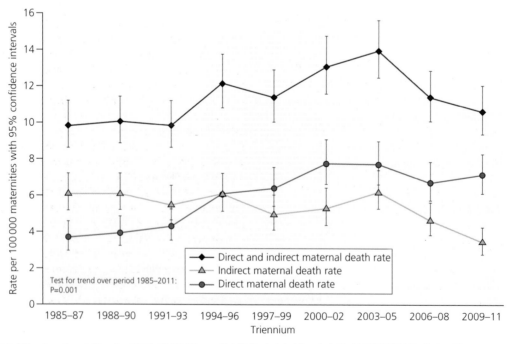

Fig. 34.3 UK maternal mortality rates (1985–2013). Source: Knight M *et al.* (eds) on behalf of MBRRACE-UK. *Saving Lives, Improving Mothers' Care – Surveillance of maternal deaths in the UK 2011–13 and lessons learned to inform maternity care from the UK and Ireland Confidential Enquiries into Maternal Deaths and Morbidity 2009–13.* © 2015 National Perinatal Epidemiology Unit, University of Oxford.

Pre-existing health: Obesity is a major risk, particularly for cardiac and thromboembolic disease; 30% of direct deaths occurred in women with a body mass index (BMI) >30. Cardiac disease remains the major indirect cause of death.

Level of care received: 'Substandard care' was present in more than half of all deaths.

Reporting methods: The UK system is extremely robust. Many other countries consider death certificate data alone, which leads to underascertainment of cases.

Causes of maternal mortality

Globally, the main causes of maternal mortality are haemorrhage, obstructed labour, infection, severe pre-eclampsia and the consequences of illegal abortion. The causes are slightly different in developed countries: those from the UK are described below.

Direct deaths

Venous thromboembolic disease is the most common cause of direct death, in spite of increased awareness and use of thromboprophylaxis. Deaths were from pulmonary embolism and cerebral venous thrombosis. Obesity is a particular risk factor, and weight-specific dosage is required.

Sepsis (genital tract) has become less most common, but community-acquired group A streptococcal sepsis was a major contributor in recent years.

Haemorrhage remains a common cause.

Amniotic fluid embolism is described in Chapter 32.

Hypertensive disease is becoming a rarer cause of maternal death.

Other causes include disorders of early pregnancy (mostly ectopic pregnancy), anaesthesia, acute fatty liver and genital tract trauma.

Indirect deaths

Cardiac disease includes acquired and congenital cardiac disease, the incidence of which is rising among pregnant women. The importance of cardiological input has been repeatedly emphasized.

Neurological disease such as epilepsy is the second most common indirect cause.

Sepsis (non-genital tract) such as pneumonia and influenza are major causes. In 2009–11, 1 in 11 maternal deaths were from influenza; this emphasizes the importance of vaccination.

Psychiatric disease is increasingly recognized, although most died after 42 days (i.e. late). Many were suicides, and although most had a psychiatric history, this was often not recorded or recognized.

Other indirect causes include drug/alcohol-related deaths, domestic violence, epilepsy and intracerebral haemorrhage.

Principal causes of maternal death
Thromboembolism
Hypertensive disorders
Cardiac disease
Ectopic pregnancy and abortion
Haemorrhage
Neurological disease
Psychiatric disease and suicide
Infection

Intervention in pregnancy and labour

The rate of obstetric intervention differs widely in different countries and hospitals or areas. Caesarean section is the most widely scrutinized, although induction rates, external cephalic version (ECV) rates and instrumental delivery rates should also be audited. The caesarean rate at different hospitals in the UK varies from 20% to >30%, and this cannot be entirely accounted for by population differences or 'casemix', be this medical or social differences. It is further dependent on the degree of supervision by, and interest from, senior staff and on institutional culture, midwifery skills and the percentage of home deliveries. A classification system called the Robson 'Ten Groups' examined 10 different groups of women, recording both the caesarean section rate in that group and the group's contribution to the overall caesarean section rate. This has been modified below (see box). It is clear that a previous caesarean section is a major indication for another, whilst other multiparous women have a very low risk; this emphasizes the importance of avoiding the first caesarean section. Likewise, the use of induction is associated with an increase in caesarean section (although care must be taken as it is usually 'higher risk' pregnancies that undergo induction). It is only by using such classifications that attempts can be made to alter practice.

Reasons why the caesarean rate is high

Attempted reduction of perinatal and maternal risks: Most breech babies and the majority of women with one previous caesarean section undergo caesarean section; these together account for the majority of elective caesarean sections (not in labour). Cardiotocography (CTG) in labour is widely used to try to avoid severe hypoxia, yet it is known to increase the risk of emergency caesarean section. Clearly, as severe adverse outcomes become rarer, the 'net' to prevent them is spread wider.

Clinical skill: This contributes in the management of labour and interpreting CTG, and skill at instrumental delivery or twin deliveries.

Fear of litigation: This is widely cited as contributory.

Maternal fear of labour: This contributes to prolonged labour though fear and anxiety, but also to maternal request for caesarean section. If a mother knows the chances of having a very long labour and *then* a caesarean section are high, it is not surprising if she requests an elective one.

A belief that caesarean section is the answer to most problems: Yet most adverse perinatal outcomes and maternal ones are not related to labour.

Classification of caesarean section		
*Indication**	*Approx. cs rate (%)*	*Approx. % of total cs (%)*
Previous caesarean section	70	20–25
Term breech presentation (if external cephalic version available)	95	15
Nulliparous: cephalic, spontaneous labour	10	10
Nulliparous: cephalic, induced labour	20–25	10–15
Elective term cs (not breech or previous cs)	(100)	5
All multiparous women, cephalic, in labour	2	5
Preterm babies	40	5–10
Multiple pregnancies	60	5–8
Pure 'maternal request'	(100)	<5
Other	–	<5

cs, caesarean section.
* Modified from Robson (2001).
† Individual units vary greatly.

Further reading

Centre for Maternal and Child Enquiries (CMACE). *Perinatal Mortality 2008: United Kingdom.* CMACE: London, 2010. Available at: http://www.publichealth.hscni.net/sites/default/files/Perinatal%20Mortality%202008.pdf (accessed 25 July 2016).

MBRRACE-UK. *Saving Lives, Improving Mothers' Care. Lessons learned to inform future maternity care from the UK and Ireland Confidential Enquiries into Maternal Deaths and Morbidity 2009–2012.* Available at: www.npeu.ox.ac.uk/downloads/files/mbrrace-uk/reports/Saving%20Lives%20Improving%20Mothers%20Care%20report%202014%20Full.pdf (accessed 25 July 2016).

MBRRACE-UK. *Perinatal Confidential Enquiry. Term, Singleton, Normally-Formed, Antepartum Stillbirth.* 2015. Available at: https://www.npeu.ox.ac.uk/downloads/files/mbrrace-uk/reports/MBRRACE-UK%20Perinatal%20Report%202015.pdf (accessed 25 July 2016).

MBRRACE-UK. *Perinatal Mortality Surveillance Report 2016: UK Perinatal Deaths for Births from January to December 2014.* Available at: www.npeu.ox.ac.uk/mbrrace-uk/reports (accessed 25 July 2016).

Robson MS. Can we reduce the Caesarean section rate? *Best Practice and Research. Clinical Obstetrics and Gynaecology* 2001; 15: 179–194.

Birth statistics at a glance

Stillbirth	Fetus born dead at 24+ weeks
Neonatal death	Neonate dies <28 days after delivery (early is <7 days)
Perinatal mortality	Stillbirths plus early neonatal deaths; if 'corrected' excludes congenital anomalies
Main causes	Unexplained antepartum, intrauterine growth restriction, preterm labour, congenital anomalies, antepartum haemorrhage, intrapartum hypoxia, pre-eclampsia
Rate	7–10 per 1000 (~1%) (UK)
Maternal mortality	Mother dies during or within 42 days of pregnancy from any cause related to (direct) or aggravated by (indirect) the pregnancy or its management, but not from accidental or incidental causes
Main causes	Direct: venous thromboembolism, sepsis, hypertensive disease, haemorrhage, amniotic fluid embolism, ectopic pregnancy
	Indirect: cardiac disease, neurological, sepsis (non-genital including influenza) and psychiatric disease
Rate	11.4 per 100000 (~0.01%) (UK)

CHAPTER 35

Legal (UK) and ethical issues in obstetrics and gynaecology

An awareness of the medical law is essential in all areas of medicine, particularly in obstetrics and gynaecology. Not only is medical litigation a particular problem in the specialty but there are statute laws, such as the Abortion Act, which regulate everyday practice.

Consent

Consent to procedures

The Mental Capacity Act 2005 provides clear legal guidance as to what constitutes valid consent. Firstly, a patient must have the *capacity* to consent; they lack *capacity* if they have a disturbance in their mind or brain such that they cannot understand or retain the relevant information or communicate their decision. The pain and distress caused by labour are not sufficient to find that a woman lacks capacity. Valid consent requires that it is given voluntarily and that prior to giving consent, the patient must be 'informed' of appropriate information regarding procedures or treatment. Secondly, the benefits, alternative options and risks should be discussed. Risks include those serious, even if very rare, and those frequently occurring. Possible additional treatments (e.g. blood transfusion) should be mentioned. Consent should be taken by someone familiar with the procedure and, preferably, the person performing it.

A recent case (*Montgomery vs Lanarkshire Health Board 2015*) highlighted a key area of consent law. The law now requires the doctor to take 'reasonable care to ensure that the patient is aware of any material risks involved in any recommended treatment, and of any reasonable alternative or variant treatments'. Essentially, risks of a procedure and of not doing a procedure should be discussed: only this allows fully 'informed' consent.

Refusal of medical treatment

Competent adults have the legal right to refuse medical treatment even where it is in their best interests. A number of these cases have been brought to the courts where a woman refuses to undergo a medically advised caesarean section. In UK law, the fetus *in utero* has no legal rights until the moment of birth. Therefore, even if this refusal results in injury or death to the fetus, the law should support a competent woman's right to refuse treatment.

Consent by children

Where children under the age of 16 request contraception or termination of pregnancy without their parents' knowledge, those with 'capacity' can consent to treatment. General Medical Council (GMC) guidance

Obstetrics & Gynaecology, Fifth Edition. Lawrence Impey, Tim Child.
© 2017 John Wiley & Sons, Ltd. Published 2017 by John Wiley & Sons, Ltd.

states that it is acceptable to provide these services providing the child understands the advice given and its implications and that in the case of requesting contraception, they are likely to have sexual intercourse in any event. The doctor must have tried to get the child to discuss this with a parent, be convinced that the child's physical or mental health is likely to be affected without the treatment and that it is in the child's best interests to have the treatment without parental knowledge (www.gmc-uk.org).

Clinical negligence

The vast majority of medical care is of high quality. However, patients rightly expect to receive competent medical care and if they are harmed as a result of it, the law entitles them to appropriate recompense. This is the basis of claims in negligence. For a claim of negligence to succeed, the claimant must show that:

1 the defendant (usually a hospital trust rather than an individual doctor) owed a duty of care to the claimant

2 the defendant breached that duty

3 this was on the balance of probabilities the cause of the harm (causation).

The standard of care required is governed by the *Bolam principle*: 'A doctor is not guilty of negligence if he or she has acted in accordance with the practice accepted as proper by a responsible body of medical men skilled in that particular art' (*Bolam vs Friern Hospital 1957*). This implies that imperfect medical care is not necessarily 'negligent'. However, it has been recently established (*Montgomery vs Lanarkshire Health Board 2015*) that the Bolam principle does not apply to issues of consent, as the extent to which a doctor may be inclined to discuss risks with patients is not determined by medical learning or experience.

Establishing causation is particularly difficult in obstetrics. When an infant is born in poor condition and subsequently develops cerebral palsy, it is labour, as the most recent and apparently dangerous event, that is frequently blamed. Furthermore, patients often perceive labour-related events to be preventable. Hypoxia in labour, however, probably accounts for only 10% of cases of cerebral palsy. Guidelines to help establish whether hypoxia in labour is to blame have been drawn up (*BMJ* 1999; **319**: 1054), although they bear little relationship to whether cases are settled (*BJOG* 2003; **110**: 6).

Negligence claims in the UK

Legal claims are funded in the UK by the Clinical Negligence Scheme for Trusts (CNST) insurance scheme. Hospitals pay insurance premiums to the National Health Service (NHS) Litigation Authority (www.nhsla .com), which is responsible for payments to claimants. There is a separate CNST 'standard' for obstetrics because it is a high-risk area of clinical practice. The insurance premium is dependent on claims history and the fulfilment of varied criteria, including risk management processes, minimum standards of clinical care, training guidelines and numbers of senior medical staff. Trusts can achieve three different standard 'levels' that influence the insurance premium they pay; these act as financial incentives to make changes considered beneficial to patient safety.

The CNST began in 1995 and the total value of reported CNST claims in the specialty by 2010 was £4.38 billion, twice that of claims in any other specialty. This reflects the damages in cerebral palsy cases, where the combined general and future damages for the long-term care needs of a child can be several million pounds. There is no evidence, however, that substandard practice is becoming more common. Today's patients are more informed, they expect more and they do not expect that pregnancy, as a normal life event, could go wrong. Funding options for litigation have also changed, with increased availability of legal expenses, insurance and claimants' solicitors offering conditional fee agreements.

Avoiding litigation

Besides ensuring you do your best medically, including referring to other more experienced colleagues if you are unsure, remembering the '4 Cs' will help prevent allegations of negligence (Fig. 35.1). *Consent* must be

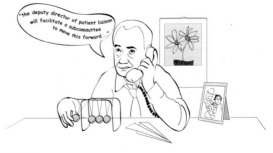

Fig. 35.1

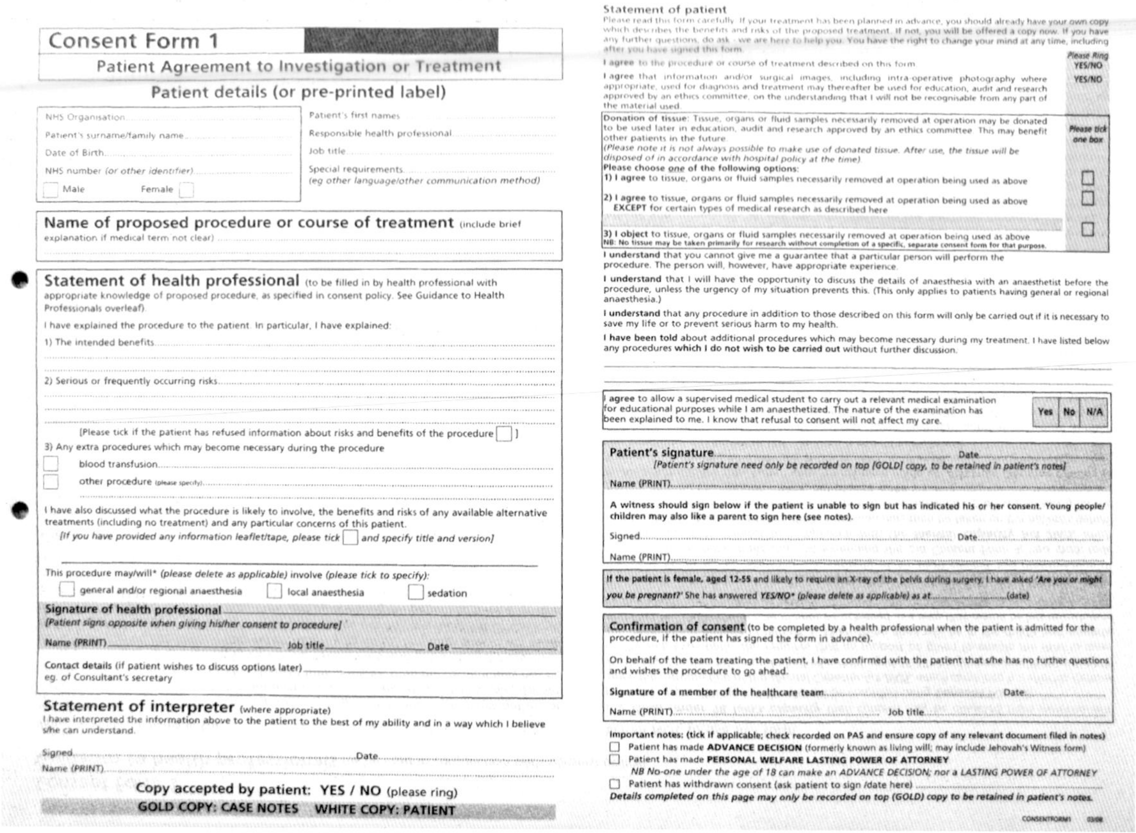

Consent Form 1

Patient Agreement to Investigation or Treatment

Patient details (or pre-printed label)

NHS Organisation

Patient's surname/family name

Date of Birth

NHS number *(or other identifier)*

Male Female

Patient's first names

Responsible health professional

Job title

Special requirements
(eg other language/other communication method)

Name of proposed procedure or course of treatment (include brief explanation if medical term not clear)

Statement of health professional (to be filled in by health professional with appropriate knowledge of proposed procedure, as specified in consent policy. See Guidance to Health Professionals overleaf).

I have explained the procedure to the patient. In particular, I have explained:

1) The intended benefits

2) Serious or frequently occurring risks

[Please tick if the patient has refused information about risks and benefits of the procedure]

3) Any extra procedures which may become necessary during the procedure

blood transfusion

other procedure (please specify)

I have also discussed what the procedure is likely to involve, the benefits and risks of any available alternative treatments (including no treatment) and any particular concerns of this patient.

[If you have provided any information leaflet/tape, please tick and specify title and version]

This procedure may/will* *(please delete as applicable)* involve *(please tick to specify)*:

general and/or regional anaesthesia local anaesthesia sedation

Signature of health professional

[Patient signs opposite when giving his/her consent to procedure]

Name (PRINT) Job title Date

Contact details (if patient wishes to discuss options later)
eg. of Consultant's secretary

Statement of interpreter (where appropriate)

I have interpreted the information above to the patient to the best of my ability and in a way which I believe s/he can understand.

Signed Date

Name (PRINT)

Copy accepted by patient: YES / NO (please ring)

GOLD COPY: CASE NOTES WHITE COPY: PATIENT

Statement of patient

Please read this form carefully. If your treatment has been planned in advance, you should already have your own copy which describes the benefits and risks of the proposed treatment. If not, you will be offered a copy now. If you have any further questions, do ask - we are here to help you. You have the right to change your mind at any time, including after you have signed this form.

Please Ring

I agree to the procedure or course of treatment described on this form. YES/NO

I agree that information and/or surgical images, including intra-operative photography where appropriate, used for diagnosis and treatment may thereafter be used for education, audit and research approved by an ethics committee, on the understanding that I will not be recognisable from any part of the material used. YES/NO

Donation of tissue: Tissue, organs or fluid samples necessarily removed at operation may be donated to be used later in education, audit and research approved by an ethics committee. This may benefit other patients in the future.
(Please note it is not always possible to make use of donated tissue. After use, the tissue will be disposed of in accordance with hospital policy at the time).

Please tick one box

Please choose one of the following options:

1) **I agree** to tissue, organs or fluid samples necessarily removed at operation being used as above

2) **I agree** to tissue, organs or fluid samples necessarily removed at operation being used as above **EXCEPT** for certain types of medical research as described here

3) **I object** to tissue, organs or fluid samples necessarily removed at operation being used as above

NB: No tissue may be taken primarily for research without completion of a specific, separate consent form for that purpose.

I understand that you cannot give me a guarantee that a particular person will perform the procedure. The person will, however, have appropriate experience.

I understand that I will have the opportunity to discuss the details of anaesthesia with an anaesthetist before the procedure, unless the urgency of my situation prevents this. (This only applies to patients having general or regional anaesthesia.)

I understand that any procedure in addition to those described on this form will only be carried out if it is necessary to save my life or to prevent serious harm to my health.

I have been told about additional procedures which may become necessary during my treatment. I have listed below any procedures **which I do not wish to be carried out** without further discussion.

I agree to allow a supervised medical student to carry out a relevant medical examination for educational purposes while I am anaesthetized. The nature of the examination has been explained to me. I know that refusal to consent will not affect my care. Yes No N/A

Patient's signature Date

[Patient's signature need only be recorded on top [GOLD] copy, to be retained in patient's notes]

Name (PRINT)

A witness should sign below if the patient is unable to sign but has indicated his or her consent. Young people/children may also like a parent to sign here (see notes).

Signed Date

Name (PRINT)

If the patient is female, aged 12-55 and likely to require an X-ray of the pelvis during surgery, I have asked ***'Are you or might you be pregnant?'*** She has answered *YES/NO* (please delete as applicable) as at* (date)

Confirmation of consent (to be completed by a health professional when the patient is admitted for the procedure, if the patient has signed the form in advance).

On behalf of the team treating the patient, I have confirmed with the patient that s/he has no further questions and wishes the procedure to go ahead.

Signature of a member of the healthcare team Date

Name (PRINT) Job title

Important notes: (tick if applicable; check recorded on PAS and ensure copy of any relevant document filed in notes)

Patient has made **ADVANCE DECISION** (formerly known as living will; may include Jehovah's Witness form)

Patient has made **PERSONAL WELFARE LASTING POWER OF ATTORNEY**

NB No-one under the age of 18 can make an ADVANCE DECISION; nor a LASTING POWER OF ATTORNEY

Patient has withdrawn consent (ask patient to sign /date here)

Details completed on this page may only be recorded on top (GOLD) copy to be retained in patient's notes.

CONSENTFORM1 03/08

Fig. 35.2 Consent form.

thorough and this, and any discussion with or examination of a patient, must be *clearly documented* (Fig. 35.2). Each entry in the notes must be legible, dated and signed, preferably with the doctor's name printed. *Communication* before and during treatment is essential, but even after an adverse event, an adequate explanation, with *candour*, may be all that patients require.

Clinical governance

The chief executive of a trust now carries responsibility for the quality of medical care. Every trust must have mechanisms to ensure the quality of care, identify faults and improve the service, and report annually on this. 'Clinical governance' has been developed, ostensibly to maximize safety, and is described as 'a framework through which NHS organizations are accountable for continuously improving the quality of their services and safeguarding high standards of care by creating an environment in which excellence in clinical care will flourish'. In English, this means 'do a good job and prove it'.

Clinical governance incorporates the implementation of evidence-based and 'effective' practice, and audit of this. Evidence-based guidelines for the management of common clinical situations exist, including from the National Institute for Health and Care Excellence (NICE: www.nice.org.uk), although these cannot cover the management of every clinical situation. It is easier to defend clinical practice if guidelines have been followed; equally, where a clear deviation has occurred, negligence is more likely to be alleged unless a clear reason for the deviation in practice is documented.

Risk management

Risk management aims to reduce risk of patient harm. Each NHS trust has an incident reporting system to report adverse incidents; these range from third-degree tears to maternal death. The organization is expected to review, learn and, if necessary, change clinical practice or systems to try to prevent these occurring again. Data on adverse outcomes for individual trusts are collected nationally (www.npeu.ox.ac.uk/downloads/files/mbrrace-uk/reports/MBRRACE-UK%20-%20 Perinatal%20Surveillance%20Report%202013%20-%20 Supplementary.pdf). In addition, the Care Quality Commission visits and assesses trusts, providing scores on aspects such as use of resources and 'quality of services'. The latter assesses a mass of criteria, including cleanliness, and is a poor measure of quality.

Complaints procedure

Successful local resolution of a complaint can reduce the likelihood of litigation, although a complaint may be a precursor to litigation. The NHS complaints procedure specifies time limits for the acknowledgement, investigation and resolution of a complaint (www.legislation.gov .uk/uksi/2009/309/contents/made). Independent advice and representation from the Independent Complaints Advocacy Service (ICAS) are available. If unsatisfied with the response, a seldom-used escalation is available. A complainant may also make a complaint about an individual to their regulatory body, e.g. the GMC.

Confidentiality

The doctor has a moral, professional, contractual and legal duty to maintain patient confidentiality. No details can be disclosed to a third party, including a relative, without the patient's consent. The Data Protection Act 1998 extends this duty to ensuring adequate protection and storage of information, such as patient records and communications. However, confidentiality can be breached in exceptional circumstances where the health and safety of others would otherwise be at serious risk. For example, if a doctor knew that their patient was at risk from an HIV-positive partner who refused to disclose their disease status, the law would support them in breaking this confidentiality.

Regulation of fertility treatment

Approximately 1 in 80 deliveries in the UK is a result of assisted reproduction. Regulation of fertility treatment and embryo research is stringent in the UK. Fertility clinics and centres performing assisted conception procedures and human embryo research must be licensed and inspected regularly. They must submit information, including success rates for their treatments, which is published. Key legal issues will be considered in this section.

Reducing multiple births

Currently, 1 in 5 *in vitro* fertilization (IVF) conceptions results in multiple pregnancy, known to have higher maternal and fetal complications. The law allows a maximum of two embryos to be replaced in a cycle unless a woman is aged 40 or over, when three embryos may be replaced. IVF clinics are now legally required to have a documented strategy to reduce the number of multiple births. In effect, this means each clinic must have set criteria which, if met, mean that women should be offered elective single embryo transfer.

Embryo testing

Preimplantation genetic diagnosis (PGD) is used in conjunction with IVF to select embryos. PGD is legal in order to establish whether an embryo has a genetic, chromosomal or mitochondrial disorder that may affect its capacity to result in a live birth. It may also be used to avoid the birth of a child who would develop a serious illness. Controversially, it is now legal to create a 'saviour sibling', a child who after birth will be able to donate HLA-matched cord blood for a sick sibling.

Embryo research

Human embryos can be used for research for no more than 14 days, or after the primitive streak has appeared, whichever is sooner. Research on embryos requires a specific licence for each project and each time patients must give written consent to their embryos being used.

Regulation of abortion

Almost 200 000 abortions are carried out in the UK each year. Although access to abortion is commonly perceived as 'on demand', the Abortion Act 1967 states that abortion is only legal if two doctors agree that a woman fits particular criteria. In practice, 90% abortions are carried at less than 13 weeks' gestation under the 'mental health' clause of the bill. Less than 1% of terminations are carried out because of the risk to the child of serious handicap and less than 0.1% of all abortions are carried out after 24 weeks' gestation. Every abortion must be notified to the Department of Health.

Some ethical issues in obstetrics and gynaecology

The spectrum of ethical debate in obstetrics, gynaecology and reproductive medicine is vast; a good start is *Medical Ethics and the Law* by Hope, Savulescu and Hendrick. In this section, a number of the most controversial topics are discussed, along with the basics of some well-established moral theories. The aim is to introduce a few of the difficult issues in this field of medicine.

Is there a right to have children?

Since the advent of IVF, it has become increasingly possible for people who cannot conceive naturally (for example, a postmenopausal woman or a same-sex couple) to have children. The UN Universal Declaration of Human Rights states that 'men and women of full age, without limits due to race, nationality or religion, have the right to found a family'. This right may be a *negative* right, a right not to be prevented from having a family. However, those who believe that the state must provide fertility treatment to all may argue that this is also a *positive* right, a right to be helped by others. The practical ethical question therefore is whether there is a duty to provide assistance for reproduction if needed.

Concern is often raised regarding the welfare of children born after assisted reproduction. In the UK, the law requires that clinics consider the welfare of any child born as a result of assisted reproduction, as well as the need for supportive parenting. However, if an embryo is created and replaced during an IVF cycle, that individual potential child could never have been born in other circumstances or to other parents. On one level, therefore, the 'welfare of the child' argument only holds weight if the life of the child would be so terrible that he or she would be better off never having existed.

Choosing embryos

Decisions about reproduction are particularly difficult in relation to inherited disease, such as those caused by single-gene disorders (e.g. cystic fibrosis). PGD allows choice, but many ethical questions arise from its use. Opponents regard it as a type of eugenics, a method of ridding the population of certain types of people. If PGD were compulsory to avoid particular diseases then this would be fair, but the reality is one of parents desperate to avoid suffering of their future children.

A common objection to the use of PGD to create a tissue-matched 'saviour sibling' is that the child created is used as a commodity. This goes against Immanuel Kant's famous view that people should never be used solely as a means but always be treated as an end in themselves. However, parents who choose PGD are undergoing costly and not necessarily successful IVF to have a tissue-matched child. They argue that the child created is wanted for the child it will be, not simply for the stem cells that may help their sibling. It is difficult to identify that harm is done to the potential child, its parents or society.

Abortion

The moral problem of abortion is one every student or doctor should consider. Ultimately, each individual must decide for themselves where the balance lies between the right of a woman to choose to end a pregnancy and the conflicting rights or interests of the fetus.

Fetal rights

Views on the moral status of the fetus are often polarized. The crucial question for many is when does an embryo or fetus become a 'person' with full moral status and rights? What defines personhood is also debatable but may include characteristics such as consciousness, self-awareness and rationality. The question as to when an embryo becomes a person has been answered in many different ways.

Many faith groups, such as the Catholic Church, argue that the potential to become a person should accord even the embryo full moral status. This view demands that in no circumstance (even pregnancy after rape) could the rights or interests of a woman over-ride the right of the fetus to life. Another view is that as the fetus develops, it has an increasing claim to life that requires ever stronger reasons to over-ride that claim. With this 'gradualist' view, it is felt that certainly in late pregnancy very strong reasons (e.g. major abnormality) are needed to terminate a pregnancy. UK law effectively follows this viewpoint. A more rigid view is that only those in possession of moral personhood can claim rights such as the right to life. This view means that at any gestation, the fetus does not have the traits to fulfil moral personhood, and thus abortion could be justified at any gestation. Critics of this suggest that this justifies not only abortion but also infanticide.

Maternal rights

Unless one believes that the fetus should be accorded full moral status, when abortion can never be justified, then the issue lies in the competing rights of the woman with those of the fetus. Autonomy is a key principle in medical ethics and most agree that individuals have the right to determine decisions about their own life. For many women, self-determination regarding when to have children or whether to choose to continue a pregnancy affected by a particular condition is an essential part of having autonomy.

Professionals' rights

For a healthcare professional, whether or not to participate in pregnancy termination is a personal decision. If urgent complications arise, however, there is a duty to treat the sick patient.

Further reading

Hope T, Savulescu J, Hendrick J. *Medical Ethics and the Law: The Core Curriculum*, 2nd edn. Edinburgh: Churchill Livingstone, 2008.
www.dh.gov.uk
www.nhsla.com
www.nice.org.uk
www.supremecourt.uk/decided-cases/docs/UKSC_2013_0136_Judgment.pdf

Gynaecology management

Management of bleeding or pain in early pregnancy

Fundamentals	Exclude ectopic pregnancy; ensure viability of intrauterine pregnancy

Causes	Ectopic pregnancy Miscarriage Molar pregnancy Gynaecological

Resuscitation	If collapse or heavy vaginal loss, intravenous (IV) access, give colloid and cross-match blood

History	Review of gynaecological history. Nature of pain and bleeding? Has intrauterine pregnancy already been confirmed? Past pelvic operations? Ectopics? Pelvic inflammatory disease (PID)? Sexually transmitted infection (STI) (i.e. ectopic risk factors)?

Examination	General	Anaemia, blood pressure (BP), pulse
	Abdomen	Tenderness, rebound tenderness
	Pelvis	Size of uterus, cervical excitation, adnexal mass/tenderness, amount of vaginal blood loss, cervical os open/closed (insert IV line first if ?ectopic), remove any products in os with polyp forceps

Investigations	Urine pregnancy test initially, serum if ectopic suspected; ultrasound scan of pelvis (trans-vaginal sonography (TVS) if <7 weeks), full blood count (FBC), 'group and save' (G&S)

Management

If threatened	Usually allow home if bleeding light
If missed	Consider surgical management of miscarriage (SMM) (previously known as evacuation of retained products of conception (ERPC)), medical or conservative management
If inevitable/ incomplete	Patient bleeding heavily: give ergometrine intramuscularly (IM), confirm no products to be removed immediately from cervical os, do SMM Patient not bleeding heavily: consider medical or conservative management
If complete	(Empty uterus, history/examination) Allow home
If molar pregnancy	Do SMM, check histology and human chorionic gonadotrophin (hCG) and refer to supraregional centre
If certain ectopic	*Acute* presentation: salpingectomy by laparoscopy or laparotomy *Subacute* presentation: surgery vs medical management. Laparoscopic salpingectomy or salpingostomy if significant pain/adnexal mass/visible FH/hCG>5000 IU/mL. Medical management with methotrexate an option if none of the above. 10% still require surgery after methotrexate

If unsure but possible ectopic (symptoms suggestive but uterus empty on ultrasound scan (USS) and no adnexal masses or pelvic free fluid (blood), termed *pregnancy of unknown location (PUL)):*

> *Acute* severe pain suggestive of ectopic (despite normal scan), do urgent laparoscopy.
> *Subacute*: check serum hCG and repeat 48 h later. If >50% decline then non-viable pregnancy. If change is between 50% decline and 63% increase then ectopic likely and management as per above. If >63% increase then viable pregnancy likely and rescan 10 days

After miscarriage or ectopic pregnancy:

Give anti-D if patient Rhesus negative. Offer counselling or referral to support group

Management of abnormal uterine bleeding

Fundamentals	Defined as any variation from the normal menstrual cycle, includes changes in regularity and frequency of menses, duration of flow or amount of blood loss. Heavy menstrual bleeding (HMB) is the most common complaint Although rare, malignancy should be excluded
Causes	PALM-COEIN ('palm-coin')
Structural	PALM **P**olyps **A**denomyosis **L**eiomyomas (submucosal and others) **M**alignancy and hyperplasia
Non-structural	COEIN **C**oagulopathy **O**vulatory dysfunction **E**ndometrial (disorder affecting local endometrial haemostasis) **I**atrogenic **N**ot yet specified
History	Review of gynaecological history. Volume/timing/scale of blood loss? Effect on daily living? Intermenstrual/postcoital bleeding (PCB)? Dyspareunia/dysmenorrhoea? Cervical smear history? Menopausal symptoms? When was last menstrual period (LMP)? Plans for fertility?
Examination	General — Weight, anaemia Abdominal — Masses Pelvis — Uterine size, consistency, mobility. Masses. Cervix
Investigations	Full blood count (FBC), consider thyroid function tests (TFTs), coagulation and urine pregnancy tests. Do cervical smear if not up to date Ultrasound scan (USS) Endometrial biopsy if scan abnormal, or if >40 years of age, or if <40 years but significant intermenstrual bleeding, failed medical treatment or risk factors for endometrial cancer (e.g. obesity, diabetes, nulliparity, history of polycystic ovary syndrome (PCOS), and family history of hereditary non-polyposis colorectal cancer (HPNCC))
Management	
If <40 years	Progestogen intrauterine system (IUS) if wants contraception, or combined oral contraception (COC) to regulate/reduce volume if wants contraception Tranexamic acid and/or non-steroidal anti-inflammatory drugs (NSAIDs) if menses regular to reduce volume and if wanting to conceive Do endometrial biopsy if medical treatments fail Endometrial ablation (after biopsy) or hysterectomy

(Continued)

Management of abnormal uterine bleeding (Continued)

If >40 years, or <40 with significant intermenstrual bleeding or endometrial cancer risk factors	Do pelvic ultrasound plus outpatient endometrial biopsy or in/outpatient hysteroscopy IUS if wants contraception COC to regulate/reduce volume if wants contraception and no contraindications Tranexamic acid, NSAIDs if regular menses to reduce volume Cyclical progestogens to regulate; hormone replacement therapy (HRT) if perimenopausal Endometrial ablation (after biopsy) or hysterectomy
If postmenopausal bleeding only	Urgent pelvic ultrasound; Pipelle biopsy ± hysteroscopy if >4 mm endometrium or recurrent bleeding
If PCB only	Do cervical smear ± colposcopy. If negative, consider cryotherapy
If malignancy	Treat appropriately (see Chapters 3 and 4)
If treatment failure	Hysterectomy, preferably vaginal or laparoscopic if possible, or embolization of fibroids

Management of the pelvic mass

Fundamentals	Exclude ovarian malignancy; remove persistent or enlarging masses unless asymptomatic fibroids or intrauterine pregnancy

Causes in postmenopausal women

Ovarian malignancy	
Benign ovarian tumour	
Fibroids	
Rarer	Abscess, bladder, gastrointestinal tumour

Causes in premenopausal women

Pregnancy	
Functional ovarian cyst	
Benign ovarian tumour	
Fibroids	
Rarer	Endometriosis, ectopic
	Abscess/hydrosalpinx
	Ovarian malignancy
	Bladder, pelvic kidney

History	Review of gynaecological history. Menstruation? Pain? Weight loss?	
	Gastrointestinal/urinary symptoms? Investigate abnormal bleeding independently	
Examination	General	Weight, anaemia, lymphadenopathy, breasts
	Abdomen	Masses, ascites
	Pelvis	Mobility, consistency of mass; separate from uterus?
Investigations	Ultrasound scan (USS). CA 125, urea and electrolytes (U&Es), full blood count (FBC), liver function tests (LFTs). Consider magnetic resonance imaging (MRI), and gynae-oncology multidisciplinary team review if malignancy suspected. Cross-match if for surgery	

Management

Premenopausal women:	
If fibroids	Manage according to symptoms and fertility plans
If non-uterine mass <5 cm	If pain/abscess, laparoscopy
	If not, reassess 2 months; if enlarged or solid/cystic, laparoscopy
If non-uterine mass >5 cm	Do laparoscopy ± laparotomy
Postmenopausal women:	
Do laparoscopy. Proceed to laparotomy unless documented history of fibroids that are not enlarging	

Management of urinary incontinence

Fundamentals	Incontinence is neither normal nor incurable, but treatment depends on the degree of inconvenience caused. The aim of the history, examination and investigations is to differentiate between urodynamic stress incontinence (USI) and overactive bladder (OAB) as the primary cause since the management differs

Causes

Urodynamic stress incontinence (USI)
Overactive bladder

Rarer	Overflow incontinence
	Fistula

History	Review of gynaecological and obstetric history. Incontinence with 'stress' or urgency? Daytime frequency? Nocturia? Enuresis? Haematuria? Dysuria? What is fluid/caffeine intake? How much is the patient's life affected? Smoker?

Examination	General	Weight, chest problems (chronic cough)
	Abdomen	Exclude masses, urinary retention
	Pelvis	Exclude pelvic mass. Look for leak when coughing, prolapse, particularly of bladder neck (use Sims' speculum)

Investigations	Do mid-stream urine (MSU) and urinalysis
	Ultrasound or postmicturition catheterization if retention suspected
	Urinary diary: nocturia with small volumes suggests overactive bladder
	Cystometry if considering surgery, for diagnosis of USI or if failed medical treatment
	Consider methylene blue/intravenous pyelogram (IVP)/computed tomography (CT) urogram if possible fistula (rare in the UK, suggested by continuous incontinence after recent pelvic surgery and/or irradiation)

Management

Optimize weight/fluid intake

If probable overactive bladder	Bladder training and antimuscarinics. If poorly tolerated then sympathomimetics. If no help then cystometry ± cystoscopic botulinum toxin injection. Consider vaginal oestrogen if postmenopausal
If USI likely	Physiotherapy (pelvic floor muscle training (PFMT)) then Duloxetine ± surgery (only after cystometry) in form of tension-free vaginal tape/transobdurator tape (TVT/TOT)

Management of vaginal discharge

Fundamentals	Discharge is usually physiological or infective. Attention to detail prevents the diagnosis of 'intractable' discharge from being made

Causes

Common	Candidiasis
	Bacterial vaginosis (BV)
	Atrophic vaginitis
	Cervical eversion/ectropion
	Gonococcal/chlamydial cervicitis
	Trichomoniasis
Rarer	Malignancy, foreign body

History	Review of gynaecological history. Ask about: Colour? Odour? Timing? Irritation? Intermenstrual or postcoital bleeding?
	Ask regarding: Pelvic pain? Sexual intercourse? Superficial and deep dyspareunia?
	Bloody discharge suggests cervicitis or, less commonly, malignancy of cervix or endometrium

Examination	Pelvis	Palpate for pelvic masses/tenderness
	Speculum	Cervix: look for eversion/ectropion
		Vaginal walls: Redness, discharge, foreign body, atrophy
	Vulva	Dermatoses, redness, fissures, ulcers

Investigations	High vaginal swab (HVS) for candida culture
	Endocervical swab for NAATS for gonorrhoea, chlamydia and trichomonas
	Cervical smear within the screening programme guidelines
	Slide and examine with wet prep microscopy and Gram stain, pH with litmus paper, do whiff test

Discharge and diagnosis

Cause	Itching	Discharge	pH	Redness	Odour	Treatment
Ectropion/eversion	No	Clear	Normal	No	Normal	Cryotherapy
Bacterial vaginosis	No	Grey/white	Raised	No	Fishy	Antibiotics
Candidiasis	Yes	'Cottage cheese'	Normal	Yes	Normal	Antifungals
Trichomoniasis	Yes	Grey/green	Raised	Yes	Yes	Antibiotics
Malignancy	No	Red/brown	Variable	No	Yes	Biopsy
Atrophic	No	Clear	Raised	Yes	No	Oestrogen

Management

If whiff test and swabs negative, infective cause unlikely

Reassure if physiological
Treat atrophic vaginitis with oestrogen cream (or consider hormone replacement therapy (HRT) if postmenopausal)
Treat cervical ectropion with cryotherapy or diathermy

If infection present:

If candidiasis	Use oral fluconazole or clotrimazole pessary
If BV	Use clindamycin cream or metronidazole
If sexually transmitted infection (STI)	Treat appropriately and arrange contact tracing

Management of the subfertile couple

Fundamentals	Investigate after one year of failure to conceive, or earlier if irregular or absent periods, female age >35 years, or history of pelvic infection or trauma in either partner. Investigations centre on: (1) ovulation, (2) sperm, and (3) female pelvis (patent fallopian tubes)

Common causes

Polycystic ovary syndrome (PCOS)
Tubal damage/pelvic inflammatory disease (PID)
Male factor
Endometriosis
Unexplained

Uncommon causes

Hyperprolactinaemia
Hypothalamic hypogonadism

Initial assessment

History		See the couple together. Offer counselling. Advise folic acid
		Review of gynaecological, medical and surgical history. Previous pregnancies, time to conceive each, and outcomes. Menstruation? Exercise? Smoking or drugs? Eating habits? Sexual intercourse frequency? (History from male if semen analysis abnormal)
Examination	General	Health, body mass index (BMI), hirsutism
	Pelvic	Look for masses, tenderness or reduced mobility
Investigations	Ovulation	Check for ovulation: mid-luteal progesterone
		If anovulatory: follicle-stimulating hormone (FSH), luteinizing hormone (LH) (days 2–5), thyroid function tests (TFTs), prolactin, testosterone, antimullerian hormone (AMH)
	Semen analysis	
	Female pelvis	Transvaginal ultrasound scan: *ovaries* (antral follicle count (AFC) and morphology, presence of polycystic ovary (PCO)) and *uterus* (fibroids/polyps)
		Fallopian tube patency (only if semen quality consistent with chance of natural conception): HyCoSy scan, hysterosalpingogram (HSG) or laparoscopy and dye

Review

Results should be ready, and treatment can begin. Two or more causes may be found

If anovulation	Normalize BMI
If PCOS	Give clomifene (or letrozole) tablets days 2–6 and check mid-luteal progesterone. Ultrasound monitoring of follicular response. 10% multiple pregnancy rate. Alternatively, metformin daily, no need for ultrasound monitoring
	If no response then metformin + clomifene, or gonadotrophin injections, or laparoscopic ovarian diathermy
	Still no response then IVF

(Continued)

Management of the subfertile couple (Continued)

If prolactin raised	Repeat and if persistent/high, do computed tomography (CT) of pituitary
	Start bromocriptine/cabergoline
If TFTs abnormal	Treat appropriately
If FSH, LH low	Start gonadotrophin ovulation induction injections. No success after 6–12 months then IVF
If FSH and LH high	Recheck and do AMH and ultrasound AFC tests. If consistent, premature menopause: offer egg donation. Then pill/hormone replacement therapy for bone protection

If semen analysis abnormal then repeat it.

If mild/moderate abnormalities	Optimize general health, avoid testicular overheating
If marked abnormality	Examine male, do FSH, LH, testosterone, prolactin, TFTs, karyotype and refer to andrologist
If oligospermic	Where no treatable cause found, consider *in vitro* fertilization (IVF) + intracytoplasmic sperm injection (ICSI)
If azoospermic	Donor insemination or surgical sperm retrieval (SSR) followed by IVF + ICSI
If ovulating and normal sperm	HyCoSy /HSG or laparoscopy and dye test

If fallopian tube damage:

If both tubes blocked	IVF
If peritubal adhesions	Surgery (divide) at time of laparoscopy, still no conception after 6 months then IVF
If endometriosis	Surgery (diathermy/laser) at time of laparoscopy, still no conception after 6 months then IVF

If all tests normal (i.e. unexplained infertility):

Try for natural conception for up to 24 months and then consider IVF

Management of acute pelvic pain

Fundamentals	Alleviate pain; identify and treat cause; consider ectopic pregnancy

Common causes

Ectopic pregnancy
Septic/incomplete miscarriage
Ovarian cyst accident
Pelvic inflammatory disease
Endometriosis
Renal tract infection/calculus
Appendicitis
Ovarian malignancy if older
None found

History		Review of gynaecological history. Timing? Nature/site of pain? Menstruation? Dyspareunia? Sexual/contraceptive history? Gastrointestinal symptoms/anorexia?
Examination	General	Appearance, shock, temperature, blood pressure (BP), pulse, anaemia
	Abdomen	Site and degree of tenderness, bowel sounds
	Pelvis	Masses, cervical excitation, adnexal tenderness, discharge
Investigations		Pregnancy test (ALL women of reproductive age), swabs for culture if negative, ultrasound scan (USS), full blood count (FBC), mid-stream urine (MSU)

Differentiation between common causes of acute pelvic pain

	Ovarian cyst accident	Ectopic	Pelvic inflammatory disease (PID)	Appendicitis
Initial pain	Unilateral	Unilateral	Bilateral	Right-sided
Bleeding	Occasional	Usual	Often	Unusual
Discharge	Occasional	Bloody	Usual	No
Fever	Low grade	No	Often	Low grade
Peritonism	Often	Often	Often	Usual
Pregnancy test	Usually negative	Positive	Negative	Negative
Ultrasound	Usually shows cyst	Empty uterus, ?adnexal mass/fluid	Normal	Normal pelvis

Management

Give analgesia, admit, nil by mouth

If probable ectopic	Laparoscopy
If ovarian cyst	Laparoscopy
If PID	Antibiotics
If unsure	Where pregnancy test negative, admit, observe, give antibiotics empirically, and do laparoscopy if no improvement

Management of chronic pelvic pain

Fundamentals	Exclude pathological causes with history and laparoscopy, offer support if apparently not pathological. Rare in postmenopausal women, so consider malignancy

Causes

Endometriosis

Adenomyosis

Chronic pelvic inflammatory disease (PID)

Irritable bowel syndrome (IBS)

Adhesions

Urinary tract: interstitial cystitis

Chronic pelvic pain syndrome

History	Review of gynaecological history. Is pain cyclical? Dyspareunia? Bowel habit and effect of opening bowels on pain (bowel endometriosis or IBS)? Discuss effect on patient's life, and stress/life events
	Ask about previous pelvic infection or surgery

Examination	General	Health, weight, appearance; mental state
	Abdomen	Tenderness, masses
	Pelvis	Tenderness, masses, endometriosis on uterosacral ligaments

Investigations	Ultrasound scan (USS), mid-stream urine (MSU) sample, magnetic resonance imaging (MRI) if ?adenomyosis or extensive endometriosis suspected, particularly with bowel involvement
	Do high vaginal swab (HVS) and cervical swab
	Laparoscopy

Management

If features of IBS	Antispasmodics and refer to dietitian ± gastroenterologist
If other symptoms or signs (e.g. abnormal bleeding)	Investigate and treat appropriately
Initially	Consider trial of ovarian suppression with combined oral contraceptive (COC) (or gonadotrophin-releasing hormone (GnRH) analogues)
	If improvement, can continue without further investigation. If no help, consider non-hormonal/gynaecological cause
	Progestagen intrauterine system (IUS) if adenomyosis or endometriosis suspected
Perform laparoscopy	If wants firm diagnosis, declines drug treatment or if drugs fails. If wanting to conceive so cannot use ovarian suppression
If organic cause	Treat appropriately
If adhesions at laparoscopy	Cut but ascribe pain to them with caution
If laparoscopy negative	If intractable pain try ovarian suppression with COC or GnRH analogues
If successful	Continue with ovarian suppression. If not possible then consider total hysterectomy and bilateral salpingo-oophorectomy if family complete
If unsuccessful	Pain management programmes, psychotherapy or counselling

Management of chronic dyspareunia

Fundamentals	Differentiate between deep and superficial dyspareunia, exclude organic, and consider psychological factors

Causes

Deep causes	Endometriosis
	Chronic pelvic inflammatory disease (PID)
	Pelvic mass
	Irritable bowel
	Ovarian cyst
Superficial causes	Vagina/vulval infection
	Surgery, childbirth
	Psychological
	Also: vulval disease, atrophic vaginitis

History	Review of gynaecological/obstetric history. Dyspareunia deep or superficial? Timing? Sexual history? Other symptoms? What is the patient's reaction to the problem?

Examination	General	Mental state
	Abdominal	Masses, tenderness
	Pelvic	If superficial, inspect vulva and vagina: pinpoint tender area
		If deep, uterine mobility, adnexal and uterosacral tenderness/thickening (?endometriosis)

Investigations	Superficial	High vaginal swab (HVS) and cervical swab
	Deep	Ultrasound scan (or magnetic resonance imaging), laparoscopy

Management

Superficial dyspareunia:

If painful ulceration	Often herpes simplex	Swab, contact tracing, aciclovir
If discoloration	Vulvar intraepithelial neoplasia (VIN)	Biopsy, then treat
If vaginal discharge	Trichomoniasis, candidiasis	Take swabs, treat
If thin red epithelium	Atrophic vaginitis	Topical oestrogen/hormone replacement therapy (HRT)
If mass	Vaginal cyst, Bartholin's abscess	Surgery
If normal	Psychological/vaginismus	Gradual dilatation; psychotherapy
If recent surgery/birth	Perineal trauma	Unless obvious abnormality, wait 6 months before surgery (e.g. Fenton's repair)

Deep dyspareunia:

Do laparoscopy	If organic cause found	Treat (fibroids/retroverted uterus are rare as causes)
	If pelvis normal	Treat as chronic pelvic pain; consider psychotherapy

Management of the abnormal smear

Fundamentals	Cervical screening reduces the incidence of cervical carcinoma. Smears identify cellular abnormalities, called *dyskaryosis*, classed as borderline, low or high grade. If borderline or low-grade changes are present then human papilloma virus (HPV) is tested to triage care
	Colposcopy gives the histological diagnosis of cervical intraepithelial neoplasia (CIN), graded I–III
History	Review of gynaecological history. Contraception and sexual intercourse? Menstruation? Cervical smear history? Vaginal discharge? Smoking?
Examination	To exclude coincidental disease or advanced carcinoma

Management

If smear is:

Borderline or low-grade dyskaryosis	HPV negative: back to routine recall
	HPV positive: colposcopy
High-grade dyskaryosis	Do colposcopy
Cervical glandular intraepithelial neoplasia (CGIN)	Colposcopy; hysteroscopy if cause not found

If colposcopy suggests:

CIN I/HPV	Do biopsy, repeat smear in 12 months
CIN II–III	Large loop excision of transformation zone (LLETZ)
Invasion	Diagnostic cone biopsy

If histology shows:

CIN II–III	Repeat smear and HPV in 6 months. If both normal then back to routine recall. If either or both abnormal then repeat colposcopy
Invasion <3 mm (stage 1a(i) carcinoma)	Do cone biopsy
Deeper/lymph invasion	Treat as cervical carcinoma

Obstetric management

Management of common problems in the antenatal clinic

Fundamentals

Listen to the patient
All mothers should have basic assessment including blood pressure (BP), urinalysis and symphysis–fundal height (SFH) recorded. Beware of unexplained proteinuria or reduced fetal movements

Management

If reduced fetal movements:
Basic assessment. Note SFH.
Do cardiotocography (CTG): look for reactivity (accelerations)
Second and subsequent presentations: arrange ultrasound scan (USS) for growth and amniotic fluid volume. Advise about continuing surveillance of movements. Deliver by caesarean section if CTG abnormal

Possible ruptured membranes (spontaneous rupture of membranes (SROM)):
Ask regarding contractions and colour of the fluid. Check presentation. Check for infection, particularly if preterm
If history equivocal, do sterile speculum examination to look for fluid and perform point of care test (e.g. Actim PROM).
Avoid digital examination unless contractions or CTG abnormal
If SROM confirmed, subsequent management depends on gestation: if >37 weeks, consider induction of labour

New hypertension, but BP <160/110mmHg, no proteinuria:
Possible early/mild pre-eclampsia. Recheck BP and urinalysis twice a week and refer for USS
Do full blood count, urea and electrolytes, liver function tests, uric acid
Consider sFlt-1/PlGF assay; treat BP ≥150/100mmHg

Hypertension, BP ≥160/110mmHg ± 1+ proteinuria:
Admit to hospital, give antihypertensive and manage as pre-eclampsia. Check protein/creatinine ratio (PCR)

No hypertension, ≥2+ (new) proteinuria:
Manage as for new hypertension. Check PCR. Consider sFlt-1/PlGF assay

Symphysis–fundal height >2cm below number of weeks at 24 weeks or more:
Arrange USS for size and amniotic fluid volume, and umbilical artery Doppler (± middle cerebral artery Doppler at >34 weeks) if small for gestational age confirmed
Consider coexistent pre-eclampsia

Transverse lie:
Check previous scan to determine that the placenta is not low lying
If <37 weeks: review at 37 weeks
If ≥37 weeks: do USS ± admit to hospital

Breech at/after 37 weeks:
Refer for USS and consider external cephalic version

Pregnancy at 40+ weeks:
Recheck gestation. Offer cervical sweep at 40+ weeks. Offer induction of labour between 41 + 0 and 42 + 0 weeks

Suspected polyhydramnios:
Do USS: if confirmed, look for fetal anomaly on ultrasound and exclude diabetes

Management of the small for gestational age (SGA) fetus

Fundamentals	Perinatal mortality is higher with birth weight <10th centile, but babies whose growth has slowed are also at risk	
Common causes	Constitutional factors Idiopathic Maternal disease, e.g. pre-eclampsia Smoking Multiple pregnancy	
History	Review of obstetric and medical history. Previous birth weight? Smoking? Complications (e.g. pre-eclampsia, threatened miscarriage)? Vaginal bleeding? Fetal movements? Assess risk factors for SGA including pregnancy-associated plasma protein A in first trimester, abnormal uterine arteries	
Examination	General	Blood pressure (BP) and urinalysis
	Abdominal	Symphysis–fundal height
Investigations	Ultrasound scan (USS); umbilical artery (UmbA) Doppler; middle cerebral artery (MCA) Doppler	

To identify the small for dates fetus

'Low-risk' pregnancy	Measure symphysis–fundal height. If ≥2 cm less than gestation or <10th customized centile, refer for USS and UmbA Doppler
'High-risk' pregnancy	As above with serial USS measurement of fetal growth and umbilical artery Doppler from 26–28 weeks, then at 32 and 36 weeks (frequency depends on risk)

Management

Consider non-placental cause, e.g. chromosomal abnormality, cytomegalovirus infection

If ultrasound shows:

Size >10th centile	Continue usual antenatal care	
Size <10th centile	If <37 weeks	Do UmbA and MCA Doppler Look for fetal/maternal disease, e.g. pre-eclampsia
	If >37 weeks	Consider delivery (induction) or wait if MCA and UmbA Doppler (CPR) normal and >3rd centile

If size <10th centile, <37 weeks and Doppler shows:

Normal resistance	Repeat USS and UmbA Doppler every 2 weeks ± MCA Doppler after 34 weeks	
High resistance	Repeat USS. Weekly antenatal care and estimated fetal weight. Twice-weekly UmbA Doppler Deliver by 36 weeks, consider caesarean section (CS)	
Severe abnormality (absent/reversed end-diastolic velocity)	If >32 weeks	Deliver, usually CS after steroids
	If <32 weeks	Fetal Doppler, steroids, daily computerized CTG, fetal medicine opinion to time delivery by CS

Management of hypertension in pregnancy

Fundamentals	Hypertension is blood pressure (BP) ≥140 mmHg systolic or ≥90 mmHg diastolic	
	Pre-eclampsia is common, is unpredictable and can kill the mother and fetus. Monitor both	
Causes	Pregnancy induced	Pre-eclampsia and transient
	Underlying (long term)	Essential and secondary
History	Review of obstetric history. Did hypertension predate pregnancy/20 weeks? Risk factors for pre-eclampsia?	
	Headache? Epigastric pain?	
Examination	General	Recheck BP and urinalysis. Look for epigastric tenderness, oedema, radiofemoral delay and renal bruits
	Abdominal	Symphysis–fundal height
Investigations	Do urea and electrolytes (U&E), full blood count (FBC), liver function tests (LFTs), uric acid, urine protein:creatinine ratio (PCR) (if >trace proteinuria)	
	Ultrasound scan (USS) for growth, umbilical artery (UmbA) Doppler, cardiotocography (CTG)	
	If long-term hypertension, electrocardiogram (ECG) and thyroid function tests (TFTs)	

Management of pre-eclampsia

As outpatient	If BP <160/110 mmHg, and no protein on urinalysis or PCR <30
	Do twice-weekly BP and urinalysis, fortnightly USS for fetal growth and UmbA Doppler
Admission	If BP ≥160/110 mmHg or hypertension as above *and* significant proteinuria (PCR >30 mg/mmol, 2+ protein on urinalysis), or if symptoms or fetal compromise (severely abnormal umbA Doppler)

Treat BP if:

BP ≥150/100 mmHg: use labetalol 1st line, nifedipine 2nd line, IV labetalol 3rd line

Delivery:

If eclampsia	Give magnesium sulphate, stabilize, restrict fluid, CTG. Deliver. Intensive monitoring
If other complications	Stabilize, restrict fluid. Consider magnesium. Computerized CTG. Deliver by caesarean section (CS). Intensive monitoring
	If severely abnormal UmbA Doppler, CS by 32 weeks
If no complications	If proteinuria and >34–36 weeks, admit, daily computerized CTG, induction
	If proteinuria and <34 weeks, steroids, monitor daily as inpatient including CTG, deliver (usually CS) if deterioration
	If no proteinuria and BP <150/100 mmHg, consider delivery after 37 weeks
After delivery	Treat BP ≥150/100 mmHg, fluid balance; FBC, U&E, LFTs.
	Keep checking BP daily until 6 days postnatal

Management of abnormal or unstable lie at term

Fundamentals	Only abnormal after 37 weeks: exclude pathological cause Although 85% spontaneously turn to cephalic and deliver normally, can lead to cord presentation or prolapse if membranes rupture or at the onset of labour and uterine rupture
Common causes	Lax multiparous uterus Abnormal uterus Pelvic obstruction, e.g. placenta praevia Polyhydramnios
History	Review of obstetric history. Diabetic? Multiparous? Placental site on anomaly scan?
Examination	Abdominal Palpation of lie, liquor volume, fetal size Vaginal (If not placenta praevia) Exclude pelvic mass
Investigations	Ultrasound scan (USS) for liquor volume, fetal/uterine abnormality, placental site
Management	
If lie unstable <37 weeks	Recheck at 37 weeks Inform woman of need for prompt admission to hospital if membranes rupture or when labour starts
If lie unstable >37 weeks	Admit and stay unless cephalic for >48 h
If lie never longitudinal	Admit from 37 weeks and caesarean section (CS) at 39 weeks
Intrapartum management	If spontaneous rupture of membranes, vaginal examination to exclude the presence of a cord or malpresentation Vaginal and pelvic assessment including excluding cord presentation Consider external version to correct lie – a stabilizing artificial rupture of membranes should be done with caution Bladder distension can cause a changing fetal lie; encourage the woman to void before performing any procedures If the lie is not longitudinal and cannot be corrected – caesarean section

Management of breech presentation

Fundamentals	Breech presentation at term is associated with increased risk External cephalic version (ECV) reduces the incidence of breech presentation and caesarean section (CS)	
Causes	Idiopathic Abnormal fetus Pelvic obstruction Twins Uterine anomaly	
History	Review of obstetric history. Check gestation	
Examination	Abdominal	Confirm presentation
	Vaginal	(If not placenta praevia)
Investigation	Ultrasound scan (USS) to confirm, look for abnormalities, placenta praevia and suitability for ECV	

Management

If <37 weeks	Review at 37 weeks	
If >37 weeks	Counsel, and attempt ECV if no contraindication	
If contraindication to ECV	CS at 39 weeks, check presentation first	
If ECV successful	Manage as normal, avoid induction of labour for 48 hours post ECV if possible	
If ECV unsuccessful	If 'suitable' vaginal birth, estimated fetal weight <3.8 >2.5 kg, neck not extended, not footling	Offer vaginal birth if expertise available
	If unsuitable vaginal birth	CS at 39 weeks, check presentation first
Intrapartum	No proven advantage of emergency CS where breech diagnosed in advanced term labour: manage on individual basis Preterm breech may be advisable to deliver by CS unless advanced labour	

Management of antepartum haemorrhage

Fundamentals	Resuscitate mother first, beware concealed haemorrhage, deliver baby if fetal distress or heavy maternal blood loss
Common causes	Placenta praevia Placental abruption Undiagnosed
History	Review of obstetric history. Is placental site known? Pain (constant/contractions)? Volume and colour of blood loss?

Examination		
	General	Colour, pulse, blood pressure
	Abdomen	Tenderness, uterine activity, size and presentation, head engagement
	Pelvis	Vaginal examination (if placenta praevia excluded)

Investigations	Cardiotocography (CTG) (immediate), ultrasound scan (USS) to determine placental site/fetal viability
	If heavy bleed: catheterize and record hourly urine output Full blood count, group and cross-match. Coagulation screen. Urea and electrolytes

Management

Resuscitation	IV access. Analgesia The shocked patient must receive full resuscitation: enact massive haemorrhage protocol: call for senior help, anaesthetics and haematology. See postpartum haemorrhage (PPH) section for further information

Placenta praevia:

Shock/heavy bleeding or >37 weeks	Caesarean section (CS). Give blood
	Risk of PPH
Blood loss stopped, <37 weeks	Give steroids if <34 weeks, anti-D if Rhesus negative
	Keep in hospital; CS at 39 weeks

Placental abruption or undiagnosed bleed:

CTG abnormal	Emergency CS. Give blood
Fetus dead	Anticipate coagulopathy and transfuse blood and fresh frozen plasma
	Induce labour. Intensive monitoring
CTG normal, >37 weeks	Induce unless small painless bleed
CTG normal, <37 weeks	Steroids if <34 weeks, anti-D if Rhesus negative
	Serial USS

Recurrent small painless bleeds without placenta praevia:

Inspect cervix, consider colposcopy. Serial USS

Management of prelabour rupture of the membranes

Fundamentals	Beware of infection; if infection present, deliver whatever gestation	
Causes	If <37 weeks as for preterm labour Idiopathic Infection Polyhydramnios	
History	Review of obstetric history. Known group B streptococcus (GBS) carrier? Gestation? Colour of fluid? Contractions? Consider risk of infection especially if preterm	
Examination	General	Temperature, pulse, blood pressure
	Abdomen	Lie, presentation, engagement, tenderness
	Vaginal	If diagnosis uncertain, pass sterile speculum to look for amniotic fluid Only if abnormal lie or presentation, perform digital examination
Investigations	Point of care diagnostic test, e.g. AMNISURE, if diagnosis uncertain	
<37 weeks	Cardiotocography (CTG), full blood count (FBC) and C-reactive protein Ultrasound scan (USS) for growth, presentation, liquor volume if preterm	
>37 weeks, low risk	Intermittent auscultation only	
>37 weeks, high risk	CTG, FBC and CRP USS for growth, presentation, liquor volume if preterm	
Management		
If infection	(1+ of fever/maternal or fetal tachycardia/abdominal tenderness/offensive liquor) antibiotics and deliver whatever gestation	
If meconium	Induce labour, CTG until delivery	
If <36 weeks	Do 4-hourly pulse, temperature and fetal heart rate. Give steroids if <34 weeks Give erythromycin for 10 days up 37 weeks. Induce labour at 36 weeks	
If >36 weeks	Immediate induction slightly reduces risk of maternal postnatal infection but may prefer to wait If waiting, check temperature 4 hourly. Give antibiotics in labour if known GBS carrier	

Management of induction of labour

Fundamentals	Induction can fail. Easier to do in multiparous than nulliparous. Induced labour is more painful than spontaneous labour
Common indications	Prolonged pregnancy Prelabour term spontaneous rupture of membranes (SROM) Medical conditions in pregnancy (e.g. diabetes, hypertension) Intrauterine growth restriction (IUGR) Multiple pregnancy
History	Review of obstetric history. Check gestation, indication
Examination	Abdominal Check longitudinal lie and cephalic presentation
	Vaginal To assess cervical dilatation
Investigation	Cardiotocography (CTG)
Management	
Cervix ≤2 cm dilated or parity ≤2	Give prostaglandin E$_2$ usually in morning; reassess 6 h later
	If cervix unchanged and first baby, repeat prostaglandin once
	Otherwise, artificial rupture of membranes (ARM), oxytocin if no labour in 2 h
Cervix dilatation ≥3 cm or parity ≥3	Do ARM and await labour. Oxytocin if no labour in 2 h. Offer epidural before starting Syntocinon
In labour	Anticipate slow progress initially and maintain encouragement. Treat as high risk (use CTG) depending on indication, and if >1 dose of prostaglandin or if oxytocin given

Management of slow progress in labour

Fundamentals	Slow progress is <2 cm cervical dilatation in 4 h in all women or slowing of the rate of progress in all women Oxytocin shortens the length of the labour but does not affect mode of birth Beware slow progress in multiparous/previous caesarean section (lower segement caesarean section – LSCS)

Causes

Powers	Inefficient uterine action
Passenger	Very large baby, occipito-posterior (OP) position, brow or face
Passage	Cephalo-pelvic disproportion

History

History	Review of obstetric history. Parity? Induction?
	Look at partogram: rate of cervical dilatation (<2 cm in 4 h or slowing), rate of descent of head
	If slow progress in second stage, has passive stage been ignored? Oxytocin used?

Examination

Examination	General	Temperature, pain relief, hydration, adequate support, pattern of fetal heart rate
	Abdomen	Note fetal size, degree of engagement
	Vaginal	Cervical dilatation, station of head, position and attitude, moulding
Investigations	Cardiotocography (CTG)	

Management

First stage:

Consider	Parity Cervical dilatation and rate of change Uterine contractions Station and position of presenting part The woman's emotional state

Offer the woman support, hydration and appropriate, effective pain relief

If nulliparous	Do artificial rupture of membranes (ARM); start oxytocin if no further dilatation 2 h later
If multiparous	Do ARM; start oxytocin 2 h later if no malposition

Increase oxytocin every 30 min until 4–5 contractions in 10 min. Offer epidural before starting oxytocin

Both	If cervical dilatation has increased by <2 cm after 4 h of oxytocin, consider CS. If cervical dilatation has increased by ≥2 cm or more, advise 4-hourly vaginal examinations

Second stage:

If nulliparous	Anticipate if head high/epidural present: start oxytocin and delay pushing by 1 h
If multiparous	No oxytocin: anticipate malposition or presentation
Both	Push for 1 h; then reassess to ensure progress Allow up to 2 h active second stage in women with first babies Allow up to 1 h active second stage in women with second and subsequent babies If birth not imminent, operative vaginal birth if prerequisites met; CS if not

Management of suspected fetal distress in labour

Fundamentals	Resuscitate mother first Most suspected fetal distress cases are false alarms Beware confusing maternal and fetal heart rates Consider fetal blood sampling (FBS) unless bradycardia, when act quickly
Causes	Cord compression Chronic fetal compromise Prolonged labour; rapid labour Acute intrapartum events, i.e. cord prolapse, uterine rupture, abruption
History	Review of obstetric history and labour: is it high risk, induced? Are there risk factors for intrauterine infection? Is there evidence of prolonged labour? Why is fetal distress suspected (i.e. abnormal cardiocotogram (CTG) or pH of FBS) Flat on her back? Epidural or oxytocin? Frequency of contractions? Vaginal bleeding (suggests abruption)

Examination		
	General	Take blood pressure, temperature, pulse
	Abdominal	Uterine tenderness, scar tenderness (if previous caesarean section - CS)
	Vaginal	Assess for cord prolapse and assess progress of labour

Management

Resuscitation	Lie mother in left lateral, Treat reversible causes, stop any oxytocin infusion. Intravenous (IV) fluid especially if recent epidural	
If cord prolapse or bradycardia	Urgent delivery (CS or operative vaginal birth depending on stage of labour)	
Assess other CTG abnormality particularly baseline rate and variability Note also type of decelerations (if any) Use FIGO/NICE CTG classification		
If pathological CTG abnormality	Do FBS and analyse pH	
	If pH <7.20	Urgent delivery
	If pH <7.25, ≥7.20	Repeat FBS at 30 min
If CTG abnormality worsens/persists	Repeat FBS at 30 min. Do not usually do more than 2 FBS	
Intrauterine infection causes a fetal tachycardia but can cause fetal compromise with a normal pH		

Management of maternal collapse

Fundamentals	Request senior help early and involve anaesthetic staff. Haemorrhage is the most common cause	
Causes	Haemorrhage	Intra-abdominal/revealed
	Sepsis	
	Also	Eclampsia or severe pre-eclampsia
		Pulmonary or amniotic fluid embolus
		Maternal cardiac disease
		Hypoglycemia
		Drugs both illicit and prescribed
		Epilepsy, cerebral venous thrombosis
Resuscitation	Clear airway, oxygen. Ensure uterus does not compress inferior vena cava (aortocaval compression)	
	Cardiopulmonary resuscitation (CPR) if necessary	
	NB: if antenatal >20 weeks, do immediate CS if CPR >2 min	
	Intravenous (IV) access	
	Magnesium sulphate if eclampsia	
History	Review of obstetric and medical history. Eye-witness account? Ante/postpartum? Vaginal bleeding? Pain? Seizures? Review drug chart (opioids? Magnesium?)	
Examination	General	Colour, pulse, temperature, blood pressure, sweating
		Lungs/heart
		Assess whether hypovolaemia or cardiorespiratory embarrassment, glucose stix if diabetic
	Abdominal	Uterine and abdominal tenderness; fetal lie
		If postpartum, uterine size
Investigations	Cross-match, clotting, full blood count, urea and electrolytes, liver function tests	
	Lactate. Cardiotocogram if fetus undelivered	

Management

If sudden cardiorespiratory embarrassment:
Consider pulmonary embolus, amniotic fluid embolus or cardiac decompensation in cardiac disease. Still consider volume loss

If sepsis:
Take blood cultures, lactate then administer broad-spectrum antibiotics, IV fluid and oxygen. Watch urine output, lactate, and observations
Source control including delivery if chorioamnionitis

If seizures:
Consider eclampsia, epilepsy or cardiorespiratory embarrassment

If hypoglycemic:
Give IV glucose and/or glucagon

If hypovolaemia (but reconsider sepsis):
Enact massive haemorrhage protocol: call for senior help, anaesthetics and haematology

Antepartum	If bleeding heavy	Placenta praevia or abruption likely
	If not but pale/tachycardic with abdominal pain	Abruption/uterine rupture likely
Postpartum	If bleeding heavy	Atonic uterus/retained placenta, or laceration likely
	If not, but pale/tachycardic	Uterine rupture or atonic uterus full of blood

Management of massive postpartum haemorrhage

Fundamentals	Defined as estimated blood loss >1000 mL with ongoing bleeding. Replace volume, stop bleeding, correct or prevent coagulopathy. Call for senior and anaesthetic/haematological help early

Causes

Most common	Uterine atony including retained placental parts
	Perineal/vaginal trauma
Also	Cervical laceration
	Uterine rupture
	Coagulopathy

Resuscitation	Is placenta delivered? If not, do so
	Lie patient flat, give oxygen
	Intravenous (IV) access, colloid or uncross-matched blood if *in extremis*
	Compress uterus bimanually. Empty bladder

History	Review of obstetric history. Pain? Mode of delivery?

Examination	General	Pallor, pulse, blood pressure
	Abdominal	Size of uterus, abdominal tenderness
	Vaginal	For bimanual compression. Exclude uterine inversion
		Palpate abdomen and inspect for vaginal tears

Investigations	Check full blood count (FBC), clotting, cross-match

Management

Enact massive haemorrhage protocol: call senior help, anaesthetics and haematology	
Replace volume while controlling haemorrhage	Up to 2 litres warmed Hartmann's solution
	Up to 1–2 litres warmed colloid until blood arrives
	Blood if cross-matched
	If cross-matched blood is still unavailable, give uncross-matched group-specific blood OR give 'O RhD negative' blood
Correct coagulopathy	Fresh frozen plasma (FFP) 4 units for every 6 units of red cells
	Cryoprecipitate if fibrinogen low
If perineal/vaginal trauma	Compress immediately with swab and suture ASAP
If uterus poorly contracted	Give ergometrine and oxytocin infusion.
	Remove placental tissue manually if present
If bleeding persistent	Examination under anaesthetic: uterine cavity, cervix and vagina
If uterine atony confirmed	Intramuscular prostaglandin F_{2a} if oxytocics fail
If uterine bleeding persists	Laparotomy, consider brace suture/tamponade with balloon/embolization/hysterectomy or ligation of the internal iliac arteries
After	Check clotting, FBC. Aim for Hb 8 g/dL. Watch fluid balance and oxygen saturation
	Oxytocin infusion

Principles of blood volume replacement

Blood loss is often underestimated

The uterus is a muscle and cannot contract unless adequately perfused. Severe shock/anemia lead to uterine atony

Normovolaemia is the priority

Stop the source of bleeding

Use FFP: 4 units for every 6 units of packed cells

Management of preterm delivery

Fundamentals	Most common cause of childhood handicap	
Aetiology (note: these overlap)	Infection	Vaginal, e.g. bacterial vaginosis (BV), sexually transmitted infections, unknown urinary tract infection (UTI)
	Cervix	'Incompetence', usually idiopathic
	Fetal 'survival' response	Pre-eclamptic toxaemia (PET), intrauterine growth restriction (IUGR), placental abruption
	Multiple pregnancy	Higher risk with increasing number
	Uterine abnormalities	e.g. fibroids, congenital abnormalities
	Polyhydramnios	e.g. congenital abnormalities, diabetes
	Other associations	Male gender, low social class, extremes of age
	Iatrogenic delivery	Usually PET or IUGR
Screening	On history; transvaginal sonography (TVS) of cervical length; fibronectin assay	
Prevention	Antibiotics if BV or UTI Cervical suture: usually ultrasound indicated Reduction if high-order multiple pregnancy (>2) Progesterone supplementation: from history or cervical length	
Features	Abdominal pains, rupture of membranes, per vaginam (PV) bleeding, sepsis	
Investigations	Ultrasound, cardiotocography (CTG), high vaginal swab (HVS) for infection Fibronectin assay/TVS of cervix to confirm diagnosis	
Management		
	Establish gestation accurately Discuss prognosis for baby with family and establish their wishes Steroids if <34 weeks, tocolysis (e.g. nifedipine) to delay labour if no chorioamnionitis Magnesium for neuroprotection Antibiotics if in labour Electronic fetal monitoring if >26 weeks Before 26 weeks, manage conservatively Caesarean section for normal indications including breech Liaise with neonatologists/consider transfer if not in Level 3 neonatal unit At birth, allow cord to pulse for at least 30 seconds before clamping unless immediate resuscitation required	

Management of sepsis/severe sepsis

Fundamentals	Rapid (1) assessment of severity and (2) treatment prevents mortality	
	Sepsis	Infection with systemic inflammatory response
	Severe sepsis	Sepsis with end-organ dysfunction including hypotension or lactate >2 mmol/L
	Septic shock	Severe sepsis unresponsive to initial treatment; or lactate >4 mmol/L
Causes	Antenatal	Chorioamnionitis Group A streptococci (GAS) Urine infection Influenza Also: chest infection, thromboembolism
	Postnatal	Uterine infection Urine infection GAS Wound infection Also: chest, perineal infection, mastitis, thromboembolism, influenza
Organisms	GAS, *E. coli*, also *Strep. pneumoniae*, *Staph. aureus* including methicillin-resistant SA (MRSA), group B streptococcus, influenza A (H3N2) and influenza B	
History	Review of obstetric and medical history. Mode of delivery? Prolonged spontaneous rupture of membranes? Pain? Cough? Shortness of breath? Dysuria?	
Examination	General	?Temperature <36/ >38, pulse >100, blood pressure
	Abdomen	Uterine or loin tenderness
	Vaginal	Uterine tenderness, cervical os open?
	Other	Breasts, legs, chest, perineum/wound, intravenous (IV) sites
Investigations	Routine	Full blood count; blood, urine and high vaginal swab cultures Venous lactate
	±	Ultrasound of uterus if postnatal Sputum, wound swab cultures; venogram

Management

Principles	'Sepsis 6'
Take (<1 h)	Blood cultures, venous lactate, regular observations including urine output
Administer (<1 h)	Antibiotics, IV fluid (30 ml/kg), Oxygen
Re-evaluate	Repeat lactate. If >4 mmol/L or hypotension unresponsive to fluid, consider inotropes/ intensive therapy unit transfer Request senior and microbiological input Ensure bacterium sensitive to isolated organism (multiple resistance increasingly common)
If chorioamnionitis	Antibiotics, induce labour or caesarean section
If endometritis	Antibiotics, review after culture sensitivity. Do evacuation of retained products of conception if not improving <24 h or retained products
If wound infection	Keep clean and give antibiotics. Consider exploration/debridement
If chest infection	Antibiotics and arrange physiotherapy
If mastitis	Antibiotics and consider possibility of breast abscess requiring drainage

Appendix 1

Common drugs: safety and usage in pregnancy and breastfeeding

Drug	Risk*	Conclude	Alternatives	Breastfeeding
Antibiotics				
Metronidazole	Possible increased risk of preterm labour	Caution	Clindamycin	Safe
Penicillins	Nil known	Use if indicated	N/A	Safe
Erythromycin	Nil known	Use if indicated	N/A	Safe
Cephalosporins	Nil known	Use if indicated	N/A	Safe
Augmentin	Possible increased neonatal risk if preterm birth	Caution	Penicillins	Safe
Tetracyclines	Discolour teeth if 2nd trimester	Avoid	Erythromycin	Safe
Trimethoprim	Folic acid antagonist	Avoid	Cephalosporins	Safe

Fundamentals: bacterial infection in pregnancy requires treatment

Drug	Risk*	Conclude	Alternatives	Breastfeeding
Analgesics				
Non-steroidals (normal dose)	Closure of fetal ductus arteriosus. Fetal oliguria. Possible cerebral haemorrhage	Caution (avoid for analgesia). Monitor fetus with ultrasound	Paracetamol	Safe
Aspirin (low dose)	Nil known	Use if high risk of pre-eclampsia	N/A	Safe
Paracetamol	Nil known	Safe	N/A	Safe
Opiates	Maternal/fetal dependency	Only if severe pain or drug dependency	(Methadone if opiate addict)	Beware accumulation

Fundamentals: best use paracetamol, plus codeine if more severe

Drug	Risk*	Conclude	Alternatives	Breastfeeding
Anticoagulants				
Warfarin	Teratogenic. Fetal haemorrhage	Only if artificial heart valves (seek advice)	LMWH	Safe
LMWH (e.g. fragmin)	Maternal bleeding in OD. Safe for fetus	If indicated	N/A	Safe

Fundamentals: anticoagulation is probably underused in pregnancy, warfarin only used in exceptional circumstances

Drug	Risk*	Conclude	Alternatives	Breastfeeding
Antihypertensives				
ACE inhibitors	Fetal renal failure. Teratogenic (3% risk)	Avoid	Methyldopa. Nifedipine	Captopril safe
Methyldopa	Nil known	Best 1st line	N/A	Safe
Beta-blockers	Possible IUGR if early	Caution, 3rd line	Methyldopa	Safe
Ca antagonists	Nil known	Best 2nd line (e.g. nifedipine)	N/A	Safe
Thiazide diuretics	Maternal hypovolaemia	Avoid	Methyldopa	Safe

Fundamentals: severe hypertension in pregnancy is common and life-threatening and requires treatment

(Continued)

Common drugs: safety and usage in pregnancy and breastfeeding (Continued)

Drug	Risk*	Conclude	Alternatives	Breastfeeding
Endocrine/hormone treatments				
Thyroid hormone	(Replacement therapy)	Use if indicated	N/A	Monitor thyroid
Propylthiouracil	Fetal hypothyroidism (rare)	Use, minimum dose	N/A	Monitor thyroid
Carbimazole	Fetal hypothyroidism (rare), aplasia cutis	Use, minimum dose	Propylthiouracil	Monitor thyroid
Insulin	(Replacement therapy) Maternal hypoglycaemia	Use with usual precautions	N/A	Safe
Metformin	Probably safe, few data	Caution	Insulin	Safe
Fundamentals: treatment of underlying disease greatly reduces maternal and fetal risks				
Immunosuppressants				
Ciclosporin	Nil known	Continue, monitor levels	N/A	Probably safe
Azathioprine	Minimal	Continue if indicated	N/A	Safe
Prednisolone	No fetal effects Maternal gestational diabetes, hypertension	Use minimum dose	N/A	Safe
Fundamentals: treatment of underlying disease (e.g. transplant) imperative and greatly reduces maternal and fetal risks				
Psychiatric medications				
Tricyclics	Largely safe	Use if high risk of relapse	Fluoxetine	Safe
SSRIs	Paroxetine teratogenic (3% risk), others probably safe	Use if high risk of relapse (avoid paroxetine, fluoxetine probably best)	Fluoxetine	Safe
Lithium	Teratogenic (cardiac) (10% risk)	Use only if high risk of relapse	Difficult	Watch for toxicity
Neuroleptics	Possible very mild teratogenicity, largely unknown	Usually continue because of risk of relapse (avoid clozapine)	Difficult	Probably safe
Fundamentals: psychiatric disease is a major problem during/after pregnancy so treatment may need to continue				
Antiepileptics				
Sodium valproate	Impaired childhood cognition, teratogenic (4–9% risk)	Minimize combinations Consider change if <12 weeks	Carbamazepine N/A	Safe
Carbamazepine	Teratogenic (1–3% risk)	Usually continue	N/A	Safe
Lamotrigine	Teratogenic (1–5% risk)	Usually continue	N/A	Safe
Fundamentals: best sorted preconceptually. Seizure control imperative, but minimize combinations and doses. High-dose folic acid				

Common drugs: safety and usage in pregnancy and breastfeeding (Continued)

Drug	Risk*	Conclude	Alternatives	Breastfeeding
Other drugs				
Steroids (lung maturation: betamethasone and dexamethasone)	Nil known with single course	Use if high risk for preterm labour Betamethasone best	N/A	N/A
Beta-agonists	Nil known at antiasthmatic doses	Use if indicated	N/A	Safe
Ursodeoxycholic acid	None known	For cholestasis	N/A	Not indicated

ACE, angiotensin-converting enzyme; IUGR, intrauterine growth restriction; LMWH, low molecular weight heparin; OD, overdose; SSRI, selective serotonin reuptake inhibitor.

*Note background risk of congenital malformations 1–2%.

Appendix 2

Normal maternal ranges in pregnancy

Full blood count

Hb	10.5–14.0 g/dL	Levels higher if routine supplementation given
WBC	5.0–11.0 g/dL	Levels unchanged in pregnancy, but rise in labour
Platelets	100–450 × 10⁹/L	Slight drop towards term

Note: High Hb associated with worse perinatal outcomes. Rapid drop in platelets suggestive of complications in PET

Thyroid function

Free T4	11–22 pmol/L	Slightly lower in early pregnancy
Free T3	43–5 pmol/L	Slightly lower in early pregnancy
TSH	0–4 mU/L	Aim for 1.5–2.0 if replacement therapy

Note: Undertreated and subclinical hypothyroidism associated with cognitive deficit in childhood

Renal function

Urea	2.8–3.8 mmol/L	Lowered in pregnancy
Creatinine	50–80 mmol/L	Lowered in pregnancy
Uric acid	0.14–0.35 mmol/L	×100 should be <gestation in weeks after 20 weeks
Na⁺	135–145 mmol/L	Unchanged in pregnancy
K⁺	3.5–4.5 mmol/L	Usually slightly low in pregnancy
Protein excretion	<0.3 g/24 h	Slightly raised

Note: Increased renal excretion in pregnancy. High creatinine/uric acid common with PET

Liver function

ALP	<500 IU/L	Raised in pregnancy
ALT	<30 IU/L	Slightly reduced in pregnancy
AST	<35 IU/L	Slightly reduced in pregnancy
Albumin	28–37 g/L	Slightly reduced in pregnancy

Note: Rapid rise in liver enzymes common with complications of PET

Other

ESR	>30	Elevated; no clinical use in pregnancy
CRP	<8	Unchanged by pregnancy
Glucose	<6.0 fasting	Slight fall in pregnancy
	<8.0 after food	

Note: Tight glucose control improves outcomes with maternal diabetes

ALP, alkaline phosphatase; ALT, alanine aminotransferase; AST, aspartate aminotransferase; CRP, C-reactive protein; ESR, erythrocyte sedimentation rate; Hb, haemoglobin; PET, pre-eclamptic toxaemia; TSH, thyroid-stimulating hormone; WBC, white blood cell.

Index

Note: page numbers in italics refer to figures.